K.T. MACLAY'S
TOTAL
BEAUTY
CATALOG

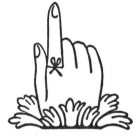

TEXT DESIGN BY
JOSEPH R. MESSINA

Coward, McCann & Geoghegan, Inc.
New York

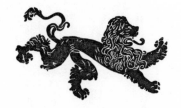
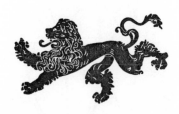

Published by Coward, McCann & Geoghegan, Inc.
200 Madison Avenue
New York, N. Y. 10016

Library of Congress Cataloging in Publication Data
Maclay, K   T
K. T. Maclay's total beauty catalog.

1. Beauty, Personal. 2. Beauty, Personal—
Equipment and supplies—Catalogs. 3. Cosmetics—
Catalogs. I. Title. II. Title: Whole beauty catalog.
RA778.M1487   646.7'2   77-21522
ISBN 0-698-10835-3

Printed in the United States of America

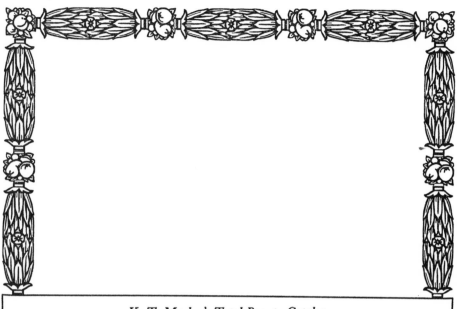

K. T. Maclay's Total Beauty Catalog
is dedicated to Linda, who thought it up;
to Jane, who thought I could do it;
to Pat, who warned me;
to David, who kept me going;
to Sabina, my most enthusiastic critic;
to Norman, without whose knowledge and support and
inspiration this never would have happened;
and to all the friends who held my hand and contributed their time,
talent, good thoughts and love.

ktm

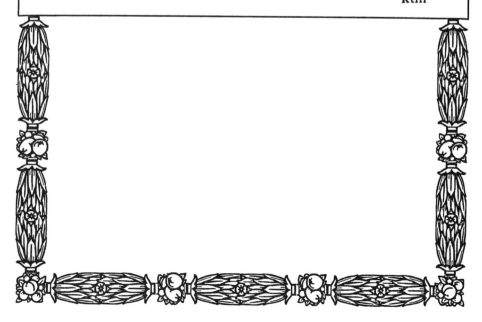

BEFORE YOU GO ANY FURTHER—HERE'S A VERY IMPORTANT MESSAGE ABOUT PRICES

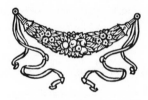

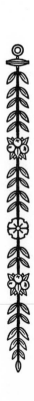

Next to the unbelievable quantity and variation of products on the market today, price ranks as the most confusing element in the beauty industry. It's theoretically possible to buy the same brand-name hair product for 89¢ (at a discount drugstore), $1.25 (at a beauty supply house) and $2.25 (at a downtown department store).

While great economy is possible, a senior vice president at a major cosmetics firm once told me that if he tried to sell a $10 face cream for 15¢, he wouldn't be able to give it away. If, on the other hand, he raised the purchase price of the same cream to $15, there'd be lines of anxious customers fighting each other to get their hands on it.

Obviously, as price increases (in this business) so does desire. The difference is in thinking of yourself as a 15¢ face—or as a million-dollar property.

The prices in the *Total Beauty Catalog* were current at the time the book was assembled and are included *for comparison only*. There is NO GUARANTEE that ANY price listed here will bear any resemblance to the selling price of the product or service by the time you need it.

Please take this warning in the benevolent spirit in which it is offered and check competitive prices before buying anything.

CONTENTS

TAKING IT OFF

Welcome to Fat City—and Be Careful 9

Crash Diets I Have Known and Loved 10

The Total Picture 11

Dictionary of Nutrition 12

Metabolics 12

Ms. Crenshaw's Natural Way to Super Beauty 12

Figuring Made Simple 14

Two From Dr. Stillman 14

Dr. Atkins' Eat Fat—Get Thin Program 15

Boon For the Business Lunch 15

Collector's Item 16

Doctor Solomon's Easy, No-Risk Diet 16

The (100% Genuine) Mayo Clinic Diet 17

Free Booklet 17

1950's Nostalgia 18

Name-Droppers' Delight 18

Cellulite 19

How To Be Cellulite Free Forever 19

Let Them Eat Cake 20

Here's A Diet That'll Really Keep You Hopping 20

Fat Can Be Beautiful 20

The Ever-Popular Grapefruit Diet 21

It's All In the Mind 21

Obesity Loves Company 24

Taking It Off With Tops 24

Whittling It Away With Weight Watchers 25

Coping With Compulsion At Overeaters Anonymous 25

Doing It In a Diet Control Center 26

Jaw Wiring—A Rash Solution 27

Pennsylvania Doctors Prove Eating's Okay! 28

GETTING IN SHAPE

Uh, One . . . And Uh Two, And Uh Three . . . Stretch 30

Warning About Exercise 31

One Wondrous Book About Walking 31

Executive Woman's Guide to Cross-Country Jogging 32

Two Items About Running 34

Easy Does It 34

Inactivity Will Kill You 34

Aerobics in Dallas 35

You Are How You Move 35

Free and Inexpensive (But Valuable) Stuff You Can Get From the President's Council on Physical Fitness 36

Miss Craig's 21-Day Shape-Up Program 37

Occidental Face-Saving 38

Bringing Up Baby 38

Exercise Fun For the Entire Family 39

Let's Hear It For the Grown-Ups 39

Ten-Shun! 39

Om, Om on the Range 40

Tai Chi For Everybody 40

Belly Dancing in Memphis 41

Belly Up to the Barr, Girls 41

While We're on the Subject of Belly Dancing 41

The Well-Equipped Sportswoman's Gym (Notes on the Home Front) 42

Equipment K.T. Maclay Would Have In Her Home Gym If She Had the Money 42

Get Yourself a Punching Bag 44

Sophisticated Exercising: The Extraordinary Exercycle 45

This is Not a Picture of a Man Caught in a Printing Press 45

84 Years of Experience 46

Touché 46

Fencing Equipment 46

Luxury Exercise 46

Barbara Perlman Delivers 47

Convenience Exercise 47

Special Deals 47

Tap Is Back 48

Always Wanted a Dancer's Body? 48

Dance Your Troubles Away 48

Bodyworks 48

Karate 49
Distaff Defense 49
The Friendliest Chorus Line in New
    York 49
Don't Forget About the Women's Y 50
And Now a Word About the YMCA 50
California Yoga 51
Ron Fletcher's Body Contrology Helps You Get
    It All Together 52
The $1,000 Exercise Party 52
Jumping Rope 53
Nostalgia and Derring-Do 53
Status (and Other) Jump Ropes 54
Health Clubs Are Getting the Fat Off the
    Land 55
Where Is Everybody? 55

Beauty and Pleasure Through Health 55
K.T. Maclay's Advice on Choosing a Health
    Club 56
Checklist of Things to Think About While
    Touring a Health Club 58
Ethical Practices 59
Help For the Weary Traveler 59
Hotels With Health Clubs 59
Spas For All Seasons 61
Intimate Details of a First-Time Mind Boggling
    Spa Experience 62
Bruce Becker's Advice to the Novice Spa
    Person 72
These Spas Will Be Happy to Send You
    Brochures and Information 74

TAKING CARE OF YOUR SKIN, FEET AND FINGERNAILS

Fascinating Formula 405 127
Baby Yourself—Free Booklets From Johnson &
    Johnson 128
Vonderful, Versatile, Vaseline 128
Getting Totaled at Saks, by C.B. Abbott 129
Beautiful Hands Are Happy Hands 131
What a Palmist Sees When He Looks at Your
    Nails 131
The No-Polish Polisher 132
How I Got the Hundred-Dollar Hands:
    Confessions of a Hand Model, by Suzy
    Kalter 132
The Dallas Nail Bounty or How Your Nails
    Can Earn You $$$$$ 134
Several Sinfully Self-Indulgent Ways to Have
    Fabulous Feet 134
Beauty Books to Keep in Your Kitchen 135
It's a Long Long Time From May to Sep-
    tember 136
Cornucopia of Cosmetics from the Corner
    Store 137
Oily/Bumpy Skin Treatments 137
Treats to Make Normal Skin Nicer 138
Dry Skin Defense Against the Moisture-
    Robbers 138
A Bagatelle of Baths 139
Miscellaneous Groceries For Mouth, Eyes,
    Fingernails and Wrinkles 139
Reexamining the Marvels of Massage 140

K.T. Maclay's Philosophical Approach to Skin
    Care 103
Maclay's Simplified Guide to Skin Type 105
A Quick Glance at the Treatment Biggies 105
Adventures Among the Skin People, by Gillian
    Eltinge 113
The Eltinge Guide to Elegant Esthetics 113
Other Beauty Biggies You Might Want to
    Investigate 118
On the Subject of Youngness: Books by a
    Down-to-Earth Doctor 119
Sand Rash? Windburn? Chapped Lips? Tennis
    Toe? 120
Interesting Ways to Get Your Skin Clean 120
Luxury List: The Most Expensive Cleansers
    and Toners on the Market 121
Some Very Special Face and Body Soaps 121
The Most Incredible Piece of Literature Ever
    Printed On a Six-by-Six Piece of Paper: The
    Dr. Bronner Peppermint Soap Label 122
Bonne Bell Wants You to Know 123
Creamy Cleanser With Extra Added Attrac-
    tions 123
Buff It Off 124
Newfangled Facial Care 124
Horrifyingly Expensive H_2O 124
The Marvels of Masqueing 125
Ever Wonder How a Prune Got to Look That
    Way? 126

SMELLING MARVELOUS

More Power to the Perfumed Pulse!   76
Speaking of Power   77
The Nose Knows   77
Scentual Terms You'll Want to Know About   78
Affordable Deliciousness   80
Five Sure-fire Ways to Shop for Scent   81
Bone Up On the Best of Families   81
Men Test the Perfumes You Wear—Here's One Man's True Story   84
A Question of Image   84
Perfume Your Light Bulbs—Other People Do   84
K.T. Maclay's Fabulous Fragrance Directory   85

Getting the Perfume to the Pulse Point   95
Key West Fragrance Factory Lets You Mix Your Own   96
Body Scents   96
How I Didn't Become A Master Perfumer   96
Some of the Costliest Components in the World   99
Not Kidding Around   100
Oil of Everything   100
What the Elves Hid In the Perfumer's Workshop   100
Giving Birth to Charlie   101
A Modern Morality Tale, Describing the Dangers and Benefits of Perfume   102

BEING CAREFUL ABOUT SUN WORSHIP

Caution: Tanning May Be Hazardous to Your Health   141
Danger: Pay Attention   143
Mother Maclay's Sensible Sun-Care Program   144
Total Beauty Catalog Directory of Who's Doing What About Suncare   145
Sun Blocks   145

Special Sunscreens For Lips, Ears, Nose and So On   146
Sunscreens (for Medium Protection)   147
After-Sun Special   148
Synthetic Tanners   149
Bronzers To Be Used Instead of Makeup or With It   149

BEING RECONSTRUCTED

Phyllis Diller Says "Do It!"   151
Stop! Take This Important Test   151
The Exciting Story of My Operation, by Stephen Lewis   151
You Don't Have to Wait Till You Look Awful—A Top Dermatologist Talks About Plastic Surgery   154
The Operations   158
What to Read Before You See the Doctor   160
Big-Name Plastic Surgeons Around the World   172
"Elizabeth's" Eye Life (A Pseudonymous Report on One Woman's Surgery)   163

Famous People Who Have Not (Nor Do They Plan To) Have Plastic Surgery   164
Free Pamphlet on Plastic Surgery   164
Have You Ever Thought About Having Everything Done at Once?   164
"Plastic Surgery" in Glorious Technicolor   165
The Painful Truth About My New Chin, by Karen West   166
Getting It Done For Less   167
The Less-Than-$15 Face Lift   167

MAKING UP

Three Gossipy Books on the Beauty Business 196

Free Catalog Hits 198

How I Found My Million Dollar Face in a Five-and-Ten-Cent Store, by Bambé Levine 198

The Practical Advantages of Playing Around 199

Factory Fact-Lets 201

Phyllis Posnick's How-Not-to-Make-Mistakes Manual 202

Five Popular Misconceptions About Eye Makeup 202

Million-Dollar Woolgathering 203

Mrs. S's Bluesky Makeup Notebook or, What's In Store for the Day After Tomorrow? 204

Your Chance to Become the High School Cover Girl of the Year and Win $1,000, Too! 205

Men Who Work in the Business 205

More Books 206

Marvels of Modern Magazines 208

The Cosmopolitan Beauty Philosophy 208

Jet-Set Beauty Booklets 208

Cinandre's Selection With a Sensible Price Tag 209

What To Do If Your Favorite Product Is Discontinued 209

Hooray for Hollywood!—In New York 210

Gloria Natale (The Makeup Lady) Tells All 210

Dynamite Drugstores 213

HANDLING YOUR HAIR

Up From Confusion 170

Katherine Everett Doesn't Need to Wear Curlers to Bed 170

Shampooing 171

Wash and Wear Hair 171

Set Your Hair With Jello 171

Gonna Wash Them Rocks Right Out of My Hair 171

Pampering Poor-Pearl Hair 172

Several Sensuous Ways to Get Your Scalp to Tingle 172

Shine On Silver 173

Mint Condition 174

Two Vegetarian Answers To the Conditioning Dilemma 174

Why Not Use Rosemary Instead of a Conditioner? 175

Down With the Oilies 176

Haircutting and Hairdressing 176

The Engineered Haircut 176

What Are Those Superstar Hairdressers Really Like? 177

Getting Clipped, by Dale Burg 179

How Much Do You Love Your Haircutter? 180

Growing . . . Growing . . . Grown 180

Styling It Yourself 181

Yes . . . But Can You Blow Your Hair Dry? 181

Help Is On the Way 182

Gum In the Pigtails? 182

Keeping That Afro Attractive 182

Hair Begins at Forty 182

Want That Gray to Go Away? Take Vitamins! 183

Where Were You During the Belle Epoch? 184

And Now a Word From Mr. Hair Spray 185

Beauty-Supply Houses: Heaven's Gift to the Hair Nut 185

Getting The Brush 186

My Kingdom for a Fine-Tooth Comb 186

Some Combs Are Just for Show 187

Left-Handed Implements 187

Harriet's Home Hair-Coloring Handbook 188

The Ever-Popular "Does She or Doesn't She?" Question 190

Create a New Light In Your Life 191

Haircolor Hotline 192

Interview With Little Orphan Annie 192

Blue Is the Color of My True Love's Hair 193

COMPLAINING—WHERE TO TURN WHEN SOMETHING GOES WRONG 214

APPENDIX A—List of Major Cosmetics Manufacturers 219

APPENDIX B—List of Fragrance Manufacturers 222

APPENDIX C—Publishers Whose Books Appear in These Pages 223

TAKING IT OFF

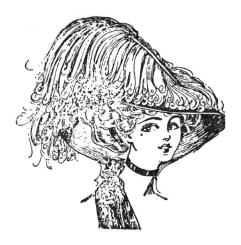

A day can be brightened by seeing someone just a little plumper than you are.
—Democrat-Union, Lawrenceberg, Tennessee

Welcome to Fat City—and Be Careful

At last count there were 17,294 ways to lose weight listed in the public records. Fifty-one of these diets involved grapefruit and eggs. If you want to lose weight, there is help (or at least information) everywhere you turn. You can fast, drink nothing but liquids, put staples in your ears, or even have your jaw wired. The following pages will introduce you to some of the most famous, most talked about, most effective, most interesting and most bizarre ways to shear off extra poundage. Some of these diets are controversial. Some (depending on your condition) might even be dangerous.

None of this information, interesting as it may be, is intended as medical treatment or advice. Should you decide to go on a diet (any diet), please, *please* call your doctor, ask him or her about it and keep in touch with your physician until you've reached and maintained your desired weight. Any less prudent approach to dieting would do both you and your diet a great disservice.

Quick Guide to Popular Diets

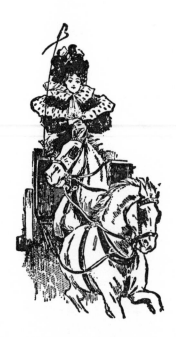

Crash Diets I Have Known and Loved

Fad diets, I am convinced, DO have their place in life. They are interesting, offbeat, exciting and great fun to talk about. They can quickly carve off several extra, unwanted, unnecessary pounds. They can even convince you that having a svelte new body is worth the trouble of adopting and maintaining a nutritionally sound maintenance program, and sticking to it for the rest of your life.

But intrigued as I am with each new, nifty diet gimmick, I have to keep reminding myself that there *are* perilous drawbacks. Some diets can cause you to unwittingly digest portions of your own body. If you digest your heart, you can have a heart attack. If you digest your kidneys, you become a prime candidate for kidney failure. If you stay on a no-protein diet long enough, you can simply disappear.

The side effects of other diets can cause such unattractive, unwanted and unhealthy reactions as gout, pain, dehydration, headache, fatigue, depression, constipation, diarrhea or hardening of the arteries. Dieting can be dangerous for diabetics or pregnant women. As far as I'm concerned, selling one's soul to be thin is one thing, but gout, heart attacks and kidney failure are quite another.

The warnings in every diet book that tell you to check their precepts with your physician are there to protect you. But you have to remember that those warnings are only effective if you pay them heed. Ignoring the signals can be (and too often is) deadly. There is only one sure, sane, safe, time-tested method for being practically positive that you're dieting wisely. That is to check ANY diet (no matter how sound it looks to you, or how many of your friends have become sylphlike by following it) with your doctor, then follow his or her directions. There are as many crash diets as there are people who have failed or gotten bored to tears with "regular" diets. Contrary to popular opinion, crash diets have several very good things going for them—the first and most important of which is that they are weird. They break your ordinary pattern of eating. Most of them are one-food programs, which means that there's very little to think about, prepare, serve or clean up after.

Second, crash diets can be effective almost instantly. I don't know anyone who isn't heartened by losing five or six pounds in a week. So these quick and visible results give you the courage to go on to well-rounded maintenance diets that, granted, may take longer, but will eventually get you to where you want to be.

I am a veteran of many of these crash diets myself, so it is in the spirit of universal thinness that I now review ... CRASH DIETS I'VE KNOWN AND LOVED.

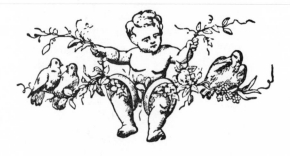

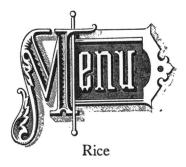

Rice

Betty Hughes (TV personality and wife of ex-New Jersey Governor Richard Hughes) and Burl Ives have lost tons by eating nothing more than cooked rice (⅓ of a pound at each meal), unsweetened fruit juice, real fruit (in limited quantities) and tea. Mrs. Hughes says that the rice begins to taste like Kleenex after a bit, but also assures us that it's worked wonders for her. This is a diet that has to be closely supervised. For detailed information, check with the Duke University School of Medicine in Durham, North Carolina.

Oh yes, another nice thing about this diet is that it's inexpensive. Dirt cheap, actually, as a 12-ounce box of River Brand Natural Brown Rice can be yours for 43¢.

Bananas and Milk

A raw banana and 8 ounces of whole or skim milk or yogurt, six times a day, plus a heavy vitamin supplement, does the trick here. This diet is rumored to be safe for one or two weeks only. Again: check with your doctor.

Ice Cream

The Baskin-Robbins way to lose ten pounds in five days. Eat a cup of any flavor ice cream three times a day (or half a cup six times a day) and you still consume less than 870 calories in all. When I was in high school, I used to spend a week or so on this diet every three months. It worked fine, but after about the second day I would have killed for a hot, juicy, rare ham-burger and some crisp salad. By the way, you can get 24 ounces of Baskin-Robbins "Nuts To You" ice cream for $2.95.

Yogurt

It's the same principle as the ice cream diet, but better for people who can't tolerate sugar. You can have a pint of *plain* yogurt six times a day. Remember that's PLAIN yogurt. Commercially flavored yogurt just about doubles your calorie intake. Eight ounces of Dannon Plain Yogurt costs 35¢.

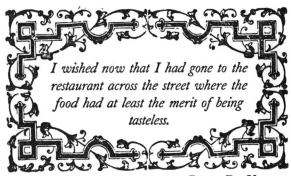

I wished now that I had gone to the restaurant across the street where the food had at least the merit of being tasteless.

—PETER DE VRIES,
Comfort Me with Apples

THE TOTAL PICTURE

For more intense information on information on crash diets, fad diets and good, old-fashioned, regular diets, get a copy of *Rating the Diets* by Theodore Berland and the editors of *Consumer Guide.*

The book is a fascinating, carefully researched, clearly set out explanation of just about every diet known to humans. It's a must for any cautious, curious or downright confounded dieter. In addition to dietary solutions to fat problems, this valuable collection of information discusses diet doctors, starvation, surgery, exercise and psychological solutions like Overeaters Anonymous. It's also crammed full of helpful charts and tables on topics ranging from "Exercise Equivalents of Food Calories in Minutes," which tells you how long it takes to burn the stuff off your body, to an extremely detailed table of "Nutritive Values of the Edible Parts of Foods."

I borrowed my copy of *Rating the Diets* from the desk of an extremely generous editor at *Weight Watcher's Magazine,* but you can get your own copy by sending $1.95 to:

RATING THE DIETS
c/o Consumer Guide
3323 W. Main Street
Skokie, Illinois 60076

Dictionary of Nutrition

For anyone interested in how the food they eat is used and used up, the *Dictionary of Nutrition* is a handy reference book to have around the house. The concise, accessible format sets out all the latest authoritative information on vitamins, minerals and nutrients, along with their important properties, uses, dosages and dangers. Both common and technical terms are defined; the composition of over four hundred foods is listed and you have only to flip to the appropriate word or phrase to uncover a wealth of objective nutritional information.

DICTIONARY OF NUTRITION
by Richard Ashley and Heidi Duggal
Pocket Books (Paperback, $1.95)

Metabolics

Understanding your metabolism (what your body does with the food you feed it) is crucial to anyone serious about healthy dieting and sensible weight control. Dr. Lamb, the author of *Metabolics,* is against low-carbohydrate and fat reducing programs. He does, however, propose a revolutionary new concept for dieters that counts "overhead" calories—the calories we burn up while our bodies snooze in a hammock. Dr. Lamb puts it this way:

The calories you use at rest are the overhead expense of running your body. The calories you eat are your total income of energy. The calories you use in physical activity are taken from those left after the overhead-calorie expense. Any calories left over after both overhead and spending, are stored as fat.

Doctor Lamb doesn't follow the standard eat less–exercise more path, which is exactly what makes him so refreshing; he simply tells you how to regulate your body so you use more calories at rest.

For the whole story, as well as an interesting, easy-to-follow book on the subject, get:

METABOLICS
by Lawrence E. Lamb, M.D.
Harper & Row (Hardcover, $9.95)

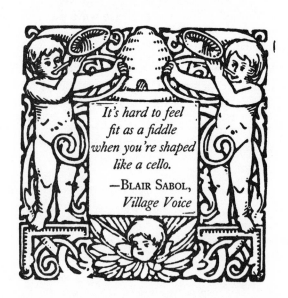

It's hard to feel fit as a fiddle when you're shaped like a cello.
—BLAIR SABOL, *Village Voice*

Ms. Crenshaw's Natural Way to Super Beauty

Remember, ask your doctor about any diet you plan to follow.

Natural Way to Super Beauty is truly a *super* beauty book that lays out all the ground rules for the amazing Lecithin, Cider Vinegar, Vitamin B$_6$ and Kelp Diet. An amazing diet it is, too. So much so that it caused a run on natural food stores the likes of which nobody'd seen since Dr. Taller sent everyone running out to buy safflower oil. This time, however, we were all hot on the trail of those four magic thinner-downers.

Lecithin: An emulsifier with a very high phosphorous content that seems to keep fat in a liquid state so that it rolls off your body. It's also a natural diuretic. One to two tablespoons of lecithin granules a day sprinkled over wheat germ or disguised in a glass of orange juice is what Ms. Crenshaw's plan calls for. You do all this not to lose *weight* specifically (your 1000-calorie-a-day diet does THAT) but to *shift* your weight around to where you want it. (Personally I think I want it where Raquel Welch has it, but that's another story.)

Cider Vinegar: One teaspoonful in a glass of water after every meal—because fat and vinegar don't mix (just like oil and vinegar don't). According to Ms. Crenshaw, the vinegar has a tendency to "win out." This also causes the fat to roll off. Remember to brush your teeth after every vinegar dose. This is very important, because vinegar can blacken your teeth and the last thing you'd want to do is become ugly in the process of becoming svelte.

Kelp: Kelp is seaweed which you can get in compressed tablets from your health food store. Take five or six tablets with your vinegar drink after meals—I'm not exactly sure why, but it's part of the program.

Vitamin B$_6$: A magic vitamin that balances sodium and potassium in the body and therefore helps regulate your body fluids.

Ms. Crenshaw (who is a fashion and beauty reporter for the *New York Times*) discovered this natural-food supplemented lo-cal diet plan after years of *sturm und drang* and paranoia. *Natural Way to Super Beauty* is her very own personal book in which she tells you all about it. It's like having her right there in your living room. You'll be happy you did, too, because (aside from the fact that she weighs about a hundred pounds soaking wet, with her shoes on) she's a fascinating lady. So what if she's a little crazy about getting her weight down? So what if she'll brook no slaggards? So what if she insists you stick to the rules (*all* the rules) always and forever ... and requires you to keep copious *written* records of every calorie that finds its way past your bicuspids? Reading the book will excite you and scare you and inspire you to lose weight and get healthy and beautiful in the process.

By the way, there is a hundred-page reference guide smack in the center of the book called the "Everything Chart." What it does is break down the calorie, carbohydrate, protein, saturated fat, vitamin and mineral content *per serving* of all the foods anyone is likely to eat.

This is not a reference book. It's meant to be read from cover to cover. You'll enjoy every minute of it ... the book, that is. As for the Lecithin, Cider Vinegar, Vitamin B$_6$ and Kelp Diet, just keep in mind that what's good for Ms. Crenshaw might not be right for the rest of us.

NATURAL WAY TO SUPER BEAUTY
by Mary Ann Crenshaw
David McKay Company (Hardcover, $9.95)
Dell (Paperback, $1.75)

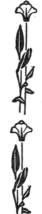

Two men are sitting in a cafe, and a camel walks past.
"What does that make you think of?" says the first.
"Food," says the other.
"Since when are camels used for food?"
"I haven't eaten today, everything makes me think of food."
—Sufi story

quoted by Adam Smith, *Powers of Mind*

CALORIE COUNTERS

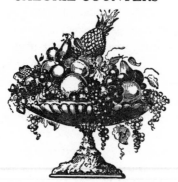

Figuring Made Simple

Got room on a counter top? Why not get a Diet Computer, complete with scale and calorie cards, to cut your figuring problems down to a minimum?

DIET COMPUTER
Approximately $14.95
Hammacher Schlemmer
147 East 57th Street
New York, New York 10022

Two From Dr. Stillman

Dr. Stillman says about his high-protein (water) diet that if you follow it to the letter, you can lose between seven and fifteen pounds the first week and five pounds every week thereafter until you reach your proper weight. The basis for all this weight loss is that your body uses up lots of energy to break down protein. Therefore, if you eat lots of protein (the reasoning goes), you'll burn up more fat and store less of it. If you also cut back on carbohydrates while you're eating all this protein, you will eventually melt fat out of your fat-storage centers and get thinner.

It seems like a terribly exciting concept. You can eat all the lean meat, fish, poultry, eggs and low-fat cheese you like. You have to cut bread, booze, milk, cream and sugar out of your life altogether—but after a while, I suppose, you get used to it. Oh yes, you'll also need a multi-vitamin supplement, and you have to drink eight full glasses of water a day. This is eight full glasses of H_2O in addition to any other liquid (tea, broth, club soda) you drink, which is probably why Dr. Stillman's *The Doctor's Quick Weight Loss Diet* is also known as THE WATER DIET and why those of us who've tried it now make wide passes around the water taps, or check in advance to see that there will always be a ladies' room handy.

THE DOCTOR'S QUICK WEIGHT LOSS DIET
by Irwin Maxwell Stillman & Samm Sinclair Baker
Dell (Paperback, $1.25)

Here's the Second Dr. Stillman Diet

A low protein–vegetarian approach to dieting off inches that bans meat, milk, cheese, fish and all the other sources of protein we've been taught to think of as standard diet fare. On *The Doctor's Quick Inches-Off Diet,* you eat only vegetables, fruits, soups, juices, an occasional bowl of cereal and a mandatory vitamin supplement. How many calories do you think there *are* in a truckload of lettuce?

THE DOCTOR'S QUICK INCHES-OFF DIET
by Irwin Maxwell Stillman & Samm Sinclair Baker
Dell (Paperback, $1.25)

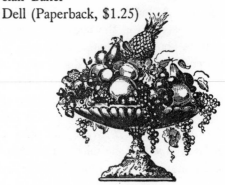

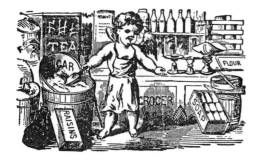

Dr. Atkins' Eat Fat– Get Thin Program

No more starving on minicaloric diets! Have mayonnaise and cheesecake! Have mayonnaise *on* cheesecake if you want to. Think of it: bacon, eggs, cream cheese, lobster with drawn butter—the saturated, cholesterol-loaded, patent-leather works.

Dr. Atkins says fat people can't handle carbohydrates. So what he does is start his diet plan with one week of NO carbohydrates at all. No vegetables, no fruits, no sugars, soft drinks, bread, pastry, ice cream or even chewing gum for heaven's sake.

On this high-fat, low-carbohydrate regime, men can expect to lose seven pounds, women five pounds at the end of Week One ... at which point you step to the next plateau. Add five grams of carbohydrates each day for five days. You test your urine regularly with a urine test-stick or tablet, which you can get at any drugstore. The color of the test stick, after testing, will indicate whether the body is still burning off fatty tissue. When people go on a no-carbohydrate diet, the body goes into a state called ketosis, which means that there are unburned chemicals (called ketones) left behind in the urine while the body is burning fat. If ketones are present, your urine test-stick will turn purple, and, according to Dr. Atkins, as long as your test stick turns purple, you can continue to add carbohydrates and *still* lose weight. You can add a smidge of cantaloupe or a little wine, a tomato, several pea pods or even a sliver of cheesecake. As long as you keep burning fat, you will continue to lose. What you're really doing, according to the good doctor, is switching fuel; you're burning fat instead of carbohydrates. And all the while you're eating high-fat foods that keep you feeling full and satisfied—no more hunger pangs. Once you reach your ideal weight, there's a maintenance program that lets you slowly sneak in some starch while still living off the fat of the land. The Atkins diet, as attractive as it may sound, has been criticized for recommending such high levels of cholesterol.

Who's right? Whose advice should you follow? Your doctor's (of course).

DR. ATKINS' DIET REVOLUTION:
THE HIGH CALORIE WAY TO STAY
THIN FOREVER
by Robert C. Atkins
David McKay Company (Hardcover, $6.95)
Bantam (Paperback, $1.95)

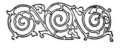

Boon For the Business Lunch

Wow! A low-carbohydrate program that lets you be wicked while losing weight. Imagine a dinner of succulent squab ... fresh green broccoli nestled in hollandaise ... and a perfect, elegant, educated but sprightly Chateau Lafite Rothschild champagne—and all of it on your DIET!

Well, that's what *The Drinking Man's Diet* promises, and whether it delivers or not, it was still one of the most popular and most talked-about diets of the 1960s.

THE DRINKING MAN'S DIET
Gardner Jameson & Elliot Williams
Cameron & Company (Paperback, $1.00)

Collector's Item

If you want a copy of Dr. Taller's celebrated *Calories Don't Count* diet, you'll simply have to rummage around in the attic for it.

My mother and many other friends who tried this high-fat program in the middle sixties still swear by it and insist on telling me stories about Dr. Taller himself. He was, it seems, eating five thousand calories a day, keeping his cholesterol level normal and still losing weight. My guess was that he was a Martian. *His* premise (on the other hand) was that if you eat the right fats, you stimulate production of certain hormones that work to get rid of your stored fat. He also strongly suggested that you take two tablespoons of polyunsaturated oil before every meal. Unfortunately, he chose to promote the CDC (Calories Don't Count) brand of safflower-oil capsules along with his book. This was the point at which the federal government stepped in, convicted him on six counts of mail fraud and stopped the presses.

CALORIES DON'T COUNT
by Herman Taller
Simon & Schuster (Out of Print)

Doctor Solomon's Easy, No-Risk Diet

The plan is easy. You can even have pretzels, ice cream or chocolate-chip cookies and not feel that you're cheating. You can indulge in all your favorite foods. You can have a constantly varied, constantly interesting menu as many as six times a day. You can eat ANY food on the Easy No-Risk master list (in the recommended quantity) and never count a calorie. All the boring computation work has already been done for you.

The plan works in "shares," which, when translated, means the precomputed amount of each average serving of food. For example: A one-ounce serving of beef, veal, lamb, pork or liver equals one Protein Share. But, so do five small oysters, or one ounce of cheese. Since you are allowed six Protein Shares a day, you can have either one six-ounce steak, or three ounces of lamb, ten small oysters and two ounces of cheese to make up your protein quotient. You're allowed six Protein Shares, three Fruit Shares, two Dairy Shares, three Fat Shares, five Bread Shares and as many free-lance vegetables as you can handle. You can even drink occasionally by exchanging two and a half Fat Shares for a one-and-a-half-ounce jigger of Scotch, or by foregoing one slice of bacon for an eight-ounce glass of white wine.

If you follow the No-Risk plan to the letter, you consume 1,200 calories per day, never feel hungry and satisfy all your nutritional requirements. You can tack the lists of food shares up on your refrigerator door, then mix and match constantly—or simply follow Dr. Solomon's mouth-watering weekly menu plans. For the really serious dieter there's even a section devoted to "Diet Meditation" advice, which uses behavioral therapy and meditation techniques to help you stick to your weight-loss program.

If you're tired of figuring out just how many calories or carbohydrate grams you're getting in your Quarter Pounder, perhaps it's time to look into one of the easiest, tastiest diets around.

DOCTOR SOLOMON'S EASY, NO-RISK DIET
by Neil Solomon, M.D., Ph.D., and Mary Knudson
Coward, McCann & Geoghegan
(Hardcover, $7.95)

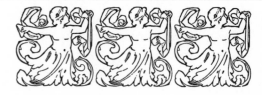

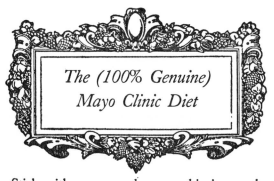

The (100% Genuine) Mayo Clinic Diet

Stick with me now, because this is a rather complicated mathematical proposition. The main thing here is to lower calories. According to the Mayo Nomogram, you begin by figuring out your daily total calorie intake on the basis of fifteen pounds less than you now weigh. You then (with the aid of the chart, a pencil and paper, and perhaps your handy pocket calculator) find the basal calorie count that fits that desired weight, then subtract from that figure the number of calories you plan to stay on for the duration of your diet. This gives you a figure that equals your "calorie deficit," which is the amount of calories you'll be cutting out of your daily meal plan. By multiplying this figure by 0.002 you can tell how many pounds you can expect to lose per week. You should then reassess your daily calories according to your real weight every nine weeks.

Oh, and while you're at it, you should also be keeping a detailed chart recording your accurate weight-loss curve. Whew! A calculator helps, but I've already lost several ounces just with the paperwork.

THE MAYO CLINIC DIET MANUAL
W. B. Saunders Co.
Philadelphia, Pennsylvania 19105
(Softcover, $6.45)

NOTE: The *Mayo Clinic Diet Manual* is also available at medical bookstores or can be mail-ordered from:

BARNES & NOBLE BOOKSTORES
MEDICAL DEPARTMENT
105 Fifth Avenue
New York, New York
$6.45 plus 75¢ for mailing
(New York residents, please add sales tax)

The Low Calorie Diet

I can only assume that *The Low Calorie Diet* went into its twenty-fifth printing in 1974 because it was so full of good recipes and good advice that people just kept wanting it. Eating is, after all, a legitimate pleasure. And, as far as I'm concerned, anyone who can help keep it that way for those of us who miss each tiny fattening calorie is doing the world a favor.

Marvin Small does other favors in this nice little book. One is using brand names for packaged foods. The other is enclosing a tear-out calorie counter right smack in the center of the book. This handy pamphlet is just the right size to throw in a handbag and consult before going over the caloric edge at the company picnic.

THE LOW CALORIE DIET
by Marvin Small
Pocket Books (Paperback, $1.50)

But Jesus, when you don't have any money, the problem is food. When you have money, it's sex. When you have both it's health, you worry about getting ruptured or something. If everything is simply jake then you're frightened to death.
—J. P. DONLEAVY, *The Ginger Man*

Free Booklet

The American Heart Association will send you a free booklet of low-fat recipes if you send them a self-addressed, stamped envelope. Just write to:

AMERICAN HEART ASSOCIATION
FREE LOW-FAT RECIPES
44 East 23rd Street
New York, New York 10010

In Spain, once a woman is married, she never again has to fight the dinner table ... So our women eat and love their children and go to the movies and gossip and put their faith in the Church, and to hell with dieting, and you won't find a more contented group of women in the world.
—A Spaniard's view of married Spanish women, as recounted by James A. Michener

1950's Nostalgia

Polly's Principles is a book you have to get, if only for the pictures. There are thirty-two pages of them, covering Polly Bergen's rise to fame and fortune from the age of two right up through the present. Besides the spectacular photographs, the book is an odd but interesting blend of biography and beauty information. My favorite chapter is the one that includes Polly's own diet: "Eating is Controlled Cheating."

While it is basically a maintaining diet, you *can* lose weight on it. You start by eating exactly as you always have during the first week of the Cheater's Diet. The only difference is that you cut all your portions in half. This gets you used to seeing less food on your plate and prepares you for Week Two. During Week Two you delete everything that's superfattening from your meals ... but double your portions of things like meat, eggs, cheese, vegetables and fruit. This makes the plate look full and is psychologically satisfying. For Week Three the fattening things (like bread, French fries, fettuccine Alfredo and so forth) are measured at between half and three quarters of what they were during Week One.

Every fourth day or so you'll be able to have a dessert that is clearly *verboten* (an éclair, a piece of blueberry pie, raspberries smothered with whipped cream), but you will eat only half of it ... thereby cheating, feeling incredibly good, and still sticking (mostly) to the rules.

POLLY'S PRINCIPLES
by Polly Bergen
Bantam Books (Paperback, $1.95)

Name-Droppers' Delight

A nutritionist for over fifty years, and now almost eighty-two years old, Gaylord Hauser is living testimony to his theories on health and beauty. He still takes long walks each day and swims several miles in morning and afternoon sessions at his California home.

The revised and updated edition of his treasury of secrets is so rich in nutritional information it's almost fattening. Recipes and formulas for diet and good health abound. So do countless dropped names of Hauser's celebrity friends and clients, from Greta Garbo right through Albert Schweitzer. Also of interest are: "Reducing Plans From All Over the World" and a chapter called "Let's Dine Out," which lists menus OK'd for the conscientious dieter forced to dine at such chic watering holes as 21 and Mercurio's in New York, Maxim's in Paris, Chicago's Pump Room and the Alvear Palace Hotel in Buenos Aires.

GAYLORD HAUSER'S NEW TREASURY OF SECRETS
by Gaylord Hauser
Farrar, Straus and Giroux, Inc.
(Hardcover, $8.95)

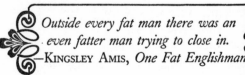

Outside every fat man there was an even fatter man trying to close in.
—KINGSLEY AMIS, *One Fat Englishman*

Cellulite

For those of us who weren't satisfied with plain old fat, *Cellulite* tells us the story of fat gone wrong. Orange-peel lumps and bumps. Jodhpur thighs that won't go away no matter how hard you diet. That's cellulite (pronounced cell-u-LEET). To counteract its ravages Nicole Ronsard has developed a program and a life-style based on bland diet, lots of water, calisthenic and yogic exercises, deep breathing, proper elimination, massage and total relaxation.

Mme. Ronsard says that "cellulite is more than simple fat. It is a gel-like substance made up of fat, water and wastes, trapped in lumpy, immovable pockets just beneath the skin." The cellulite diet, then, is one that focuses on purifying the body and ridding it of toxic wastes.

Mme. Ronsard disparages the use of table salt, the drinking of anything stronger than diluted coffee (except when in company, or on special occasions where *one* drink or one glass of wine is permitted). She is also against smoking cigarettes or hanging out in smoky atmospheres (like OTB offices or the city desk of a local newspaper).

The six-point cellulite program must be followed faithfully, and you must want to solve your cellulite problems enough to make the program AND the diet a part of your life for the REST of your life. You must also be prepared to give up crossing your legs and wearing girdles, because both cut down on vital circulation.

I'm especially intrigued with the Ronsard view of cellulite massage, the fine points of which include stroking, kneading, knuckling, *S* formation and wringing. You do all these things to and for yourself. "There's nothing hedonistic or luxurious about this at all," she tells us. "Rather, it is a very businesslike method of loosening your lumps." I'm inclined to agree with her.

For the full story of cellulite, be sure to see this classic book.

CELLULITE: THOSE LUMPS, BUMPS AND BULGES YOU COULDN'T LOSE BEFORE
by Nicole Ronsard
Bantam (Paperback, $5.95)

How To Be Cellulite Free Forever

This is not the original Nicole Ronsard book, but it covers much the same territory. It's smaller than the original edition, so you can throw it in a handbag and read it on the bus. Susan Winer (the author) uses a slick checklist, question-and-answer style, and includes a brief discussion of medication that can help cure cellulite, as well as a very specific chapter on camouflaging the cellulite you may not be able to get rid of.

Ms. Winer's method rests on a four-step program involving a high-protein, low-sodium diet supplemented by lots of water, a more relaxed life-style, massage and consultation with a doctor who may prescribe something to get those bulges off.

The book also has a nifty chapter on exercise, with the kind of line drawings that (through ingenious use of dotted lines) make the models appear to have more than the ordinary number of limbs.

There are also some scrumptious-sounding diet-menu plans.

HOW TO BE CELLULITE FREE FOREVER
by Susan Winer
Dell (Paperback, $1.50)

Let Them *Eat Cake*

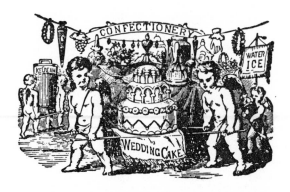

For some people, less is better. For the author of *Fasting: The Ultimate Diet,* nothing at all is best. It's cheap, effective and neat. You save money on groceries, save time washing dishes, look and feel better and lose weight into the bargain. To do this you drink nothing but water. You eat nothing at all.

Fasting is not starving. You are fasting as long as you are not eating and experience no *real* hunger. You are simply living off your reserves. Starving begins when those reserves are used up. People who fast have lost up to twenty pounds in a week or knocked off ten pounds during a weekend.

Again, this is a very controversial diet (or nondiet). Your body goes through drastic physical changes when you fast. Nausea, vomiting, low blood pressure, lightheadedness and coma are some of the unattractive side benefits of starvation. Once more, check with your doctor!

Mostly, the Cott concept can be summed up in two words: don't swallow. More information, however, and lots of stories about celebrity fasters from Gandhi to Upton Sinclair rest between the covers of:

FASTING: THE ULTIMATE DIET
by Allan Cott, M.D.
Bantam (Paperback, $1.75)

Here's A Diet That'll Really Keep You Hopping

According to Dr. Reuben's book *(The Save Your Life Diet),* the trouble with most low-calorie diet plans is that they're also low in roughage. This deficiency can cause all sorts of problems, from constipation to heart attacks and cancer. The doctor's plan is simple. Add natural high-fiber food to your diet and protect yourself from six of civilization's most serious diseases while you lose weight. The quickest way to explain the diet is simply to say: eat bran.

The benefits of following the Reuben program include economy (you can add a sufficient quantity of bran to your life-style at a cost of only 2¢ a day), satisfaction (a person on a high-roughage diet feels satisfied and full before he or she overeats), weight loss (there is some evidence that a diet rich in roughage impairs the ability of the small intestine to absorb calories) and regularity. The book makes a convincing case for restoring fiber (the one major ingredient missing from ALL modern diets) to our eating patterns. There are three "High-Roughage Reducing Diet Plans" in the book, long lists of foods to seek out and foods to avoid, and many tempting "High Roughage Recipes" and "Menu Hints" prepared by Barbara Reuben, M.S.

THE SAVE YOUR LIFE DIET
by David Reuben, M.D.
Random House (Hardcover, $7.95)

Fat Can Be Beautiful

A positive word for the sixty million obese Americans—Dr. Friedman (who wrote *Fat Can Be Beautiful)* points out that twenty million of them are *born to be fat,* predestined to fatness because of genetic, metabolic and biochemical factors beyond their control.

The most important part of this book is that Dr. Friedman explains how fat people can and should stabilize their weight and forget about the overpublicized ideal of slimness.

The book is rife with exercises, sexual hints, fashion pointers and sensible eating guides with which overweight people can be every bit as attractive and happy as their lithe compatriots.

FAT CAN BE BEAUTIFUL
by Abraham I. Friedman, M.D.
Berkley Publishing Company
(Hardcover, $6.95)

Enclosing every thin man, there's a fat man demanding elbow-room.

—EVELYN WAUGH, *Officers and Gentlemen*

The Ever-Popular Grapefruit Diet

Frequently masquerading as the Mayo Diet (which it isn't), the Grapefruit Diet has been passed from hand to hand on smudgy Xerox paper for as long as I can remember. What you do is eat half of a grapefruit with each meal and in place of other sorts of snacks (like that bag of Fritos, for instance). In addition to the grapefruit, you may breakfast on an egg, or some cottage cheese or a piece of toast, and black tea or coffee. Lunch features lean meat and a vegetable. Dinner looks very much like lunch but is eaten later in the day. The erroneous though highly touted premise for the grapefruit diet was that the fruit had an enzyme in it that sped up and intensified the fat-burning process in your body. Although the enzyme theory is pretty much recognized as hooey, half of a grapefruit can cure a stomach pang at fifty paces and is therefore (since it costs you only 50 calories) nice to use as snack food.

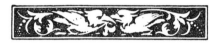

I eat merely to put food out of my mind.
—N. F. SIMPSON, *The Hole*

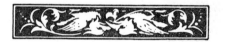

It's All In the Mind

Well, maybe it's not ALL in your mind, but *some* of it is. So, if you're serious about losing the extra set of handles around your middle, or you want to be the girl everyone refers to as "that svelte number," you might consider positive thinking.

The positive approach has made people successful, happy, serene and rich. If such difficult tasks are simple for the positive thinker, weight loss should be a snap.

The following information is a transcript of The Voice Of Unity's Radio broadcast of Thursday, September 5, 1974. It's part of the radio ministry of the Unity Center For Practical Christianity. Unity, by the way, is a nonsectarian movement dedicated to discovering and releasing the divine potential in humankind. The concept behind each radio broadcast is that you can change your life by altering your thoughts. In this particular context, you can also change your body by adopting the same methods.

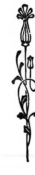
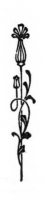

Dear Eric Butterworth:

I would like to ask you about a very tenacious subject of negativity in my consciousness, and I would appreciate any light that you may be able to offer.

I have always had a problem with being overweight. And even though I am now rather slender, I still tend to think of myself as a potentially fat person, rather than as a now-slender person. The worry that I may change from being a potentially to an actually overweight person is, it seems, always lurking in my consciousness.

I have been praying about this, but I strongly suspect that thought levels in this area need to be raised to a higher level of consciousness so that I can gain a new perspective on the whole matter. I would be grateful for your insight and guidance in the direction of discovering the Truth in this situation.

Yours truly,
A.S.P.

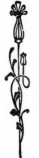
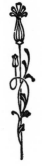

We're always happy to receive letters from our listeners, and, when possible, devote our morning broadcast to the issues that are raised. Certainly, one of the major concerns of our day is losing weight. And this listener's letter immediately goes to the heart of this widespread problem. She is not only concerned with losing weight, but with how to get the image of oneself as being slender.

Medical science has reached a consensus that what we have always considered to be a normal weight is also a "well-ness" sustaining weight. When we increase our bulk, we also increase the possibility of various kinds of physical disorders. It is absolutely imperative that we keep ourselves in balance in terms of weight. But knowing this, how do we go about it?

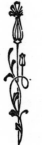
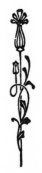

Certainly, there is more to losing weight than dieting. As many of us have discovered, the key to successful dieting is determination and self-discipline, and you can often exercise these traits as successfully even without a prescribed diet. Oh, diets are good. And, leaving nutritional controversies aside for the moment, they serve a useful purpose. But by dieting alone, we can accomplish little of lasting effect. We need to go within ourselves for real change, as with any problem.

Why do we experience a nagging hunger for food? What controls our appetite? The control is in our mental state. When you crave certain foods, it is because your mental attitude has created a demand for the food that will make your body reflect the state of your consciousness.

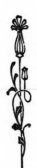
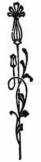

When my children were young, I experienced the typical parental concern about their eating proper foods, and often we would ask the doctor what we should do when the boys wouldn't eat what they "should." He would say, "Don't worry about it. A child has a natural guidance within his body, and he will naturally be led to eat the right things when he needs them, so leave him alone." It's marvelous to know that we are born with an inner intelligence that tends to draw to the body the things it needs, when it needs them. But when the body matures, and there is no special need for extra amounts of certain vitamins and minerals, then the body tends to follow the pattern that we set for it in our consciousness. And that's when the problem starts.

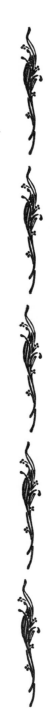

Each of us has a mental image of ourselves in the subconscious, and the foods we eat are used by our body cells to outpicture this image. Our body cells are willing servants of the mind. And if the mind sees itself in a certain way, the body is going to do everything it can to live up to that image. If necessary, your system will cause you to crave whatever it needs to reproduce it.

This is why dieting seldom produces the desired results. You may starve yourself and lose a few reluctant pounds, but if your image is too stout, you will eventually give in to your appetite and eat what you crave, becoming as stout as ever.

Remember the nursery rhyme? "Jack Sprat could eat no fat, his wife could eat no lean; And so betwixt the two of them, they licked the platter clean." You can be sure that Jack was skinny as a rake, and his wife was pleasingly plump. Thin people usually do not eat enough of the fat-producing elements, and may even dislike them!

This is not as naive and Pollyanna as you might think. Science has proven that *meditation can change physical functions.* So THINK THIN! When you are thinking fat, the craving for rich foods only increases as you eat them. But when you think thin, the craving disappears. You will be satisfied for a normal time between meals. Simply think thin and you will find yourself eating less than you did when you worked so hard to try to do without it.

Take time to be still and actually visualize the weight being sluffed off. Visualize yourself gradually becoming that slim & trim, sylph-like person you would like to be. Take this into your consciousness, and in a very few weeks, you can forget about the problem of weight. Because you will have changed from within, and that is the only place where change can ever be effective!

Here is a spiritual prescription that will help you to think thin. Take once a day. It's your new mental diet!

"I am a strong, confident, disciplined child of God. I am established today in the awareness that my body is the Temple of the Living God. All the functions of my body are harmonized and every organ is doing its perfect work in a perfect way. I am receptive and responsive this day to Divine Intelligence within me which knows the needs of my body temple. I will eat sensibly, exercise regularly, and rest sufficiently. I am free from hidden hungers that might lead to excess in eating or drinking. God's love deep within me satisfies my longing heart, and fills my soul and body with all that it requires to make my life full and complete. My appetite and assimilation of food are in divine order, and my body manifests the symmetry and perfection of God, whose expression I am. I see myself in the mirror of Truth, beholding the perfect, ideal form and shape that I desire to express in my body. I see myself thin and healthy and satisfied. Today, I will think thin!"

If you're intrigued by this extremely practical approach to positive thinking and you'd like to know if there's a Voice of Unity on the air in your area, or if you'd like to get involved with the Unity Center in your community, please write:

UNITY CENTER
143 West 51st Street
New York, New York 10019

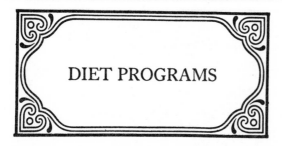

DIET PROGRAMS

Obesity Loves Company

Sometimes it's rough to diet alone. Let's face it, sometimes it's rough doing anything important without constant support from friends and well-wishers. Or, let's just say it's *easier* for some of us to get control of ourselves in congenial company. Which is probably why groups like Overeaters Anonymous, Weight Watchers and TOPS have become so very popular.

If you've been sitting there eating yogurt, gaining weight and asking yourself where you could go for help, here's the inside information on four of the most talked-about diet programs in operation today.

Taking It Off With Tops
(Take Off Pounds Sensibly)

Tops is a noncommercial, nonprofit weight-control organization founded in 1948 by a hefty Milwaukee homemaker named Esther S. Manz.

The TOPS theory is that obesity is a medical problem. It asks members to get their individual weight goals and diet recommendations from their personal doctors. While the goal and the method come from your doctor, TOPS gives you a warm, supportive atmosphere and an incentive program that makes "Queen for a Day" and the Miss America Pageant look like Little League. It is basically a do-it-yourself program with doses of group therapy, recognition and creative competition added to spur its members on to skinniness. In the words of TOPS founder and president: "Your doctor provides the diet; TOPS provides the 'do-it.'"

TOPS currently has more than 300,000 members in more than 12,000 chapters in the United States, Canada and twenty-seven other countries. In 1974 these chapters had a documented weight loss of 1,069 tons. That makes 2,138,363.20 pounds. It probably hasn't occurred to the TOPS hierarchy, but it haunts me that out of that 2,138,363.20 pounds you could theoretically construct about 14,255 brand new people.

Be that as it may ... TOPS members stay in contact with each other all week long, not just at meetings. Letters and personal visits, postcards and phone calls all play vital parts in battling fatness. The meetings themselves are convivial to the extreme. Sometimes they feature a professional speaker; at other times, there are games, contests, sing-alongs, skits and entertainment (all related, believe it or not, to weight control). There is even a TOPS songbook.

Recognition is a very important part of the TOPS philosophy, which treats losers (weight losers) like royalty and honors them by crowning them kings and queens in their various areas. There are also TOPS trophies, charms for TOPS charm bracelets, Century Club medallions (for 100-pound losers), KOPS (Keep Off Pounds Sensibly) diplomas for those who reach their weight goals ... rallies, recognition days and even a TOPS annual convention.

Membership in TOPS costs $7 annually for the first two years, $5 annually thereafter. This fee includes a subscription to *TOPS News*, the monthly membership magazine. There are no weekly weigh-in fees. You can get more information about TOPS by writing:

TOPS Club, Inc.
P.O. Box 07489
Milwaukee, Wisconsin 53207
Phone: (414)482-4620

Whittling It Away With Weight Watchers

My friend Bonnie came from a family of eaters. To give you some idea of what things were like at her house, it was nothing for one of her uncles to polish off eight dozen almond cookies after dinner. Naturally, Bonnie was overweight. The nasty part was that she'd diet all the time, then break training and gain it all back. She yo-yoed around for years until she finally joined WEIGHT WATCHERS and went from a pudgy 173½ to a sleek 144 pounds in ten weeks. The good news is that she's kept herself skinny for five years now and still feels wonderful about it. She says she owes her new, slim shape to the WEIGHT WATCHERS balanced eating plan, the friendly atmosphere at the WEIGHT WATCHERS meetings and the gentleness and understanding of the program in general.

Interested? If so, you've got to be at least ten pounds overweight first. Past that one stipulation, WEIGHT WATCHERS is a three-in-one program:

1. The Basic Plan teaches you how to satisfy your appetite with the right foods.
2. The Leveling Plan helps you through the last ten pounds to your goal weight and prepares you for . . .

3. The Maintenance Plan, which gets you back to your favorite foods in proper quantities, without putting weight back on your body.

The WEIGHT WATCHERS clerk keeps all records for you, helps you with your registration fee and your $3 weekly meeting fees. There are no contracts and no extras. And your weekly fee entitles you to go to as many meetings as you like during that week.

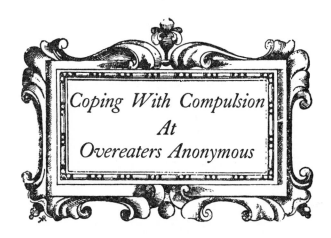

Coping With Compulsion At Overeaters Anonymous

OVEREATERS ANONYMOUS helps compulsive overeaters deal with their problems. OA works a day at a time (just like Alcoholics Anonymous) and gets you together with people who share your experiences and your difficulties so you can work together to control your cravings.

There's no *joining* OA, in the traditional sense of the word. There are no contracts and no membership fees. Contributions are strictly up to you. There are OA chapters all over the country (they're listed in the White Pages of the phone book), but if you'd like a booklet explaining more about the OA program, send a self-addressed stamped envelope and 20¢ to:

OVEREATERS ANONYMOUS
World Service Office
3730 Motor Avenue
Los Angeles, California 90034

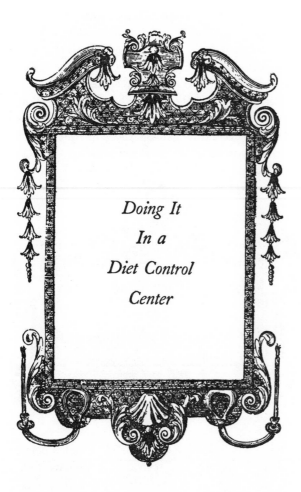

Doing It
In a
Diet Control
Center

nal Weight Watchers diet—the Diet Control Center programs offer opportunities to warm a gourmet's heart. There are no weigh-in fees, no minimum number of pounds to lose before you join. Membership is $6 and there is a $2.50 weekly meeting fee thereafter. For more information write or call:

DIET CONTROL CENTERS, INC.
Union, New Jersey
(201)687-0007

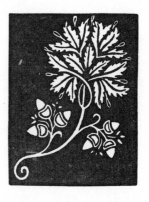

Dinner at the Huntercombes' possessed "only two dramatic features—the wine was a farce and the food a tragedy."
—ANTHONY POWELL,
The Acceptance World

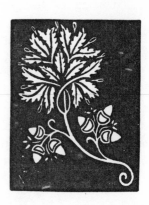

Diet Control Centers were founded by a woman who truly believed that happiness was a bagel and lox with lots of cream cheese. Not the way to get thin, you'd think. But Jacqueline Greenspan and several close friends who also had penchants for ethnic delicacies like spaghetti and meatballs and garlic bread and wine knew you could loose weight and still enjoy eating. The key was controlled portions, isometric exercises and help from people with similar problems who also wanted to stay thin forever.

There are Diet Control Centers in eight states: New York, New Jersey, Connecticut, Massachusetts, Pennsylvania, Florida, California and Wisconsin. Based on the New York City Board of Health's Obesity Clinic Diet—the same diet that provided the groundwork for the origi-

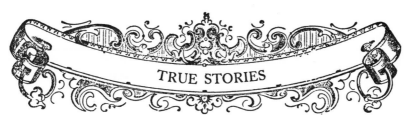

Jaw Wiring—A Rash Solution

Dear K.T.,

Of course I'll tell you how I lost all that weight.

I started going to a psychiatrist recommended by my New York shrink and, together, we worked out the ultimate weight-loss program: I had my jaw wired shut.

First, I should say that Malibu was the ideal location for my weight-loss campaign. Because even though there are several excellent restaurants right on the beach, they pretty much specialize in seafood or rumaki and, if you remember, I've always been the steak, potatoes and éclair type.

But to get back on the track—I'd heard about jaw wiring and had wondered whether it would work for me. In fact, I wondered about it for a good long time until I asked my psychiatrist about it, and after a few weeks of soul searching (and rummaging through the ice box) we decided to go ahead. My doctor (nice lady that she is) made the arrangements with the dentist and the nutritionist, and on February 2, the old choppers were temporarily decommissioned.

I had the operation at the dentist's clinic, needed only a local anesthetic and was out in just over half an hour. The dentist put wires around my incisors, left me about ¼" gap for inserting straws, aspirin, water pik and so on, and that was it.

I went back to him every week so he could unwire me for cleaning and exercise. I know this sounds terribly extreme, but it wasn't all that traumatic. Honest! The wires were no more troublesome than the braces I wore in the seventh grade. To the casual observer, I had nothing more than a slight case of Miss Porter's School Lock-jaw. (Try talking for a while with your teeth closed and you'll see what I mean.)

The real problem was staying away from solid foods. Agonizing. Can I tell you about how many dreams I had about Big Macs? The nutritionist had me on roughly a thousand calories a day. We met twice a month for consultation, examination, moral support and menus, but all I can say is that even sirloin gets tedious in a liquid state—and I can only hope that I've seen my last liver malted.

Thank God for weekly psychotherapy. And then, of course, there was this instant gratification: The pounds started dropping off immediately. If you remember, I was hitting the scales at about 250 pounds (at my fattest) and when the wires came off in October, I was a svelt 133. I've maintained the new weight so far, but it is (and I assume it will always be) a constant effort . . . so I'm going to Weight Watchers regularly and kind of loving it. Exercising, by the way, is so much easier now that I'm thin enough to see my toes. I'm on the floor twice a day and into the pool every other day for toning. Every time I see myself in a full-length mirror, I'm amazed that I've actually got a waistline! And hips! And ankles! I'll be back in New York soon to buy a new wardrobe (whoopee!) so I'll see you then. . . .

Love, Eileen

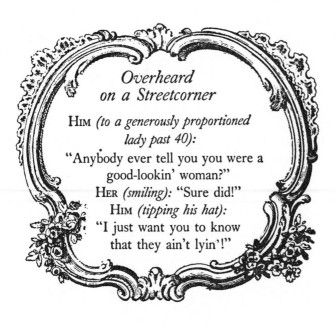

Pennsylvania Doctors Prove Eating's Okay!

I talked with Dr. Henry Jordan (cofounder of the Institute for Behavioral Education) on a day when I was feeling fat all over. My armpits didn't have creases in them. I was struggling to get the zipper on my slacks closed. Although I wasn't any thinner after my conversation with the man, I did feel much better about the possibility of losing weight.

Here's what Dr. Jordan told me:

"When Dr. Leonard Levitz and I founded the University of Pennsylvania Obesity Clinic in 1971, we did so because we believed that people could be helped to reeducate themselves to lose weight and stay slender.

"One of the things we'd discovered, for example, was that people who are obese aren't necessarily any different from normal-weight people in terms of their eating habits. But for some reason, whether they are metabolically different, or they tend to be more sedentary, obese people get into trouble with food more easily.

"Obesity is a very difficult thing to define. A lot of people say that a person isn't really obese unless they're at least 20 percent above their ideal weight (as measured against the standard weight tables). Actually, it's perfectly possible for someone to be 20 percent heavier than the table says they should be, yet still not be obese.

"We used to treat only people who were 20 percent or more above their ideal weight. At that time, our average female patient weighed about 200 pounds, our average male patient around 240 or 250. Since that time we've found that there are a large number of people who are very, very concerned about that additional 15 or 20 pounds they've put on over a period of time. They're worried about continually gaining. They've been gaining 5 pounds a year for the last three years, for example, and they want to put a stop to it.

"Now our patient selection is based not on absolute body weight, but more on the patient's concern about body weight. There are many people around who weigh 200 pounds and who don't consider themselves to have a weight problem. There are, however, other people who weigh 140 pounds and would be infinitely happier if they weighed 120.

"The Institute for Behavioral Education in King of Prussia, Pennsylvania, is an outpatient clinic geared to change eating and activity habits without locking a patient into a rigid 'do-or-die' situation. We consider eating and voluntary physical activity to be *behavior patterns* people can change and control. We work in groups of seven or eight people who meet each week for an hour and are under the direct supervision of a professional therapist.

"The minimum period of therapy is twenty weeks, because we feel we need to see people under a variety of circumstances. We want to get an overview of their routines. We want to see them while they're at work, to see what happens to them when they go on a vacation or experience a job change, or have to go through a life crisis.

"Each unsettling event in a patient's life means that the patient has to develop skills with which to cope. You may be controlling your eating very well in January, for example, but in June, when suddenly the kids are on vacation and the center of activity switches from the living room into the kitchen, and all that food is available and beckoning, all those good mid-winter eating habits can go directly down the DisposAll—and bingo, you've slipped back into your old, familiar pattern.

"Successful control of eating has a lot to do with pleasure and satisfaction. Oddly enough, most of our patients' major problems aren't the result of eating in response to anxiety or depression, but come, rather, from boredom, coupled with the easy availability and constant exposure to food.

"The classic example is that of the woman who finds herself stuck at home with her kids. She doesn't get out of the house much, even to walk the dog or stroll around the park. She spends a lot of time in the kitchen, because that's where the nerve center of the household is. She has the phone in there, and the dishwasher, and the television. Maybe she even pays bills in the kitchen, or waters the plants or whatever. And, of course, that's where all the *food* is—those see-through cake boxes and inviting little jars of salted nuts. The refrigerator door is always handy. So are the cabinets. Any woman in that situation is likely to eat her way through the day without noticing it.

"One of the biggest jobs we do at the institute is to change eating habits by changing life-styles. A patient who comes to us finds his or her attitude about food changed. We try to get away from the guilt and remind people that the greater pleasure you have in eating, the greater your weight loss can be. We get our patients to spend more time eating. To be more aware of how and when they eat. To slow down, sit down and take some time to really enjoy their food, and to make a deliberate decision that the food they're going to eat is the food they really like.

We're increasing the pleasure factor, which increases satisfaction, and paradoxically, produces greater weight loss."

The total cost of the twenty-week program at the Institute for Behavioral Education is $575. That's for the first five months. For the follow-up phase of the program, which varies in length but may last another seven months, the cost is $25 per session. Patients may come every two weeks, or once a month, or in some cases only every three months.

To contact the Institute, write:

> Institute For Behavioral Education
> Valley Forge Towers
> Suite 105
> King of Prussia, Pennsylvania 19406

Or if you'd like to read some more about the theory and program in the comfort of your own kitchen, get a copy of a book called:

> EATING IS OKAY
> by Henry A. Jordan, M.D.; Leonard S. Levitz, Ph.D.; and Gordon M. Kimbrell, Ph.D.
> Rawson Associates (Hardcover, $7.95)

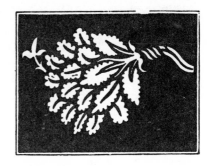

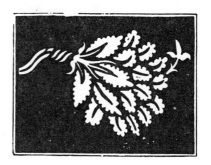

GETTING IN SHAPE

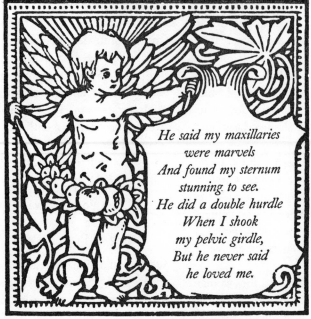

He said my maxillaries
were marvels
And found my sternum
stunning to see.
He did a double hurdle
When I shook
my pelvic girdle,
But he never said
he loved me.

—COLE PORTER, "The Physician"

Uh, One . . . And Uh Two,
And Uh Three . . . Stretch

One subject all the experts seem to agree on is EXERCISE. We're a sedentary nation, they say, and if only we realized that physical exercise could help keep us young, healthy, shapely, fit, sexy, trim and happy, we'd do a lot more of it.

What the experts do *not* agree on is what type of exercise we should be doing. Some people swear by calisthenics before breakfast. Others would rather swing on trapezes, hang upside down from rings, work out to Stevie Wonder records, or keep exercise bikes in their offices.

A simple, brisk two-mile walk does the trick for some of us, while others insist on two hours of ballet. There are books that say we can be totally fit if we spend thirty minutes a day at it. But there are also books that say all we need is seven minutes a day, or thirty minutes a week. Certain women would be total wrecks without their lunchtime visits to the health club. Many women (who would be completely content if they never saw the inside of their neighborhood exercise spa) just couldn't do without several sets of tennis three times a week. I even know one woman executive who had such a tight schedule that she ended up building a gym in her second bedroom so she could remind her muscles what they were there for, without wasting any valuable travel time. Her gym equipment, she tells me, includes a professional punching bag, which gives her a great sense of well-being after a full, frustrating day at the office.

Some of the exercise programs I've listed here are free, fun and readily available to everybody. Others require lifetime dedication or scads of available cash. But there are lots of ways to exercise that fall right in the middle of those two extremes, so read on and enjoy.

Warning About Exercise

"I would think, one of the most important things to tell people is not just to go out and DO IT. But, to think about it a little, read about it a little and maybe talk to some people. Because it's awfully easy to start doing things that can hurt you.

"There's a very easy assumption that ANY exercise is good. That's NOT TRUE. If there isn't some balance in what you do, or some idea of how to start off and not ruin yourself, you can either hurt yourself right away, or you can set yourself up for getting hurt later.

"I got it all in bits and pieces in the most complicated possible way, after ripping various things in my legs, and I have no way of gauging just how much of the answer I have now. But I'd firmly advise not only checking with your doctor before you start any exercise program, but getting ahold of as many books and magazines and trainers who know what they're talking about as possible before you begin. But, WHATEVER YOU DO, find out as much as you can before you actually start doing it and then, do it gradually. *Don't wait till you're in pain to wonder where it went wrong."*

—FRANCIS DANIEL

One Wondrous Book About Walking

Walking, in case you hadn't thought about it recently, is a marvelous, inexpensive, interesting way to exercise. And there's this fabulous book called *The Magic of Walking,* which (if you have any interest in walking at all) you should get immediately and stash in a guest room, or curl up with on the next long, rainy weekend. The book covers where to go, what to wear, and what to take with you when you walk. It also sets out all the classic rules for the ancient sport of walking.

If you're an armchair walker, the book includes a glorious ramble through the literature of walking. You'll find yourself in the company of such novelistic talents as Charles Dickens, Vladimir Nabokov, Ray Bradbury and Oliver Wendell Holmes.

For the more active the authors prepared an unprecedented walker's guide to hundreds of superb country trails and city explorations in every region in the United States and some great historic walks in Europe, Scandinavia, Canada and the British Isles.

THE MAGIC OF WALKING
by Aaron Sussman & Ruth Goode
Simon & Schuster (Hardcover, $7.50;
Paperback, $2.95)

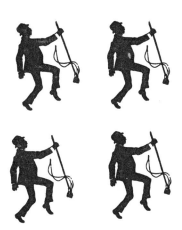

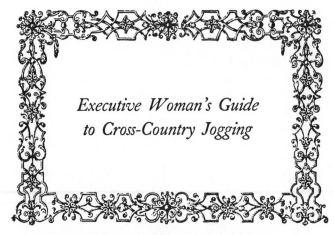

*Executive Woman's Guide
to Cross-Country Jogging*

These locations have been suggested to us by our male executive friends who travel a lot and have spent some time searching out what amount to joggers' heavens. Serious joggers insist you should never travel without your sweatsuit.

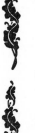
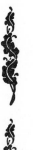

ATLANTA	Piedmont Park (3 miles north of downtown)
BOSTON	Boston Common
	Banks of the Charles River
	Boston Public Garden
CHICAGO	Grant Park
	Lake Front
CLEVELAND	Edgewater Park (turf)
	Municipal Stadium
	Case Western Reserve University (4 miles from downtown)
	North Marginal Drive (beginning at East Ninth Street)
DALLAS	Turtle Creek Boulevard (start at Downtown YMCA)
	Shores of White Rock Lake
	Aerobics Activity Center ($3 fee)
DETROIT	Belle Isle ($6 round-trip cab from downtown)
HOUSTON	Allen Park
	Memorial Park

LOS ANGELES	Santa Monica beaches
	Griffith Park
	Los Angeles City College campus
	UCLA campus
MIAMI	University of Miami campus
	Key Biscayne stretch from Crandon Park to Cape Florida lighthouse
	Birch State Park (Fort Lauderdale)
NEW YORK	Central Park Reservoir
	East River Park, FDR Drive
	Riverside Park
PHILADELPHIA	Rittenhouse Square (best before rush hour)
PITTSBURGH	Point Park State Park
PORTLAND	N.E. Marine Drive
SAN FRANCISCO	Golden Gate Park
SEATTLE	University Arboretum (10 minutes from downtown by car)
WASHINGTON, D.C.	The Ellipse (behind the White House)

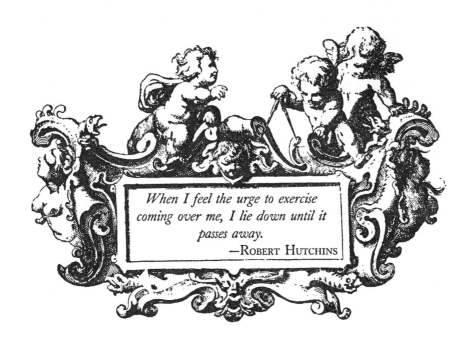

When I feel the urge to exercise coming over me, I lie down until it passes away.
—ROBERT HUTCHINS

JOGGING

Two Items About Running

1. If you have questions about special diets or shoes, or how to handle mad motorists and unleashed dogs, you can get answers from an interesting magazine devoted to runners and running. To subscribe, write:

   Runner's World Magazine
   World Publications, Box 366
   Mountain View, California 94040

2. The Road Runners Club of America publishes a newsletter, a schedule of events and holds runners' clinics before important meets. For more information write:

   Road Runners Club of America
   P.O. Box 881
   FDR Station
   New York, New York 10022

EXERCISE METHODS

Easy Does It

Profusely illustrated with black and white photographs of a healthily *zaftig* young woman in leotards, Beverly Barr's book *I'd Like to See Less of You* makes good on her promise of giving us seventy-five fast, easy-to-follow, all-purpose exercises.

In addition to the basic seventy-five, which can be done without "huffing, puffing, pushing or pulling," there are special exercises for skiers, golfers, swimmers, tennis buffs and pregnant women.

The book is written *very* simply, which lessens confusion. Each exercise has an explanation of the parts of the body it's meant to improve ... and is so well designed that if you read it once and set a paperweight on the operative page to keep it open, there is no way you can do the work badly.

I'D LIKE TO SEE LESS OF YOU
by Beverly Barr
Atheneum (Hardcover, $7.95)

Inactivity Will Kill You

Dr. Laurence Morehouse and Leonard Gross think that's awful—so they have written a book for men and women who want to live long, healthy lives and "not be so damned tired at the end of the day." The message is, "You don't have to kill yourself to stay in shape." They say, "Fitness is a piece of cake" and you can have all you want of it for thirty minutes a week of uncomplicated, thoroughly agreeable exercise.

Dr. Morehouse says you can *choose* to be a fifty-year-old person who looks sixty-five or a fifty-year-old person who looks (and feels) thirty-five. His method (which is very easy and also fun and can be done by anybody at any age) is based on principles used in the Apollo space program. It says that exercise shouldn't be controlled by time, distance or physical load (or any other EXTERNAL scale) but rather by the degree of physiological effort expended. This is measured by pulse rate. Dr. Morehouse and Mr. Gross then go on to explode fifteen myths about fitness. They also encourage fattening up before going on a diet, and they set out a very interesting list of pointers for living called GYMLESSNASTICS. These include such commonsense moves as: Don't lie down when you can sit, don't sit when you can stand, and don't stand when you can move.

As Dr. Morehouse says: "You can achieve and maintain fitness in just twice the amount of time you require to brush your teeth. You need about fifteen minutes a week to brush your teeth. You need about thirty minutes a week to be fit."

TOTAL FITNESS IN
30 MINUTES A WEEK

by Laurence E. Morehouse, Ph.D., and Leonard Gross
Simon & Schuster (Hardcover, $6.95)
Pocket Books (Paperback, $1.95)

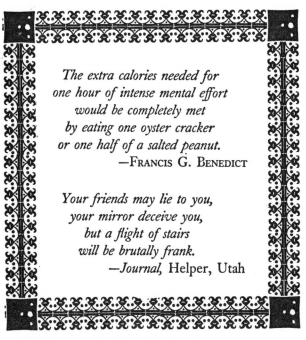

*The extra calories needed for
one hour of intense mental effort
would be completely met
by eating one oyster cracker
or one half of a salted peanut.*
—FRANCIS G. BENEDICT

*Your friends may lie to you,
your mirror deceive you,
but a flight of stairs
will be brutally frank.*
—*Journal,* Helper, Utah

Aerobics in Dallas

Aerobics is a system of physical conditioning exercises meant to strengthen your heart, lungs and circulatory system. The Aerobics Activity Center, while it isn't a prettifying place, is unique and quite famous. It's also a fine place to exercise. The facilities include: two outdoor walking/jogging tracks, an indoor running track with an electronic pacing system, an aerobics arena, an aquatics room, an exercise room and lots more. The only requirement for membership is a recent physical, including a stress electrocardiogram. The fees are as follows:

	1 Year	6 Months	3 Months
Men	$450	$250	$150
Women	$275	$150	$100
College Students	$150	—	$100

If you'd like more information or a brochure, write or phone:

AEROBICS ACTIVITY CENTER
12100 Preston Road
Dallas, Texas 75230
Phone: (214)233-4832

You Are How You Move

Dr. Neil Solomon had written two successful books on diet and weight control when he finally realized that most people, when they say they want to lose weight, are really saying that they want to LOOK BETTER. In other words, we want to be thinner AND trimmer, and to get there we have to exercise.

So Dr. Solomon began to take a good, hard look at the various exercise systems around, and found that most fad exercise programs were lacking something. Belly dancing, for example, is a very sexy way to move around, but many of the classical positions make for back strain and can even stretch the abdominal muscles (how many flat-bellied belly dancers have you seen lately?). Yoga, while it is great for the heart and lungs, tends to be somewhat boring. What's more, yoga postures, which were invented by men to be used by other men, can be particularly uncomfortable for women to get into.

Even sports like tennis and golf and swimming aren't perfect exercises, because you can be an expert three-days-a-week tennis player and still be stiff or frozen in certain segments of your body.

Realizing that there was a need for a nonboring, easy-to-accomplish, safe exercise system that was equally applicable to men, women, children and oldsters, Dr. Solomon and his body-awareness-expert sister (Evalee Harrison) developed something called DOCTOR SOLOMON'S PRACTICAL EXERCISE PLAN FOR TOTAL BODY FITNESS AND MAINTENANCE, and wrote a book about it.

All I can say is that I have nothing but vast respect for Dr. Solomon's work. His no-nonsense approach to the perils of fad exercise made me think twice about many of the exercise methods I've been involved in. I learned why I should never drink cold water after strenuous exercise (the liquid passes down the esophagus right in front of the heart, and the sudden chill can even stop the heart if it's cold enough). I took his body awareness test honestly and found that I was not on proper speaking terms with my rib cage, and that there were other areas of my body suffering from disuse.

Dr. Solomon's plan takes fifteen minutes a day, three days a week. And I can do all the work to the sound of my local rock station, so it's painless. As a matter of fact, I even enjoyed it.

Would you like to look and move more gracefully? Would you like to get rid of those saddlebag thighs, or that nagging back pain? How about feeling better, being sexier and fighting fatigue? Would you like to be able to do all these things? If so, run out and get a copy of *Doctor Solomon's Practical Exercise Plan.* It is just what the title says it is: practical. It is also sane, informative and interestingly written. All exercises are performed from a basic "stem" position and are graded in difficulty so that you can proceed at your own rate. They've been thoroughly tested on more than five thousand people, from six-year-old kids to ninety-four-year-old grandparents. The program worked for them and it can (if you stick to it) work for you.

DOCTOR   SOLOMON'S   PROVEN
MASTER PLAN
For Total Body Fitness and Maintenance:
15 Minutes-A-Day
 3 Days-A-Week
by Dr. Neil Solomon and Evalee Harrison
G. P. Putnam's Sons (Hardcover $7.95)

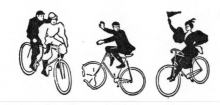

There are 7 million joggers, 15 million regular cyclists, and 15 million serious swimmers among America's 110 million adults.

Free and Inexpensive (But Valuable) Stuff You Can Get From the President's Council on Physical Fitness

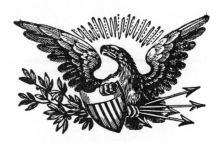

Presidential Sports Award

A national sports participation and incentives program for anybody fifteen years old and over. Awards available in forty different, popular, participant sports, from archery to weight training. For your FREE Presidential Sports Award Log Books and Qualifying Procedures, write:

PRESIDENTIAL SPORTS AWARD
P.O. Box 129
Radio City Station
New York, New York 10019

Presidential Physical Fitness Award

A national testing and incentives program for boys and girls ages ten to seventeen. FREE SCORE SHEETS AND APPLICATION FORMS for schools, clubs, and scout troops. Write:

President's Council on Fitness and Sports
Washington, D.C. 20201

An Introduction to Physical Fitness (S/N 017-000-00122-1, 60¢).

Self-testing activities, graded exercises and jogging guidelines. Information on exercise and weight control. For adults. 28 pages.

Adult Physical Fitness
(S/N 040-000-00026-7, 70¢).

Explains health and other benefits of regular, vigorous exercise. Progressive, five-level programs for men and women. Sections on weight training, water activities and daily fitness opportunities. 64 pages.

The Fitness Challenge in the Later Years
(S/N 017-062-00009-3, 75¢).

For older men and women. Exercises and activities carefully selected to combat problems of aging and to promote flexibility, balance and cardiovascular fitness. Includes self-scoring system. Large type, clear illustrations, 28 pages.

Vim (S/N 040-000-00029-1, 40¢).

For teenage girls. A basic exercise program, special "figure builders," performance goals for girls who like a challenge and physical fitness tips. 24 pages.

Vigor (S/N 040-000-00030-1, 45¢).

For teenage boys. Same as above, except that a section on weight training and "physique builders" replaces the "figure builders." 24 pages.

Important Notice

A 25 percent discount is allowed on orders of one hundred or more copies of a single title mailed to one address.

Prices shown were those in effect on August 15, 1975. Prices of government publications are subject to change without advance notice. The price charged for your order will be that in effect when your order is processed.

To get your booklets, SEND your check or money order (payable to the Superintendent of Documents) and the names and numbers of the books you want to:

Assistant Public Printer
(Superintendent of Documents)
Government Printing Office
Washington, D.C. 20402

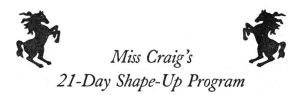

Miss Craig's 21-Day Shape-Up Program

When all the other kids in her neighborhood were practicing scales on the violin or diligently applying themselves to completing their homework, Marjorie Craig was out playing football. Or baseball. Or skiing. Or skating. Or sloshing around in snowshoes.

Now, decades later, Miss Craig is a bestselling author and the a-number-one exercise expert at the Elizabeth Arden Salon in New York City.

Still one of the bounciest women in the beauty business, her books have been praised both by the country's leading orthopedists and by the women who have reaped tangible rewards by diligently following her exercise suggestions.

Miss Craig, who brooks no slaggards, takes a very firm stand on flash-and-dash exercise. She doesn't believe in it. "Every woman should do at least a half hour of planned exercise every day of her life to get at all her muscles and improve her posture. But she should be careful about precisely how she does exercises, or she'll end up creating problems she never bargained for." That's how Miss Craig feels about it, and why her carefully developed programs never force your muscles beyond where they want to go. She never asks you to do a standing exercise with your legs pushed back, for example, because a simple maneuver like bending over to touch the floor (with your legs stiff) can cause you to throw your back out.

Posture is just as important to Marjorie Craig as is safety. That's why for the last forty years she's been teaching women to stand with "a tuck." A "tuck," in Craig terminology, is part and parcel of perfect standing posture.

"Problems," she says, "come from what happens when you ignore the tuck. For instance, most people stand with the pelvic girdle tilted forward. That makes the stomach hang out in front and the hips stick out in back. It increases your lumbar curve, throws your knees back and locks them into place. This is not only wrong, it's bad for you."

In the correct Miss Craig Standing Posture, your pelvic girdle tilts BACKWARD, bringing your fanny under and your stomach in. The curve in your back decreases, your knees bend slightly, your ribs come away from your stomach, your ears come up away from your shoulders, and suddenly you look a lot leaner.

The results of the Craig method should begin to be strikingly obvious in twenty-one days; thus the title of her first book: *Miss Craig's Twenty-One Day Shape-Up Program for Men and Women.* The book is profusely illustrated, replete with exercises for better posture, exercises for all spots on the body, special exercises for people who want to concentrate more on one place than they do on another, special exercises for tired muscles, and a wonderful postpregnancy workout.

MISS CRAIG'S TWENTY-ONE DAY SHAPE-UP PROGRAM FOR MEN AND WOMEN
by Marjorie Craig
Random House (Hardcover, $6.95)

Occidental Face-Saving

Just before Marjorie Craig wrote *Miss Craig's Face-Saving Exercises,* she dragged out her old anatomy book and reaffirmed her belief that all those little facial muscles had specific jobs to do. Problems begin when, because living conditions now are somewhat different from what they were in the Garden of Eden, those muscles aren't getting their proper allotment of work.

Miss Craig puts it this way: "The muscles of the face are attached from bone to other muscles in the skin. They're expression muscles, and you have to use them and give them exercise just the way you do all your other muscles. For example,

the big obliquus oculi that surrounds your eye was put there to close your eye and block out all light. So the proper exercise for the obliquus oculi would be to close your eyes ... squeeze them tight ... release the squeeze ... then raise your eyebrows. Your big eating muscle and the muscle that moves your jaw from side to side were made for biting and grinding hard food. Since our food today is soft, we don't spend enough time exercising these two muscles properly—so we get jowls."

If you'd rather not let your face muscles crumble from disuse, you can avail yourself of the complete Craig exercise program by getting hold of a copy of:

MISS CRAIG'S FACE-SAVING EXERCISES
by Marjorie Craig
Random House (Hardcover, $5.95)

Bringing Up Baby

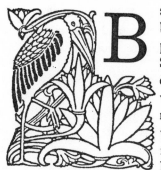

Babies doing knee bends? Tiny tots doing push-ups? "Sure!" says Suzy Prudden. "You don't just suddenly develop a healthy body in middle age. We're born with the bodies that carry us through life, and I believe we should begin building those bodies through exercise from infancy. Physical fitness should be started in the crib and *cultivated.*"

Daughter of physical culturist Bonnie Prudden, Suzy not only survived but benefited from her own exercising childhood, and has gone on to teach physical fitness to mothers and babies in the Suzy Prudden Studios in New York, Boston, Chicago and Los Angeles. According to Suzy, some mothers start gentle workouts with week-old infants. Such simple, affectionate exercises as knee bends and arm crosses help the babies learn muscle coordination and tension release, while increasing their sense of love and self-confidence. Parents who start this kind of program eventually find themselves on the lawn doing sitting foot bounces and arm swings with their toddlers, or balancing a six-month-old child on their knees while the child tries to imitate an airplane. The bonus is that everybody benefits. Family bonds and bodies strengthen, and exercising becomes a giggle. For Suzy Prudden's complete book of baby exercises be sure to get:

CREATIVE FITNESS FOR BABY
AND CHILD
by Suzy Prudden & Jerry Sussman
Morrow (Hardcover, $6.95)

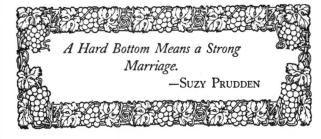

A Hard Bottom Means a Strong Marriage.
—SUZY PRUDDEN

Exercise Fun
For the Entire Family

A firm believer in physical fitness as a family enterprise, Ms. Prudden insists that exercise should be fun, and gives us exercises for every stage of life. To this end, she's designed a whole series of enjoyable exercises that helps build and maintain strong, lean, vital bodies. There are exercise-games for adults to play with their kids (like row your boat, push and pull, and paint the wall) and warm-up exercises for swimming, skiing, tennis and riding. There are facial exercises to help combat hard times, stress and tension, and some interesting sexercises for husbands and wives to practice.

Ms. Prudden writes charmingly, gives clear, easy-to-follow directions for each maneuver, and poses for all the thousands of illustrations.

SUZY PRUDDEN'S FAMILY FITNESS
BOOK
by Suzy Prudden & Jerry Sussman
Simon & Schuster (Hardcover, $8.95)

Let's Hear It
For the Grown-Ups

Remember Bonnie Prudden? (Suzy Prudden's Mommy?) The woman who invented "Sexercises"? Remember her zippy explanations of the hows and whys of physical fitness on "The Home Show"? Or her later appearances with Dave Garroway on "Today"? Well, even if *you* don't remember her, she was as much a part of my adolescence as Fire and Ice lipstick and the hair color that promised only my hairdresser would know for sure.

Now the new revised and enlarged edition of *How to Keep Slender and Fit After 30* is out in paperback. It came out just in time for me, too—chock-a-block with graphs, tests, personal anecdotes and photos of a still-slender Bonnie Prudden twisting herself into pretzel stretches, working out with dust mops and file cabinets, and demonstrating all the principles in her super-duper all-around exercise book.

HOW TO KEEP SLENDER AND FIT
AFTER 30
by Bonnie Prudden
Pocket Books (Paperback, $1.75)

Ten-Shun!

The *Royal Canadian Air Force Exercise Plans for Physical Fitness* were originally published as two separate pamphlets by the Office of the Queen's Printer in Canada. The Pocket Books edition of this RCAF way to keep fit keeps all the rough-hewn military style of the best government pamphlets. There is a wonderful non-slick quality to the silhouetted figures doing exercises, and a strange, antique look to the cartoons that pepper the pages. There are also some very important looking charts. Everything is goal oriented, so you can chart your progress right there in the book.

There are two RCAF plans: the XBX twelve-minutes-a-day plan (for women) and the 5BX eleven-minutes-a-day plan for men. How do they work? Easily, but with great precision. There are four charts of ten exercises in the XBX plan. The exercises are arranged so that they become progressively more difficult. Exercises on each chart are always performed in the same numerical order, for the same amount of time. As you work your way through the charts, the number of times each exercise is done increases, and the exercise itself goes through subtle variations that make it more difficult. This is a classic exercise book, designed for the goal directed and the especially energetic.

REVISED U.S. EDITION OF THE *OFFICIAL* ROYAL CANADIAN AIR FORCE EXERCISE PLANS FOR PHYSICAL FITNESS
Pocket Books, (Paperback, $1.50)

Om, Om on the Range

There are scads of yoga books around, but *Nova Yoga, The Yoga of the Imagination* seems to combine some pretty impressive tenets of the ancient art with the newest techniques of behavioral therapy. Therefore, it offers rewards that transcend mere shaping, toning and relaxation, delving into such areas as insomnia, compulsive eating, sexual inhibitions, excessive smoking, migraine headaches, drug addiction and crippling stutters. My favorite chapter is "How To Reach Your Center of Tranquility with Astral Projection."

NOVA YOGA
The Yoga of the Imagination
by George Francis Barth
Mason & Lipscomb (Hardcover, $6.95)

 Tai Chi (Pronounced: Tie jee) For Everybody

For those of us with a meditative bent, those of us who'd rather have another set of thumbs than do slam-bang, push-pull or calisthenic exercises, there is tai chi.

The Taoist monks in ancient China wanted to live forever, so they developed tai chi as a health-giving tranquilizer as well as a stimulating form of exercise. They also used it as a martial art, one so graceful, all-pervasive and deadly that they never had to break their thoughts while fending off bandits.

Today tai chi is done in offices, living rooms, kitchens and public parks throughout the country. The series of exercises takes only a few minutes a day. There is no special equipment to buy or carry around with you. You can perform in very little space with very little effort. In other words, tai chi is a slow, relaxed, comfortable way to keep in shape. It's also so graceful and fluid that all the exercises (when they're done right) look as though the person doing them is an underwater reed, flowing to the rhythm of the current. *Tai Chi for Health* is the definitive guide and the only English translation of the three classical writings on tai chi. It also has marvelously romantic names for each of the exercises, like: Parting the Wild Horse's Mane ... Golden Cock Stands on One Leg ... Step Back and Repulse Monkey ... Needle at Sea Bottom ... and Carry Tiger to Mountain.

TAI CHI FOR HEALTH
by Edward Maisel
Holt, Rinehart and Winston (Hardcover, $6.95)

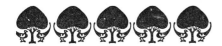

*Beauty of whatever kind, in its
supreme development, invariably excites
the sensitive soul to tears.*
—EDGAR ALLAN POE

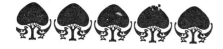

Belly Dancing in Memphis

The battle at Scheherazade is to make belly dancing a respectable pastime. Their students (secretaries, housewives and retired women looking for something interesting to do) dance for the sheer love of it. They also take advantage of Scheherazade's free programs in costume design, interesting dance procedures and various other subjects dealing with the Middle East.

A six-week belly dance course here (one night a week) runs $25. Once you reach the advanced stage, the price drops to only $18 a month, and there are no contracts to sign or hidden costs to worry about. All class rates for women over sixty-five are half-price, and if belly dancing isn't your *metier*, you might want to think about Scheherazade's courses in yoga, slimnastics or Hawaiian rhythms.

The Scheherazade people feel that belly dancing comes closer to teaching complete muscle control than any other physical activity. To make it even easier to fully immerse yourself in the art, if you're not thoroughly hooked already, they put out a catalog replete with costumes, practice records, study records and books that they sell both through the mail and on the premises in their boutique. For the catalog or for further information, write:

SCHEHERAZADE
480 Perkins EXT
Memphis, Tennessee 38117
Phone: (901)683-2454

Belly Up to the Barr, Girls

When belly dancing swept the country some years ago, some people laughed. Others sat at home and beaded dance bras. Many found themselves dancing with friends or for their husbands. Hundreds of thousands enjoyed themselves. Serena (America's foremost performer of Middle Eastern dance) has written a book that shows you how to tone and limber every succulent inch of your body, how to relax and get back in touch with yourself, how to prepare yourself for childbirth, and how to have a great deal of fun. There are over two hundred photographs, eighty-five exercises with sultry names like the Arabic Coffee Mill and the Berber Knee Walk (which is very strenuous and great for the legs and thighs). There's also a short course in playing the *zills* (finger cymbals), instructions on how to make a costume and step-by-step directions for putting on a belly dance performance of your own.

THE SERENA TECHNIQUE OF BELLY DANCING
by Serena and Alan Wilson
Pocket Books (Paperback, $1.95)

While We're on the Subject of Belly Dancing . . .

My friend Linda, the avid belly dancer of West 89th Street, was good enough to suggest that I list the following important information for belly dancers and belly dancers to be.

Belly Dance Records

The world's most complete collection of Middle Eastern recorded music lives in a dusty little office on Fifth Avenue. Mr. Guirak, who presides over all these records, will be happy to send you a catalog listing over one hundred belly dance recordings if you write to him at:

GUIRAK RECORDS
276 Fifth Avenue
New York, New York 10001

Guirak also carries professional finger cymbals ($33) and special-quality oud strings ... which I expect are for stringing special-quality ouds.

Linda (the West 89th Street belly expert) also recommends two records for beginners. They're both produced by Eddie "The Sheik" Kochak and can be ordered directly from Scepter Records.

> STRICTLY BELLY-DANCING (VOL- UMES I & II, $3.75 each)
> Scepter Records
> 254 West 54th Street
> New York, New York 10019
> Phone: (212)245-5515

GADGETS, GIZMOS AND GIMCRACKS TO EXERCISE AT HOME WITH

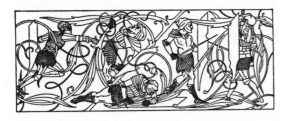

The Well-Equipped Sportswoman's Gym (Notes on the Home Front)

Naturally, home gyms, like anything else in life, can be as simple or as complex as your fantasy and your budget allows. But to give you some idea of just what the well-equipped sports-person might be able to put together from the sporting goods store and the mail order house, I include the following (purely arbitrary) list. Remember that the list provides just a sampling, and the prices are as correct as possible within a field where prices vary enormously. Basically, the watchwords in the sporting goods field are: shop around. There are bargains out there, but you'll have to look for them.

Equipment K. T. Maclay Would Have In Her Home Gym If She Had the Money

1 5′ × 10′ exercise mat	$ 56.95
1 slant board (for sit-ups)	$ 30.50
1 rubber suit (for working off water weight)	$ 31.95
1 pair 4-pound ankle-wrist weights (to make exercising more difficult)	$ 10.49
1 doorway gym bar (for chinning)	$ 6.97
1 set low parallel bars (for gymnastics)	$250.00
1 Jog Master Treadmill (for indoor jogging)	$360.00
1 pedometer (for measuring how far we jogged)	$ 11.99
1 hydraulic rowing machine (for exercising chest, legs and arms)	$129.00
1 set isotonic hand springs (for exercising shoulders and back)	$ 7.00
1 exercise bicycle	$130.00

That's what I would have in my gym, if I had the money. And what's more (unlike many of the women I know), I would run right out and get it all tomorrow. But that's only how *I* would do it. Most women I know who are involved to any extent in exercise start small. They get themselves a leotard ($7), some dance tights ($4.25), maybe even a pair of little leather ballet shoes from Capezio ($8); they join a dance class or a gym; and they call it quits. Those who don't call it quits are women who either are so hooked on exercise, or whose time is so limited, that nothing short of having a gym at home or a personal exercise program will really suit their needs.

It's *handy* to exercise on your living room floor or out in the garage. You don't have to make special arrangements, you don't have to travel. For a small initial investment you can surround yourself with all sorts of equipment, then feel perfectly free to use it at will.

My friend Betsy, for example, runs five miles every morning with the trainer of the New York Jets. Her wardrobe has pared itself down to six colorful jogging suits ($25 each) and three pairs of top-of-the-line Puma 9190 running shoes ($25.99 a pair). Anyone looking into Betsy's closet would quickly forget they were standing in her Park Avenue apartment and think perhaps that they had stumbled into the back room at Stillman's Gym. But running is important to Betsy, and being well equipped for running is part and parcel of the art.

My friend Adrienne, an executive type, didn't care a fig about running. She was more interested in where she could squeeze any exercise into her schedule than in what to wear while she was working out. So Adrienne seriously made plans to move everything she needed into a spare bedroom. She explains it this way:

"Mornings were clearly impossible for exercising. Getting the kids dressed and fed and off to school was a five-day-a-week Normandy invasion. I couldn't exercise during the day, because I was shackled to my desk at the office. Joining a health club or an exercise class wasn't really appealing either, but purely for esthetic reasons. I mean, you make an appointment to go to the gym once a week and you never do it because something else interferes that seems more important. So you put it off and it never happens. Also, I hate going to the gym and getting all sweaty and dreadful and then having to take a shower and change my makeup, put my hair back together again, pull my clothes on, and go back to the office. The only thing I really want to do after I exercise is die."

When she sat right down and thought about all this, the conclusion she came to was that having a home gym would make her life a lot easier.

"The theory was that if I could exercise at home, I could die quietly in my own bed afterward. So I started putting together the elements I thought I'd need to work out with quietly, after everyone else in the house was tucked safely between the covers. Unfortunately, that's when the problems began."

First, Adrienne wanted to have gymnast's rings ($100 the pair) so she could hang upside down from the ceiling and strengthen her stomach muscles while letting the blood rush to her head and shoulders and the tension drain out. But she couldn't do that because she had poured-cement ceilings. That was the first problem—there was just no way to install the kind of support equipment necessary. Also, the ceiling was too low to hang from unless you happened to be a six-year-old child.

Then Adrienne thought she would settle for a set of pulleys and weights ($150–$200) that would develop her shoulders and back and let her get rid of some of the aggressive energy she'd been storing up all day at the office. The problem with that was that her superintendent told her (in a rather patronizing tone of voice) that if she were to attach pulleys and weights to her plaster walls, he would lay even money that she'd pull the walls down and get her exercise picking up the pieces. So it was no go on that plan too.

Adrienne finally settled on floor mats ($34 each), which she put down in the spare bedroom, used religiously for about a month, then folded away and stored in the basement.

When I last talked to Adrienne about her home gym, she said only that it was "well intentioned." If she ever had a house in the country, she said, she'd probably have a gym in it, but she very quickly changed the subject.

Fran, on the other hand, looked at the whole topic of home exercise with her usual cool competence. In fact, she came to be the only one of my friends or acquaintances who actually pulled it together and consistently used a home exercise area.

For Fran plans for turning her foyer into a mini gym began with a minor shoulder injury and a deep-seated interest in dance. She got weights because she wanted to exercise her shoulder. She got a ballet bar and a huge 4′ × 8′ mirror when her interest switched from yoga to ballet. And, as she says: "I got some floor when I got the apartment."

I must admit that when I visited Fran's house recently, it was the mirror that intrigued me. Not only because you need a mirror to check that you're doing exercises properly and to congratulate yourself for what good shape you're in, but also because it was a fine, expensive-looking mirror, and I thought it must have set her back some to pay for it. Then Fran (who was shortening some jeans at the time) picked the mirror up in one hand and moved it into the living room to check the length of her handiwork.

"What in heaven's name is that?" I asked her.

"It's a 48″ × 96″ mylar mirror. It weighs twelve pounds and it costs $110 and I got it in the mail from Edmund Scientific Corp. (660 Edscorp Building, Barrington, N.J. 08007) and it's made to glue on the bedroom ceiling so you can watch yourself.... Oh well, it doesn't really matter what it was originally designed to do, it's great to exercise in front of."

The Porta-Bar in Fran's foyer came from a company called Ballet Bars (P.O. Box 717, Sarasota, Florida 33578) and cost her about $40.

"They're perfectly terrible if you don't have weights on them..." Fran explained as I tripped over the two $15 sandbags holding the bar down. The Porta-Bar is free-standing (the kind they used to drag out in ballet class, then move back against the wall when there was floor work to do). It's adjustable and sticks about fifteen inches out into Fran's foyer, making it extremely easy to trip over her sandbags if you're not careful.

The weights (which Fran's doctor said would strengthen her shoulder muscles) were really a set of small, solid Princess Dumbbells. They ranged in weight from a one-pound pair ($1.50) to a 10-pound pair ($15).

Being a conscientious as well as a practical woman, Fran figured her total investment, including a $34, 3′ × 6′ exercise mat on which she does floor work and stretches, came to about $250.

"Since I actually *do* exercise anywhere from two to seven times a week, depending on what else I'm doing, and I'm no longer spending $300 a year for a health club membership, and my equipment is not about to wear out before my body does, it seems to me I'm saving a tremendous amount of money."

If you're as dedicated as Fran is, or if your local Sears or sporting goods store can't handle the scope of your order, you might consider writing to Herman's, which is one of the largest sporting goods dealers in the country. They will be happy to answer your questions or send you the name of the Herman's nearest you. Just write:

HERMAN'S WORLD
OF SPORTING GOODS
2 Germak Drive
Carteret, New Jersey 07008

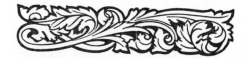

Get Yourself a Punching Bag

You'll be amazed at how happy you can feel after several aggressive minutes with a speed bag. Speed bag kits (and other interesting gym equipment) can be ordered from GEM SPORTING GOODS, and while we're thinking about it, here are some of my favorite things from the GEM catalog.

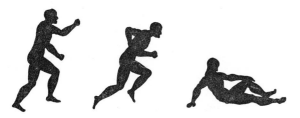

Roberts Speed Bag Set $24.95

Includes its own wooden platform, swivel- and tear-drop shaped vinyl speed punching bag. Can easily be wall-mounted at home or in the garage. Or if you're really serious about it, you can put one up in your office.

Panther Suit $31.95

Naive person that I am, I thought a panther suit was something that would make you look like a big, fierce cat. Actually, it's a rubber and nylon suit to sweat inside of while you exercise.

All-Purpose Exercise Mat $12.95

A must for doing floor work anywhere.

Doorway Gym Bar $6.97

For chinning or just hanging around from.

GEM SPORTING GOODS
29 West 14th Street
New York, New York 10011
(212)AL 5-5830

Sophisticated Exercising: The Extraordinary Exercycle

The Exercycle Corporation feels that their product is truly the "ultimate physical fitness machine" and that it is (or should be) a lifetime investment.

Simply stated, the Exercycle is a motor-guided triple-action exerciser. Its seat, handlebars and pedals all move simultaneously in a constantly changing sequence of movements. You can just sit back and let your Exercycle tone up your muscles—but you don't have to stop there. The harder you push, pull and pedal—the more you try to increase the machine's movement and speed—the more you get out of it. Fifteen minutes a day with an Exercycle can put you through all the motions of swimming, rowing, cycling, and chin-ups.

Exercycle's most popular model (THE EXECUTIVE) boasts two speeds, weight adjustment, a ½-horsepower motor and a seat cushion (for added comfort) which is listed as an extra. The EXECUTIVE EXERCYCLE lists at $775. For the name of the Exercycle dealer in your area, write:

EXERCYCLE CORPORATION
2074 Park Street
Hartford, Connecticut 06106
(203)236-0611

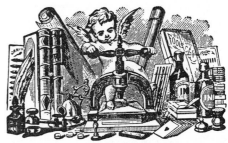

This is Not a Picture of a Man Caught in a Printing Press

This is an artist's interpretation of a man slimming, trimming and toning his body in a Nautilus Time Machine. Here we see him in a prestretched starting position on the Nautilus Super Hip and Back Machine. From this position he will move the padded resistance arm through a full 150-degree rotation. After he has done this for a while, he will have effectively exercised the strongest muscles in his body: the muscles in his hips and lower back. You, too, can have a Nautilus Super Hip and Back Machine for only $1,785. For information and a wonderful Time Machine Catalog, write:

NAUTILUS SPORTS/MEDICAL
INDUSTRIES
P.O. Box 1783
Deland, Florida 32720
(904)228-2884

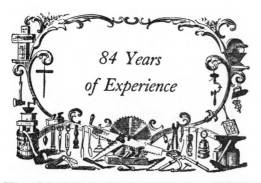

84 Years of Experience

The MacLevy people have been making heavy-duty exercise equipment since 1893. Their catalog lists everything from Abdominal Slant Boards to Vertical Knee Raise machines. Remember, this is heavy-duty equipment suitable for health clubs or the most elegantly equipped home gymnasiums. Take the Butterfly Machine, for example, the MacLevy answer to the Mark Eden Bust Improvement Course (I said it, MacLevy didn't). The Butterfly Machine weighs 220 pounds and is meant to improve your pectoral muscles, thereby increasing the apparent size of your bustline. Made out of triple chrome-plated steel, the Butterfly Machine is yours—padded with foam and upholstered in naugahyde—for $700. But why not write Mac-Levy and ask for their catalog?

MACLEVY PRODUCTS CORP.
92-21 Corona Avenue
Elmhurst, New York 11373
(212)592-6550

FENCING

Touché

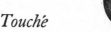

Lots of old-school fencing instructors insist on lots of hard tension in the body. Richard Rizk concentrates instead on relaxation. He makes your body "centered," as though there were an imaginary line going through you, pulling your head up and carrying your weight right into the floor for balance and strength. Fencing is a superb way to exercise while forming quick, fast, appropriate reactions, because, as Mr. Rizk says:

"There's just no second chance." Fencing is also very beautiful. In New York, call:

RICHARD RIZK (FENCING INSTRUCTOR)
Phone: (212)988-8269
10 Fencing Lessons, $50
Private Lesson, $20 per hour

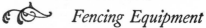 *Fencing Equipment*

George Santelli carries everything you'll need to be properly equipped for your fencing lessons, from a thumb pad right through to electrical *épée* blades . . . Santelli's has it all. If you're a beginner, you'll need a mask, a foil, a glove and a jacket—all of which you can pick up, or order through the mail, for less than sixty dollars, from Santelli. For the complete catalog, write:

GEORGE SANTELLI FENCING EQUIPMENT
412 Avenue of the Americas
New York, New York 10001
Phone: (212) AL 4-4053

EXERCISE TEACHERS WHO MAKE HOUSE CALLS

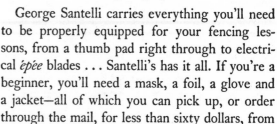 *Luxury Exercise*

Tolin Green is the wandering *wunderkind* of exercise. He is also the most expensive exercise expert in the United States. Why? Because Tolin Green makes house calls. That's right. He will bring his lithe, sinuous, well-exercised body to your house, wherever that house may be.

His terms are $100 a day plus first-class airfare and accommodations. Lucky residents of New York City can take advantage of Mr. Green's services at a more reasonable rate: $50 per session for approximately one hour (depending on your personal exercise needs) or $30 for his special series of facial exercises. Write or call Tolin Green in New York at:

TOLIN GREEN
145 West 55th Street
New York, New York 10019
(212)826-9640, 826-9666

Barbara Perlman Delivers

Barbara Perlman also makes house calls, though only in the New York area. Her system, based on yoga, stretch and dance techniques, improves stamina as well as toning and slimbering your body. She will visit hotels or give lessons at your office or in her apartment.

Ms. Perlman charges $40 for her forty-five-minute initial consultation with you, during which she discusses diet, life-style and medical history. Thereafter, a thirty-minute private lesson runs $25.

Small groups can take advantage of Ms. Perlman's services for $20 (for the first person) and $5 for each additional person. A group of three would therefore pay $30 for the lesson. Groups of eight or more pay a flat fee of $50. Write or call:

BARBARA PERLMAN
25 East 83rd Street
New York, New York 10028
(212)628-3682

DANCE YOUR WAY TO FAME AND THINNESS

Convenience Exercise

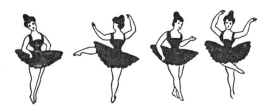

Assembly-line movements don't happen at the NICKOLAUS EXERCISE CENTERS. Here, co-ed classes of fifteen to twenty people go through a carefully developed system of body movements based on body conditioning, dance/exercise, ballet and modern dance techniques.

You work on the floor, using your own body as resistance, rather than standing and working against the force of gravity. The thirty-exercise NICKOLAUS program is designed to refresh and exhilarate without undue strain. All classes are arranged by appointment, from 9:30 A.M. to 7:30 P.M., Monday thru Friday (half-day on Saturdays).

RATES:		
	8 Classes	$ 40
	16 Classes	$ 75
	24 Classes	$110

Special Deals

First Lesson Free

Special exercises for skiers and pregnant women
PLUS:

The Quickie

Where there's a large concentration of working women among his clientele, Nickolaus has instituted a special half-hour lunchtime program that includes fifteen minutes of travel from office to Nickolaus Center, a half hour of class time, thirty seconds to grab a low-calorie, complimentary lunch of marinated chicken or seafood salad, and fourteen and a half minutes to get back to the office and catch your breath.

The Russian Ball

Gymnastic exercises to the music of Russian composers. Class includes a half hour of Nickolaus Technique followed by graceful, challenging movements that strengthen the upper body and improve posture.

Sound Body

Geared to the young, this class features a half hour of Nickolaus Technique followed by a half hour of jazz dance movements and routines done to the strains of rock music.

Magazine

Natural Living is a Nickolaus publication that comes out once a year, full of good, solid, zippy information on health, stress, exercise and vitamins. It's given free to all Nickolaus students.

NICKOLAUS EXERCISE CENTERS CAN BE FOUND AT THE FOLLOWING LOCATIONS:

NEW YORK
308 East 73 Street
(212)628-7771

10 East 45 Street
(212)986-9100

250 Third Avenue
(212)673-6960

767 Lexington Avenue
(212)838-9151

237 West 72 Street
(212)799-1030

Scarsdale, Rye, Dobbs Ferry
(914)478-0751

CALIFORNIA
9756 Wilshire Boulevard
Los Angeles
(213)274-5986

PENNSYLVANIA
Society Mill, Center City, Main Line
(215)MA 7-7125

Tap Is Back

After several decades of obscurity, the American art of tap dancing is undergoing a revival. Films showing the great tap dancers of the past—Astaire, Kelly, Rogers, Keeler and Miller—are enjoying renewed popularity and people of all ages are signing up for tap classes in hundreds of dance studios across the country.

THE BOOK OF TAP is for both the professional and the amateur. In addition to being lavishly illustrated with photographs from past and present, it has valuable instructions for beginners who want to learn how to tap from scratch ... as well as advice and comfort for professionals who want to brush up. The authors (Jerry Ames and Jim Seligman) present basic instructional material that includes an explana-

tion of basic steps for beginners as well as tap combinations for beginners, intermediates and advanced tappers, plus some really neat tap routines for everybody. In addition, there are selected lists of tap films, places to get tap paraphernalia and suggested tap records to practice with at home.

THE BOOK OF TAP: Recovering America's Long-Lost Dance
by Jerry Ames and Jim Seligman
David McKay (Hardcover, $11.95; Paperback, $6.95)

Always Wanted a Dancer's Body?

Write to Capezio Dance. They'll send you their catalog and a FREE BOOKLET called: *How to Achieve a Dancer's Body.* That's:

CAPEZIO DANCE
543 West 43rd Street
New York, New York 10036

Dance Your Troubles Away

Dancercise, the total, hour-long, head-to-toe workout set to music, is a brilliant combination of ballet warm-up exercises, yoga postures, tai chi-inspired movements and modern dance combinations. Dancercise works! And it's fun. At present, Dancercise is a totally New York phenomenon, but Jon Devlin (the dancer/choreographer who devised and developed Dancercise) has put together a "Total Exercise System" record and book that is truly the next-best thing to taking his classes. It's available for $8.70 (payable to Dancercise). Just write:

DANCERCISE RECORD AND BOOK
Viki Industries
Interstate Electronics Building
Highway 35 and Riverdale
Keyport, New Jersey 07735

Body Works

Body Works, the brainchild of jazz master Frank Wagner, is a superb way to dance away excess poundage and tension while firming up skin tone and muscles. Based on a series of nonexercise exercises known as isolations, Body Works is so easy, you hardly know you're working out. Body Works is attracting women in droves to Bergdorf Goodman in New York, where a trial class costs $5 and a series of ten lessons costs $80. If you're nowhere near the Big Apple, you can practice in the privacy of your own gracious home by getting the Body Works record ($9.95) or tape cassette (also $9.95) and a BW training manual ($12.95). Write:

BODY WORKS
Bergdorf Goodman
1 West 57th Street
New York, New York 10019

DEFENSIVE DOINGS
IN THE EXERCISE FIELD

Karate

You'd be amazed how nice people can be to you after you tell them you study karate. Not only does it firm your body, but it gives you working knowledge of a popular martial art form so you can protect yourself on the street (or at the next office Christmas party). The basic maneuvers tighten and tone your body with a benificent vengeance. Front kicks are guaranteed to work on the muscles behind your legs. Side kicks rid you of lumpy "love handles." Punching and blocking correctly can make you proud to see your arms again.

I studied at TRACY'S (which bills itself as the World's Largest Chain of Self-Defense Studios). You should be able to find one near you by checking in the Yellow Pages under "Judo, Karate and Ju-Jitsu." According to the karate grapevine, they all have pleasant, carpeted private rooms for individual lessons and comfy large areas for workouts with other students.

Distaff Defense

The Women's Martial Arts Union is a collective of feminist women training in the martial arts (karate, judo and other fighting systems). Founded in 1972, the group originally came together to exchange self-defense techniques and to establish contact between women who had been isolated minorities in separate schools and disciplines.

WMAU evolved, organized three women's martial arts conferences and attracted hundreds of women from several cities.

The conferences gave women the chance to train together, to share ideas on teaching methods, injuries, and self-defense. Now WMAU gives martial arts/self-defense demonstrations and sends speakers to schools and assorted women's events around the country.

They've also published (and are making available) two articles explaining some of the basic aspects of the martial arts and self-defense courses for those of us who know little about the subject but would like to know more. The articles ("Getting Off To A Good Start In Karate," by Nadia Telsey and Susan Ribner, 25¢, and "Self-Defense Courses or Martial Arts Courses?" 50¢) give information on choosing a good school, what to look for in price, equipment and instruction. To order the articles or request further information on WMAU, write:

WOMEN'S MARTIAL ARTS UNION
P.O. Box 1463
New York, New York 10027

 ### The Friendliest Chorus Line in New York

For women who are allergic to outsiders (or who simply don't want strangers to see them in a leotard), Sandy Berwald (of the exclusive East Side exercise-to-music studio, DANCE 'N SHAPE) is now offering "Friends Only" classes.

You get together with three or four people you know and like. Then you choose which hour and day (or days) you'd like to reserve for your private group and nobody else.

In other words, you form your own exclusive club and get all the benefits of Sandy's never-boring, ever-changing choreographed combinations of ballet and modern dance.

A phone call will reserve a "Friends Only" hour. Should there be no current availability, ask to be put on the waiting list.

DANCE 'N SHAPE
201 East 36th Street Studio 5A
New York, New York 10016
(212)689-6579
$5 (for introductory class)
$7 (per lesson)

DON'T FORGET ABOUT THE WOMEN'S

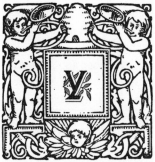

Y's are sophisticated, especially nice places to get to know. They've got dance, calisthenics and martial arts courses. You can even swim at most of them or get involved in prescription exercise or stress testing programs—or simply bake in the saunas.

The YWCA is an autonomous women's movement whose members are women and girls from twelve years old onwards. Men can take part in many of the programs at the YW, but only as associate members. And talk about convenience, there are more than four hundred YWCAs across the country. Each is a separate operation, but all of them offer some sort of wonderful exercise activity. The range of fees varies widely; in some cases class fees are extra (over and above membership), but in every case, the Y offers wonderful bargains.

New York City's Central YWCA branch lists the following off-beat classes as part of its regular program, and I'm putting them in here as a reminder that the Y is a nifty place, and to give you some idea of the value you can get for your money here.

NOTE: All classes meet for fifty minutes. Fees are individually listed and are paid in addition to a basic $12 membership fee for adult women.

AFRICAN DANCE (Beginner/Intermediate)
Rhythmic dances based on authentic African heritage, performed with live drum accompaniment. 8 sessions, $26.

BALLET (Beginner/Advanced Beginner/ Intermediate)
Basic classical ballet training and dance movement. 8 sessions, $26.

FLAMENCO (Beginner/Intermediate)
Authentic Spanish folk dance technique using rhythmic footwork and castanets. 8 sessions, $26.

JAPANESE KABUKI-STYLE DANCE
Basic technique of folkloric and classical Kabuki-style dance. 8 sessions, $26.

TAP DANCE (Beginner/Intermediate/ Advanced)
Shades of Busby Berkeley staging a comeback for fun and exercise. 8 sessions, $26.

CORRECTIVES (Beginner/Intermediate)
Small classes in exercise designed to help relieve excessive tension and improve body conditioning and posture. 8 sessions, $32.

And Now a Word About the

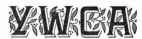

There are 18,042 YMCAs in the country, so you can find one handy almost anywhere. Membership in the Y is open to both men and women. In fact, forty percent of Y members are women. The cost of membership varies widely and is pretty much dependent on the cost of living in the area. Some Ys have a basic membership fee that covers all costs. Others operate on a basic membership PLUS an extra course fee for special courses like Scuba Diving. The basic membership fees for adults range from $20 to $200 per year, with the typical fee falling somewhere in the $50 to $60 a year area. Best to check out your own local Y in the Yellow Pages, or drop by the membership office and talk it over.

Here are some of the more interesting programs offered by the West Side YMCA in New York:

WOMEN'S WAIST WATCHERS
Forty-five minutes of dance, yoga and gymnastic exercise set to music to stretch, strengthen and tone your body. 8 sessions, $33.

YOGA (Beginners/Intermediate)
Hatha Yoga *asanas* (exercises) and yoga breathing *(pranayama)* give you a feeling of well-being while stretching and improving your coordination, increasing your vitality and preventing fatigue. 8 sessions, $33.

BELLY DANCING (Beginners)
Movement to exotic Oriental music to help define your body's curves and muscle tone. 8 sessions, $33.

MODERN DANCE EXERCISE AT LUNCH
Spend your lunch hour at the Y. Lessen muscle fag. Dance, relax and exercise. 16 sessions (two 25-minute sessions per week), $33. 24 sessions (two 25-minute sessions per week), $45.

FENCING Six Private Lessons, $15.

KARATE
Kyokusin Kai-Kan. Diplomas awarded to those who successfully complete the course and pass the test. Size, weight and sex are no object.

One lesson per week for twelve weeks, $35; two lessons per week for twelve weeks, $45.

SHAPING UP ON THE WEST COAST
California Yoga

Pat Casty moved to California from New York and immediately fell into a black depression. "Nobody ever sees you below the waist out here," she moaned. "Not unless you're on the beach or playing tennis—and by that time it's too late. I spend so much time behind the wheel of my car anyway that all my muscles seem to have settled into my backside. So I just started yoga."

At first, Pat didn't think it would work because she was convinced she needed some strenuous maneuvers like running around a track, or dancing her buns off. But two weeks with Bikram Choudray at the Yoga College of India changed all that and turned Pat into a devoted convert.

"He has people like Marge Champion in the class and there are twenty of us . . . and I should go every day because it loosens up your spine. Besides, you get ten 90-minute classes for $50 so it's really foolish not to take advantage of them."

Not only was yoga paring Pat's weight off, it was making her graceful: "You can bend down and pick up a pencil when it falls off your desk . . . You can make a good impression." She said, "At a restaurant, when you drop your silverware on the floor—I don't know, not that you go into a pretzel contortion, but somehow you're able to pick it up without making a fool of yourself."

If it works for Pat Casty, it can work for you. To find out, see:

Bikram Choudray
YOGA COLLEGE OF INDIA
9441 Wilshire Boulevard
Beverly Hills, California
Phone: (213)276-1048

Ron Fletcher's Body Contrology Helps You Get It All Together

Stop in at Ron Fletcher's little blue-doored studio on Wilshire Boulevard, and what you hear is the sound of wheezing; Sam Goldwyn, Jr., wheezing on the floor machine as he moves his knees back and forth; Barbra Streisand wheezing in the corner by the green-growing plants; Candice Bergen hanging upside down from her ankles in the front room wheezing.

Could it be *the wheezing* that causes Hollywood's Four Hundred to flock in droves to Wilshire and Rodeo? Is it THE WHEEZING?

"No!" says Ron Fletcher (ex-choreographer, dancer, gymnast and prolific student of things anatomical). "Besides," he continues, "it's not 'wheezing'—it's 'breathing.' "

Whatever you call that deep, throaty intake of breath followed by that long, loud whistling exhale, Ron's students all breathe this way as they exercise because it makes them feel better, clears their bodies of toxic wastes, gives them endless energy and carries them through their strenuous hour-and-a-half sessions of leg raises, extensions, contractions, and miniscule muscle maneuvers.

Ron Fletcher thoroughly believes in breathing (and in dance and in gymnastics and in getting the mind, the body and the spirit together). That's what body contrology is all about—an ingenious system for getting you in touch with your body so you can get more pleasure out of it. That means: better sports, better contact, better feelings and (of course) better sex.

"There's only one problem," says Fletcher. "You've got to commit yourself to working this way always and forever. Like eating the right kind of food and breathing correctly. Not everybody can make that kind of commitment. But you can tell the ones who do. They've got a certain glow about them. With some of them you can even feel it before you see them."

Whatever Contrology's got, stars are lining up

to get their hands on it.

If you'd like to invest now in YOUR charismatic futures, you can sign up for 10 personally supervised lessons ($100.) or take a single ($25.00) introductory class. You need merely make an appointment by contacting:

RON FLETCHER STUDIO FOR BODY CONTROLOGY
9549½ Wilshire Boulevard
Beverly Hills, California
Phone: (213) 278-4777

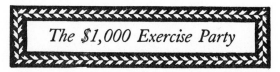

The $1,000 Exercise Party

The invitation read: You are cordially invited to appear at 9306 Santa Monica Blvd. at 8:00 P.M. on the 9th of January, 1976. Attire was casual (sweat suits). The occasion was a surprise exercise/dinner bash to celebrate the fortieth birthday of a well-known Hollywood film executive.

When the guests arrived, they were ushered into Anatomy Asylum, treated to one of Richard Simmons's special hour-long exercise classes (which, with Richard, is more like a nightclub performance you sweat through), then sent to the showers. As soon as they caught their collective breath and lowered their individual heart rates back to normal, they jogged through a connecting door (into RUFFAGE, Richard's health food–salad bar restaurant) to wolf down a dinner which included, among other things, artichokes stuffed with beluga caviar and poached salmon in a shrimp-lime sauce.

The tab for the fifty-person party ran about $1,000 (give or take a couple of hundred). Expensive? Sure, but as Richard reminded me, whipping up a special party is just part of it; you are paying for *him,* too. And HE is quite something. For one thing, he's modest; or as he puts it:

"I'm going to be a star in two years and you can all go back and say 'Gee. I remember when he taught ME a class. . . .' " For another thing, he's got all sorts of interestingly unshakable ideas about food and fat and feeling better. Here in his own words are two of them.

"There's so many quick things out there. There's quick sex and quick care and quick eyelashes. Or quick beauty, or quick bodies. You can put on an Isotoner suit and look thinner. You can get clothing specifically designed to hide your body. The only thing you can't buy frozen is *a salad*. I serve nothing but SALAD at RUFFAGE and I'm very proud of it."

Okay, Richard, what about EXERCISE?

"I don't worry about your insides as much as your OUTSIDES. I'm not worried why you hate your mother, or if you wore high heels as a kid, or if you peed in your bed. I'm not worried about those things. Forget that. If you don't like what you look like NOW ... If you're living alone ... if you have only a pet or a plant ... if you never go out ... if you eat frozen dinners ... then you're the kind of person that should come here."

By "here" Richard means THE ANATOMY ASYLUM, where classes run morning, noon and night. Private classes and big classes. Classes drowned in the sound of Ethel Merman singing "Everything's Coming Up Roses" accompanied by Richard (or one of his indomitable instructors) screaming "Harder! HAR-DER!! I want to HEAR it when you're breathing!" ASYLUM classes (which are $4.50 each) run an hour to an hour and fifteen minutes. There are usually ten people in the morning ones, thirty in the afternoons and evenings. The schedule starts at 7:30 A.M. and ends just before 8:00 at night.

All this madness can be yours at

ANATOMY ASYLUM
9306 Santa Monica Blvd.
Beverly Hills, California 90210
(213) 550-8879

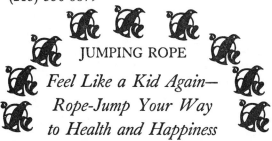

JUMPING ROPE

*Feel Like a Kid Again—
Rope-Jump Your Way
to Health and Happiness*

Next to hula hoops, I can't think of anything that took up more of my time when I was a kid, or gave me quite as much pure pleasure as jumping rope. But that's *old* news. The *new* news is that jumping rope is GOOD for you. It's easy. It's private. It doesn't take up large chunks of valuable time. And it can get you in better shape quicker than just about any other exercise. In fact, rope skipping provides the single most concentrated form of leg exercise of all, while keeping your hands, wrists, arms, fingers, shoulders, back, rib cage and nine-foot jump rope in steady motion. Even better yet, it reduces fat on thighs, legs and hips and can protect you from hardening of the arteries and heart attacks.

Jumping rope is fun. If you haven't skipped rope since you were a kid, run—do not walk—and get yourself a copy of *The Perfect Exercise*. Read it carefully. Ignore the fact that it's fun to read. Don't dwell on all the great things it tells you about the human body. Zip right past the humor and the good advice, and get into the most dynamite new exercise program to come along in years.

THE PERFECT EXERCISE
THE HOP, SKIP, AND JUMP WAY
TO HEALTH
by Curtis Mitchell

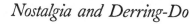
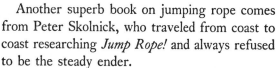

Nostalgia and Derring-Do

Another superb book on jumping rope comes from Peter Skolnick, who traveled from coast to coast researching *Jump Rope!* and always refused to be the steady ender.

The book is a collection of well-illustrated exercises, PLUS 250 rhymes guaranteed to bring it all back. Rhymes like "A my name is Alice..."; prediction rhymes, which tell you whom you'll marry; counting chants, which report the number of kisses (or whatever) given or taken ... and a whole bunch of invaluable rhymes which mock grown-ups, big brothers, the baby, teacher and anyone else who tends to make trouble. There are games, too; like Easy Ivy (for beginners) and Chinese Jump Rope, and more advanced games like the murderous Hot Pepper and Double Dutch. Jerry Darwin's photos of rope jumpers young and old, and line drawings by Marty Norman (who is awfully good at drawing feet) all play their parts in making this manual the nicest book in years for people who know it's crucial to "go all in together."

JUMP ROPE!
by Peter Skolnick
Workman Publishing Co.
(Paperback, $2.95)

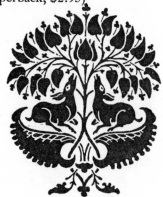

Status (and Other) Jump Ropes

I was so excited by *Jump Rope!* and *The Perfect Exercise* that I ran out to the corner card shop and picked up a fourteen-foot jump rope with plastic handles. Five minutes later, I'd shortened it to the regulation size (measured armpit to armpit while standing in the middle of it). (What you do is stand in the middle of your jump rope. From that position, if the handles reach exactly to your armpits, the rope is the right length.)

My jump rope cost all of 79¢, but it is not—as I now understand—the PERFECT jump rope. There is not enough weight to it, not enough heft. On the other hand, without this less-than-perfect equipment, I would have had to wait for the joy of skipping rope. That was unthinkable. For those of you who are equally excited about rope skipping, and equally desperate, but somewhat better equipped in the home accessories department, jump ropes can be made out of laundry line or plain old size 7 to 10 sash cord.

Dan Lurie's in New York will send you any one of four different jump ropes in the mail. Here's how they're listed in the Dan Lurie catalog:

ECONOMY SKIP ROPE	
(light weight, 7'6" cord)	$4.00
STANDARD SKIP ROPE	
(heavy weight, 8' cord)	$5.00
STANDARD SKIP ROPE	
(heavy weight, 8'6" cord, swivel handles)	$5.50
DELUXE SKIP ROPE	
(heavy 9'6" polyethylene cord, ball-bearing handles)	$7.00

To order, write:

DAN LURIE BARBELL COMPANY
1665 Utica Avenue
Brooklyn, New York 11234
(New Yorkers, add appropriate sales tax)

Curtis Mitchell recommends a skip rope with plastic fit-together handles in *The Perfect Exercise*. You can order one of these by sending $9.95 to:

E. A. JONES
Box 3164
Denver, Colorado 80201

Neiman-Marcus carries Starcase's $15 deluxe-deluxe model jump rope with an adjustable rope and handles that keep track of how many times you jump. Write Neiman-Marcus Stationery Department, adding $1.20 for postage and insurance. Or stop in at one of their branches in Dallas, Fort Worth, Houston, Atlanta, Bal Harbour, St. Louis or Northbrook (Illinois).

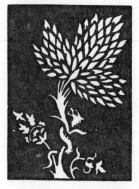 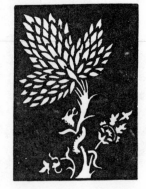

HEALTH CLUBS ARE GETTING THE FAT OFF THE LAND

Join a health club, if only for the reassurance. There are all sorts of bodies at health clubs. Some of them are bound to be in worse shape than you are. Hang around the steam room or the sauna. Check the rolls of flab. Or the breasts that are down to there—or the ladies with no breasts at all. I started to feel a lot better about my body as soon as I joined a health club. And going regularly did nothing but improve things.

—Sarah Edwards, Chicago, Illinois

Where Is Everybody?

Can't reach your friends on the phone? Maybe they're at the health club. To get your copy of a handy book that lists the names, addresses and phone numbers of 950 different health clubs from Asia to Thailand, all you have to do is send $2 to the International Physical Fitness Association and ask for their membership guide.

I found out about this lovely little guide because my membership in the New York Health Club grants me visiting privileges at any International Physical Fitness Association affiliate anywhere in the world. Many health spas throughout the country will do the same. To get your guide to participating members, WRITE:

INTERNATIONAL PHYSICAL FIT-NESS ASSOCIATION
415 West Court Street
Flint, Michigan 48502

 ### *Beauty and Pleasure Through Health*

That's what it says on the front door of the health club I belong to. It says nothing about the $345 a year membership fee, or the 10′ × 3′ swimming pool, or the 35¢ a day I tip the dressing-room attendant, or the $35 a year I pay for my own private locker. It doesn't say any of that. It says: Beauty and Pleasure Through Health.

Don't get me wrong. I really love my health club. I go there every day at lunch (or rather instead of lunch) and I steam and I swim (trying not to clonk into the other people in that miniature pool) and I sauna, and I stand under some very attractive lights that make everyone look healthy while they dry their hair and put on their makeup. And at that I'm not even taking full advantage of the club. I don't take the complete range of exercise and dance courses they offer. I don't eat in their lovely natural-food restaurant. I don't use their hundred-thousand-dollar exercise equipment. I don't even socialize particularly—but I love it anyway. What's more, for my initial membership fee I am entitled to use any one of the 950 other health clubs around the country that have a reciprocal agreement with mine. All this makes me smile just to think about it.

Other things that make me smile are the peculiar language and odd mystique you fall into when you join a health club. "Miyee Gauwd! You're wanishing!!!" says the 350-pound masseuse to a slightly overweight redhead. "How much have you lost already?" We are all preoccupied with weight and form. None of us regulars would dream of stepping on that doctor's scale in the drying area before every last hair was dry. Hair dry. No makeup. No towel. Not a single thing that might add an extra fraction of an ounce. We're also concerned with our diets: "No kidding? You've been eating nothing but brown rice and stewed fruit for HOW long???" We are amazed with ourselves. And pleased.

There is definitely something to this health-club craze. Something above and beyond the fear of coronary thrombosis and the desire to stave off the aging process as long as possible.

Nobody knows exactly, but Allied Health Associates estimates there are some two thousand health clubs carving the fat off conscientious American exercisers. Ranging from Spartan to spectacular and lightly touching all the bases in between, they're grossing well over $100 million a year—and boy, do they ever want your body!

To get it, most health clubs offer you a room full of exercise equipment, a swimming pool, a whirlpool, a sauna and a steam bath and, if you're lucky, a continuous stream of exercise classes. But be aware that health clubs are very often the material projections of their owners' personalities; so if you have the right owner, you can avail yourself of such exotic luxuries as private massages, perfumed baths, organic restaurants, mink-covered bicycle seats and oxygen to cure your hangover.

Understandably, fees for such services can be stiff: say, five hundred dollars for initiation PLUS about thirty dollars a month in dues, not counting extras like tips, locker fees or the use of the club's towels.

On the other hand, what you pay often depends on where you live—and the prices for joining a health club range all over the place. Like, for example, one club sells their two-year membership for $14 a month in Salt Lake City; but in New York City, the same club charges $27 a month for the same program. Most health clubs cost between $200 and $300 for the first year, which entitles you to use the facilities as often as you like.

Remember that you can never really be sure that the health club in your backyard is operated with the same expertise or efficiency as the health club in someone else's backyard. Even though your health club may look like part of what appears to be a national operation (a Vic Tanney's, say, or a Jack La Lanne), many health clubs are simply franchise operations, and (as with most franchises) their quality depends very much on the skill and devotion of the people who own and run them.

The best way to satisfy yourself that you'll be getting out of your health club enough benefit to offset the amount of money you're putting into it is to investigate it personally. Stick with me here; there is a Checklist of Things to Think About While Touring a Health Club coming soon.

Another good idea is to find someone who belongs now or has in the past belonged to the club you're considering. A disgruntled ex-member can open up areas of questioning you'd never consider if you weren't forced to. Likewise, a satisfied current member can point out perks and goodies you hadn't thought about that make the club even more attractive to you.

As usual, the more information you have at hand, the better equipped you'll be to make a wise decision.

Which brings us to the very important question: What should you be aware of before you sign up?

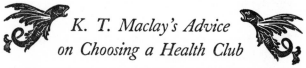

K. T. Maclay's Advice on Choosing a Health Club

Every health club I've ever been in has a person whose job it is to show you around and give you a quick, favorable impression. This means that she will nip down (or up) the stairs with you and give you a wonderfully friendly but superficial tour of her club. You have to remember that she's interested in one thing and one thing only: your membership. Selling new contracts is how her club makes its living and keeps its doors open. So while in *your* mind you are blond, five foot seven and five pounds overweight, to the person who's showing you around, you are "a contract."

There is only one way to deal with this: From the instant you walk through the front door, you must imagine that you are already a member, that you use the club every day and, in fact, that the club is your home away from home. If it IS your home away from home, and you can remember that once you sign the contract you will have a sizable investment in it, you can relax into an attitude I've come to recognize in myself as informed unreasonableness.

This means that you don't simply follow your tour guide as she trips lightly through the club like a real-estate agent, saying, "And these are the locker rooms—here's the sauna—that's the whirlpool..." and so on and so on.

Informed unreasonableness means you take your time. Ask to use the bathroom—is it clean? Go INTO the locker room and ask to see the lockers—inside. Ask about the towels. Are they in good condition? Are they frayed around the edges? Do they look like the dog's been at them? Imagine at each step of the way that this is where you'll be spending a lot of time. Ask yourself honestly, would you really *like* to spend time here? If so, all well and good. If not, you're throwing your money down the drain.

Now, ask yourself what it is you really want from your health club. Do you want to fall in during your lunch hour and take a dance class? If so, check the club's schedule. Can you get in every day and any day at lunch? Or do they have a co-ed program that means men can use the club Monday, Wednesday and Friday and women can only get in there Tuesday, Thursday and Saturday—and Sunday is a free-for-all? Is the club open late enough for you to go after work? Oh, yes, and if the club has an alternate-day program for men and women, do they have a permanent locker arrangement where you can leave your gym stuff and your swimming gear so you don't have to drag it around with you all the time? If they've got this kind of set-up, does it cost extra? Do towels cost money? Are there private dressing rooms, or do you have to struggle out of your pantyhose in full view of the pool?

Go into the sauna. Does it have enough room to lie down in, or did they build it out of an old sink closet? Are there bouquets of wet bathing suits hanging around, creating a fire hazard?

Is the health club itself physically big enough to do what you want to do in it? If your primary reason for joining is to swim, is the pool Olympic size? Or is it so small that once you put two other people in it, it will be like trying to swim in a teacup? These are important questions. If the pool is small, but you can use it on off hours when nobody's there but you, fine. But if you can only get to the club during peak-activity times—forget it.

Say you couldn't care less about the swimming pool, but you really want to use the club's dance or yoga or calisthenics classes. What's the class schedule? How long are the classes? How many other people are in them? Are they fun? Will you enjoy them—because if you don't enjoy them, you will very quickly stop going to the health club.

Now look into the showers. Are the handles coming off in your hand? Is the tile separating itself from the walls? These are not minor points, believe me. These are "quality of life" questions you have to answer before the answers to them come as a rude shock to you.

How about the steam room? Does it smell funny in there? Does it work? Is it clean? Are the other members sitting on towels? What about the gym equipment? My gym has a full complement of Nautilus and MacLevy machines that look like they came straight off the set of *2001*. But machines themselves can be dangerous. Are there attendants there to help you with your physical-fitness program? Or are there just three sets of five-pound dumbbells and a few other women struggling to work out on slant boards? Are there club hair dryers and nice makeup lights? These amenities are more important than you might think, because your health club should be an "up," and if the facilities or the physical prettiness of the place are missing, so is a large part of the experience.

What about the masseuses and the attendants? Do they look like something out of Dickens? Or are they pleasant and smiling? How much will you have to tip them to keep them happy?

Is this health club really private (open only to those bona fide members who've paid several hundred dollars) or is it open to anyone off the street at any time for the payment of five dollars to the receptionist? The exclusivity of your club is directly proportional to the rate at which things like tights, leotards and handbags disappear out of it.

What is the ambience of this health club? Is it a social, singles-bar type of place—or a grimly determined, no-nonsense, let's-get-down-to-business-and-shape-ourselves-up sort of place? Which do you want? They come in all varieties and you should (if you possibly can) use the club once before joining, just to make sure.

By now, if everything else has checked out favorably, I'm assuming that you are sitting down with a contract in your hands. Before you sign it, here are some other things to think about:

Some health clubs will let you suspend your membership if you go away for a month or so. Ask if this is possible. Otherwise you've wasted four weeks if you plan a vacation in the Galapagos. Also, ask if your club has guest privileges at other clubs throughout the country. Some do, and with no extra charge and no hassle.

Ask what the busiest times are and when the slow periods fall. I've gone to the club at times when I could fantasize that it was my own personal playground, and I've gone at other times when it was like strap-hanging in the IRT at rush hour.

One more important question to ask is whether there are any seasonal specials or discount rates available. My own club offers discounts for paying cash (actually they gave me a free month). They also have seasonal sales, like their Celebration of March Shape-Up Month and their famous discount for Buddha's birthday.

One last, superimportant point: Don't sign a contract on the spot. Most reasonable health clubs, though they hate to remove their fangs from a hot prospect, will let you take the papers home to look over at your leisure and under a bright light.

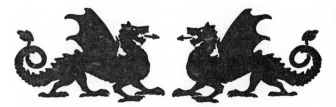

Checklist of Things to Think About While Touring a Health Club

AMBIENCE
physical appearance

atmosphere

exclusivity

other members

FACILITIES
dressing rooms

lockers

bathrooms

showers

exercise equipment

classrooms

swimming pool

sauna

steam room

whirlpool

restaurant

AMENITIES
towels

lights

soap

hand & standard hair dryers

staff

attendants

tipping

PROGRAMS
club schedule

class schedule

private instruction

special programs

BUSINESS
discounts

suspensions

access to other clubs

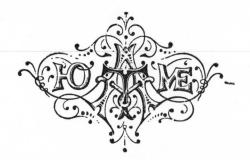

Ethical Practices

Want to know all about cancelation provisions, spa facilities, cleanliness and service? Want to know what your health club will do for you? Want to get the lowdown before you put your signature on that very important contract? Then you should have a copy of the "Code of Ethical Practices." To get one FREE from the Association of Physical Fitness Centers (which represents about 450 different health clubs), write:

Dr. Jimmy D. Johnson
Executive Director
Association of Physical Fitness Centers
5272 River Road
Washington, D.C. 20016

Help For the Weary Traveler

Tired? Miserable? Worn out from a weary day on the road? Would a half hour in the pool or fifteen minutes in the sauna set you straight? Then why not check into one of the many motels or hotels who understand your problem and have been good enough to supply health club facilities as well as comfortable accommodations.

As always, it's a good idea to check them out before you check in to make sure that all systems are still go and that the equipment and physical surroundings meet with your approval.

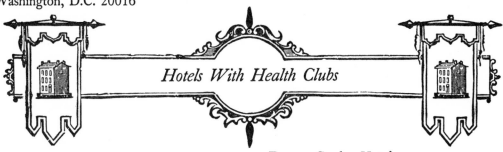

Hotels With Health Clubs

Velda Rose Motor Hotel &
Mineral Water Spa
Mesa, Arizona 85201

Arlington Hotel and Baths
Central Avenue and Arlington Park
Hot Springs, Arkansas 71901 (whirlpool thermal baths)

The Majestic Hotel & Baths
Park and Central Avenues
Hot Springs, Arkansas 71901

Velda Rose Tower & Motel
218-224 Park Avenue
Hot Springs, Arkansas 71901

Bermuda Inn
Lancaster, California 93534

Canyon Hotel
2850 South Palm Canyon Drive
Palm Springs, California 92262 (spa and sauna)

Desert Hot Springs Spa
Desert Hot Springs, California 92240

Disneyland Hotel
Anaheim, California 92802 (health club)

Erawan Garden Hotel
Indian Wells
Palm Desert, California 92260

Guenther's Murrieta Hot Springs
Murrieta, California 92362

Hotel Claremont
Ashby & Claremont Avenues
Oakland, California 94618

International Hotel Health Club & Spa
Los Angeles Airport
Los Angeles, California 90009

Spa Hotel
Palm Springs, California 92262

The Broadmoor
Colorado Springs, Colorado 80901

Hotel Ambassador
14th and K Streets, N.W.
Washington, D.C. 20005 (health club)

Hotel Continental
420 North Capitol Street, N.W.
Washington, D.C. 20001 (sauna and exercise room)

The Watergate Hotel
2650 Virginia Avenue, N.W.
Washington, D.C. 20037 (health club)

Causeway Inn Beach Resort
7627 West Columbus Drive
Tampa, Florida 33607 (sauna and exercise room)

Dupont Plaza Hotel & Apartments
300 Biscayne Boulecard Way
Miami, Florida 33131 (health spa)

Harbor Island Spa
Miami Beach, Florida 33139

Harbor Island Spa & Hotel
North Bay Village, Florida 33141

Hotel Fontainebleau
Miami Beach, Florida 33139 (spa complex)

Lago Mar Resort Club
500 N.W. 127th Avenue
Fort Lauderdale, Florida 33325 (health salon)

Lido Spa
Miami Beach, Florida 33139

Safety Harbor Spa
Safety Harbor, Florida 33572

Sonesta Beach Hotel
Key Biscayne, Florida 33149 (spa)

Sun Spa
3101 South Ocean Drive
Hollywood Beach, Florida 33019

Sheraton-O'Hare Motor Hotel
6810 North Mannheim Road
Rosemont, Illinois 60018 (spa area with sauna)

Continental Regency Hotel
500 Hamilton Boulevard
Peoria, Illinois 61652 (health club)

French Lick-Sheraton Hotel
French Lick, Indiana 47432 (mineral and steam baths)

Home Lawn Mineral Springs
Martinsville, Indiana 46151

Dawson Springs Resort Motel
Dawson Springs, Kentucky 42408

Battle Creek Sanitarium
Battle Creek, Michigan 49016

Plymouth Hilton Inn
14707 Northville Road
Plymouth, Michigan 48170 (sauna and exercise room)

Broadwater Beach Motel
Biloxi, Mississippi 48231 (health salon)

The Colony Motor Hotel
7730 Bonhomme Avenue
Clayton, Missouri 63105 (health club)

Lodge of the Four Seasons
Lake Ozark, Missouri 65049 (health spa)

Harrah's
Reno, Nevada 89501 (health club)

The Sands
Las Vegas, Nevada 89109 (health club)

Tropicana Hotel & Country Club
Las Vegas, Nevada 89109 (health club)

Resort International Hotel
Boardwalk and N. Carolina Avenue
Atlantic City, New Jersey 08404 (health club)

Gideon Putnam Hotel
Sarasota Springs, New York 12866

Spring Lake Spa
Liberty, New York 12754

The Warwick
Avenue of the Americas at 54th Street
New York, New York 10019 (health club and sauna)

Bedford Springs Hotel
Bedford, Pennsylvania 15522 (therapeutic waters)

Howard Johnson's Motor Lodge
Chatham Center
Pittsburgh, Pennsylvania 15219 (health club)

Baker Hotel
Mineral Wells, Texas 76067

The Homestead
Hot Springs, Virginia 24445 (mineral spa)

The Greenbrier
White Sulphur Springs, West Virginia 24986 (mineral baths)

Park View Inn
Berkeley Springs, West Virginia 25411 (mineral springs and baths)

Nassau Beach Hotel
Nassau, Bahamas

Harrison Hotel
Harrison Hot Springs
British Columbia, Canada

Skyline Hotel
Toronto
Ontario, Canada

SPAS FOR ALL SEASONS

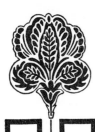
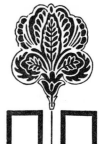

Even the most conscientious exercise or diet program can eventually grind itself into a routinized crashing bore. That's the time to take stock, check your liquid assets and look into the wild, woolly, wondrous world of the beauty spas.

In this country alone a magnificent variety of spas and retreats offers the willing mind and body a boggling assortment of alternatives. There are spas so luxurious they're like resort hotels. There are Spartan spas, specific-interest spas, health spas, nature spas and spas where you can happily go to hell with yourself.

There are spas like California's Rancho La Costa, which push their tennis pros and their country club atmospheres. There are others (like Elizabeth Arden's Maine Chance in Arizona) that promote their posh, pampered, socially exclusive privacy.

The Golden Door in California gives you biofeedback, eleven hours of strenuous exercise a day, luxurious surroundings and an 1,100-calories-a-day diet. There is even a spa in upstate

New York that won't give you stationery or allow you to smoke, drink or exercise much. Their mainstay is FASTING; about all you can expect from your time there is an impressive (though probably temporary) weight loss and several glasses of warm fruit juice.

There are spas that let you bring your entire family (except, perhaps, the dog), spas that have candy counters handy so you can cheat if you're dieting, and spas so remote or so entirely devoted to discipline that you couldn't cheat if you wanted to.

You can dress up at a spa or dress down, or dry out, or simply disappear from your husband and the kids ... or the constant phone calls that keep pestering you at the office. You can fast, frolic, feast, forage or fool around.

There are spas with doctors and spas without. There are co-ed spas for super hustling and conventlike spas for getting away from it all. Some people (like Gloria Swanson) go to spas to rest. Others (like Joanne Woodward) go to spas to "get toned." Some people go to beauty spas to *gain* weight. Some people even go for the suffering. For many, in fact, it's the shared pain, agony and deprivation of dieting in a cohesive social group that makes spa hopping unbelievably attractive.

Not all beauty resorts are plush and elegant. Some devote themselves strictly and single-mindedly to simple living. When Rancho La Puerta (in Tecate, California) began operations some thirty-seven years ago, the guests were expected to get up at five in the morning and help the founders milk the goats and chop wood for the fire.

There are some spas that trade diuretics and diet shots for exquisite atmosphere. There are others that concentrate on biocellular therapy or mud baths or chicken-embryo cocktails, or sheer starvation tactics. Some spas offer the services of a clinical psychologist to help you understand why you overeat, others get to the same place with astrological readings.

When my friend Barbara went to a spa for the first time, she didn't take any of these alternatives into consideration. Going to a spa was a matter of basic NEED for her. She simply *had* to get away. She chose the first spa she came across in a magazine, lucked into getting a reservation immediately ... and went. What happened when she got there, and how spa hopping changed her life and her outlook, has always been (for me) the representative story of what going to a top-notch beauty spa is like for most of us, in that what happened to Barbara can (and probably will) happen to you. If you're interested in one woman's story of what really goes on inside the gates of a glamour spa—read on:

Intimate Details of a First-Time Mind Boggling Spa Experience

Three days before her fortieth birthday my friend Barbara dragged her dog to Central Park and thought seriously about getting older. The snow was ankle deep that winter. The park was gray. The air quality was unacceptable. Harold, the family dog, was rambunctious. The wind turned Barbara's nose and fingertips red, causing her to think (for the hundredth time that week) about getting away.

"Someplace warm ..." she thought. "I want to go someplace warm where time doesn't matter."

Everything seemed oppressive to Barbara that morning: the cold, the park, the dog, the daily stop at the A & P, the new wrinkles she'd noticed forming little clusters at the edge of her eyes and long, worried strokes across her forehead. Her skin was dry, too. She'd seen it that morning when she got out of the bath. In fact, by the time she came home from the park, she was feeling very much like parchment.

Standing in her modern kitchen looking at the pale yellow light on the New York rooftops beyond her window, Barbara juggled the egg-encrusted breakfast dishes from the sink into the dishwasher. "I am beginning to smell ..." she thought. "I am beginning to smell like Ajax Liquid Cleanser, and spaghetti sauce, and Butcher's Wax floor polish. I'm almost forty, and I'm beginning to smell housewifey and I never thought it would be like this."

At 11:00 A.M. my friend Barbara succumbed to an overpowering tiredness. So she went to bed with a copy of *Vogue*. Snuggling in under the comforting weight of her down quilt, she propped herself up with queen-sized pillows. Her left hand occupied with a cup of warm, sweet tea, her right hand flipping idly through the pages of her magazine, at ten minutes after eleven of the morning three days before her fortieth birthday, my friend Barbara began to cry. Large, round, wet tears fell on page after page of slick color photographs of thin models wearing resort pajamas and assorted expressions of ecstasy.

"I want to be pampered..." thought Barbara as she turned the page. "I want to be pampered and taken care of and warm." And then it hit her. Right then, as though it had jumped out of the magazine and into her brain, "I will go to a spa," she thought. "I will go to a spa and let *them* worry. I will go to a spa and be oiled, and pampered, and catered to, and let them worry about being forty and dry and too heavy in the hips. I will go to the bank, and I will book myself into a spa, and I will be renewed."

And so it was that on the morning of her fortieth birthday my friend Barbara, luggage in hand, boarded American Airlines Jumbo Jet #907 for a tiny town west of the Mississippi and south of San Francisco to begin her first brush with life at a glamour spa.

Barbara was back a week later, looking marvelous. She was rested. She seemed younger. Her eyes were clear. Her hair was fuller and seemed to glint in the sunshine. Her skin looked great. And besides all that, she had a new kind of presence—that self-secure, self-sufficient, contented look that society women have. Only Barbara wasn't a society woman; she was my friend Barbara. So naturally I pumped her for details.

"What happened to you? How WAS it? What was it LIKE?" I asked.

Now Barbara, who is a statuesque woman with masses of mahogany-colored curly hair and sparkly brown eyes, has never been what you'd call reticent. So naturally she told me everything. Every once in a while she'd stop for a small sip of her vegetable bouillon or close her eyes for an instant to catch a memory as it flooded over her, but essentially what follows is Barbara's story of her first trip into spa country.

I will let her tell it to you, just as she told it to me that morning, because even now, years later, it impresses me as the sort of experience every woman can and should have the first time she goes to a glamour spa.

"Well, you know I've gotten the early plane out of New York, and by mid-afternoon, after I've had one of those plastic manicotti lunches they serve you and we're hovering over this small Western airport, I'm already in the consciousness of fear. I mean, I've spent a lot of money, and this is not a cruise or a singles weekend, and basically I'm not too sure what I've gotten myself into. So by the time I get off the plane and hear my name paged, I'm kind of shaking.

"The paging itself kind of scares me, because I've never been paged (except for a death in the family or something), but this time it's José, the chauffeur. He's a little Mexican man wearing a white uniform who takes me right in hand, gives me little gold tags for my luggage, leads me to the long, white, official station wagon and introduces me to three other women with whom I'll share the ride from the airport to the spa.

"So now it's me and José and these three other strange women from places like Indiana and Ohio and San Francisco, and they're all dressed in ultrasuede (except for one of them who already has her jogging suit on) and they all seem to know exactly where they're going. Which is my second dose of fear. They all know what they're doing because (obviously) they've been here before ... and already I'm out of it.

"We pile into the car, the four of us, and for forty-five minutes, while José drives us through these beautiful hills that look vaguely like Spain, the women are talking to one another. They're talking about the last time they were here.

They're talking about how much weight they've put on. They're talking about going on the liquid diet and how they don't want to take the da Vinci class, or the weight lifting. They're all going to go on the morning walk, but nobody wants to take afternoon yoga.

"All this is very frightening, because there I am with my two wig boxes and I don't even know where I'm going or what's going to happen to me, and I'm ·miserable because I haven't dressed appropriately. If I was really into spas I wouldn't have gotten all dressed up—I would have worn a jogging suit and maybe then I'd have something to chat with these women about—but I didn't, so I sit back and listen.

"Well, we finally get there, and all the other women bound out of the car and head for their rooms. They know where their rooms are, at least, because they've already settled that. And I'm left standing with José trying to make polite conversation.

"I'm saved (in the nick of time) by a very kind blond woman who comes out to the car and says, 'May I take your bag and help you unpack?' I demur (because God forbid this girl should see the condition of my underwear) and say, 'No, that's all right, just show me the room.'

"So she shows me the room. And the room is quite beautiful. I mean, there's a robe on your bed. And I suddenly realized that I didn't have to bring any clothing. There's a robe on the bed. There's a warm-up suit. There's slippers. There's socks. There's everything there but my right brassiere size and underpants. There's a toothbrush and toothpaste in the bathroom, and the marble-topped basin is lined with cosmetics with marvelous titles like Noon of Night Night Creme and Swan Maiden Body Moisturizer. There's even a huge cake of Neutrogena soap sitting in a little gold dish done up like a seashell. Well, I get so entranced with all these things that I forget I'm supposed to get undressed and come to get weighed and measured.

"It's about five P.M. Sunday now, and that disturbs me because I figure we've all eaten at least two meals during the day, and why should I want to get weighed and measured at five o'clock. But anyway, I figure, all right . . . Here we go. I put on the white terry cloth robe, which is big (thank God), I wrap it around me, feeling a little more secure because I figure nobody can see my problem areas, and I step outside.

"The only problem is I don't know where to go. So I go back into my room and call the desk and they send me a very sweet blond woman who leads me right next door . . . to this beautiful bathhouse.

"And here are all these women. Some are sitting in a line wrapped up in their white terry cloth robes . . . some are standing completely naked on one of two scales . . . some are being measured. And I get very nervous about this, because I don't really see that many naked women. Also, I've never really confronted my full measurements and my full height before. At the doctor's office, I can always get away with just giving him the figures off the top of my head. But I never really have to think about it. Anyway, the women are all chuckling away. They're all thin. That's upsetting. There are no obese women here. And they're all tan, and they look beautiful in their white robes. They all look like Dyan Cannon, you know? And I'm sitting there looking like Golda Meir.

"So I walk up to the weight girl and she tells me to get on the scale. She's trying to be cheerful, asking me if it's my first time at the spa, asking me if I'd prefer the left scale or the right scale. It didn't matter, because I shut my eyes anyway. Unfortunately she insisted on telling me what my weight was. Loudly. One hundred forty-five. She spoke right up so everyone else could hear her. But the funny thing was that everybody else didn't really care. Everyone else heard, but what you find out in a spa is that nobody else is really looking at you. They're only looking at themselves. Just the way YOU are. So my attention snapped back to this gorgeous, perfectly proportioned, blond physical-fitness expert who's telling me about how I'm going to look wonderful when I go home, and how it was worth coming here, and that the $1500 I slapped down was all going to be worth it. Anyway, then she puts this cold tape measure around my bazooms. And one bazoom is higher than the other and I begin to find out all sorts of things about a tape measure that have nothing to do with the actual measurement. I find out that my left thigh is really filled with cellulite. And I never noticed that. I find out that I forgot to shave my leg around the knee. And that's a whole awareness trip right there. Then, afterward, all actual numbers mean very little. So I have a 14-inch knee? Big deal. I'll never really think of myself walking around saying, 'I have a 14-inch knee.'

"When the weighing-and-measuring period is over, you go back to your room and it's kind of lonely because you haven't really made contact with any of the other women. You don't really see them because they're all in their separate rooms. So I'm sitting there on the bed, and I suddenly realize I should have brought some inspirational reading. You know, not like Harold Robbins, but something nice, to fill in those gaps ... although next to the bed is a copy of *The Art Of Loving,* which was probably left by someone who KNEW what she wanted to read.

"The room itself is kind of Holiday Inn Japanese. It's very modern and kind of stark. It's got a little altar on the right side of the bed, which you end up praying to for your pound-loss every morning. There are some fresh flowers and a little dish filled with potpourri. Outside the window you can see a very private, very tranquil, very beautiful little garden. The whole atmosphere is conducive to meditating on yourself, which you can do until about seven, when they call you to dinner with a large Chinese gong.

"At the sound of the gong you mobilize yourself for the short walk to the communal dining room, open its large double doors, and it takes your breath away. The gold silverware, the finest bone china, the beautiful crystal—you're very taken with that. And then you notice (off on the left) there's a little hors d'oeuvre table,

with a medium-sized bowl of yogurt dip. Now, I didn't know that. I thought it was real cream cheese and was horribly disappointed until I got caught up in these tiny, beautifully cut radishes. Not the normal little flower buds, these radishes were sculpted in the shape of Michelangelo's 'Head of the Young David.' I mean, whoever did these really went all out. To drink, you get a snowball with apple juice over it, which sort of vaguely looks like champagne. Everything is so beautifully served, you really aren't sure what you're eating, which I guess is the point.

"The women are chatty and just slightly uptight. They all seem to be carrying their pocketbooks to dinner. But no one's particularly dressed up. We sit down and confront the meal. It's beautiful, but there isn't much of it. I mean, there on this lovely china is one little turkey leg and four green beans and a little patch of carrot and a tiny little sneeze of a salad. You know, just a little *ka-choo* on the side. No liquid is served with dinner because it's one of the rules. So we finish very slowly because we realize we don't have very much and we're trying desperately to stretch it out. Then a little bell rings and everyone is asked to introduce herself around the table.

"Most of the other women seem to be housewives. Some of them have been here before. A lot of them are professional women—there's a lawyer, there's a doctor, there are several executive secretaries who are here for the first time—there's a nun (believe it or not) and a jewelry saleswoman from Beverly Hills whose customers chipped in and gave her this trip. Then there were a lot of mother-and-daughter acts—a seventy-year-old mother and her forty-year-old daughter, and a couple of forty-year-old mothers with their seventeen-year-old daughters along. Lots of contention there. One mother was talking and her daughter was correcting her all the time. Or the daughter was talking and the mother was correcting. Anyway, most of us looked tired and toxic that first night. I noticed it. We were all crabby about our weight and we hated sitting around in those robes.

"After dinner the staff explains what you're going to be doing through the week, and it sounds so awful. They tell you you're going to be doing sixty hours of exercise. Plus that you have to get up at five o'clock in the morning for a morning walk. Well, the last time I got up at five in the morning, I had morning sickness, so you can believe I was not looking forward to it. Besides, the thought of all those classes when they explain them is very frightening in itself. At this point I was just thinking, 'Maybe I'll just tell them I'm mentally ill, and stay in my room all week so I don't have to deal with this . . .' but sure enough, we all had to go to the family bath for indoctrination.

"The family bath is an enormous Jacuzzi set in a lovely, tiled Japanese bathhouse. You walk into this big horseshoe of a bath, which is brimming with bubbling, hot, aquamarine water. It's about 210 degrees in there and there are big, soft, plush towels stacked by the entrance. So you take a towel and you go in, and the first thing you've got to get over is shyness about your body. I realized very quickly that if I was going to experience all these spa things (like the Scotch hose and the Jacuzzi), I had to stop taking a towel all the time, or a bathing suit top; I had to stop hiding. If you spend all your energy hiding, you just don't get off on any-thing. That part was very clear. There was one woman with a mastectomy who was walking around very openly, and I said to myself, 'Here's a woman with a mastectomy who's proud of her body. What am I upset about?' So I got into the bath and watched everybody loosen up. We started talking about ourselves. About our hus-

bands and so forth. It seems that most of the women do have personal problems. But then, who doesn't? Why else would you go to a spa? You're going to relax and recuperate. You're recuperating from a stressful situation. We *all* are. So I found out that there was one woman who was drinking too much. There was one woman whose husband threatened to sue her. There was a girl who just broke up with her boyfriend. So the problems come out pretty quickly that first night in the Japanese bath.

"When we were pretty much loosened up, we went off to another little room on the side to get an acupressure massage. That alone is worth the price of admission, and it so thoroughly relaxed me that I went back to my room, put my head on the pillow and the next thing I know there's a pounding on my door to get up. And it's five o'clock in the morning. And it's time for the morning walk. And it's black out. So I put on my little jogging suit and my gloves and my socks and my running shoes, and I walk outside into this brisk gust of cold air, and I think: 'No WAY can I do this.' But there I am, huffing and puffing with five other women off to what turns out to be the end of the driveway. It just so happens that it's a mile. But the first five minutes are horrendous. Just horrendous. The second fifteen minutes, however, are *sensational.* You're breathing in real, fresh herbs from the real, fresh herb garden, and you're seeing Taco, the donkey, and the snow in the mountains. This really corny stuff starts to happen in your brain and gets you to a place where you realize you're in nature, and you start to unwind. The setting helps. You're surrounded by these incredible green woods. The air is heavy with the scent of anise. The air is so clear and the mountains are so sharp, you're sure you've never seen them before. I forgot my glasses, but for some reason it seemed that I was seeing clearly for perhaps the first time in my life. That morning walk was probably as close as I'd ever gotten to a mystical experience. Even if it did start at five o'clock in the morning.

"When it's over you go back to your room and there's a little tray there. I decided to go on the liquid diet the first day, because that's what they tell you is 'cleansing,' so there on my beautiful little bamboo tray—next to a beautiful arrangement of flowers and the beautiful Japanese napkin and my schedule for each hour, which is written out on a beautiful Japanese silk fan—there is a gorgeous crystal glass of grapefruit juice diluted with water. It's only four ounces, but it's the best grapefruit juice I've ever had. I also have some pink lemon tea and a tea bag. And a salt and pepper shaker (for what I don't know, but there they were). Naturally I ate everything. And the lemon peel. And the tea bag. The tea bag I stuck in my mouth because I thought that was good. I had a feeling it was good for my gums. Boy, was I hungry after that walk. I gotta tell ya!

"After the walk the order of the day is to change quickly into leotard and tights (which I forgot to bring), so I call the front desk and a magic little blond girl comes down with pink leotards and tights. I said, 'I don't wear pink.' She said, 'That's what you wear.' And off I go to a warm-up class. The warm-up class is basically stretching, so I feel pretty secure about it because I can still stretch and touch my toes. But the *next* two classes we really get into some heavy exercise. One is called the da Vinci class because Leonardo da Vinci devised this plan of exercising the total body. It's actually aerobics, and you're running a lot. And you're running with hula hoops (which I banged in my face) and you're running with broomsticks (with which I almost killed a classmate). One woman yelled because I banged her head with it, but everything turned out all right. The music was all Neil Sedaka and Paul McCartney. And it was really very interesting, because I learned how far behind I am in the rock world. Anyway, when the da Vinci class was over we all trotted off to a reducing class, where you just work up a sweat in your hips. Then you go in to lift weights.

"Or I should say what's left of you goes in to lift weights. Now this part is very scary for me, because I'd never lifted a weight before and I was intimidated by all that body-building equipment, but once the girl showed me how to use it, it was very easy. In fact, it turned out to be one of the best things I could do for my body, since I'd never even lifted a dumbbell before.

"When weight lifting was over, we broke for potassium broth. It was 10:45 and out came these beautiful little cups of what looks like V-8 Juice but is actually the greatest tomato juice you've ever had in your life. And pieces of cheese. String cheese. Tiny little, tiny little, thumbnail-thin pieces of string cheese. And that's all we really wanted. We couldn't really handle any more than that. It was funny. Even though we'd worked up all this sweat, we weren't really hungry.

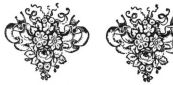

"After the broth break there was pool class, where we learned how to bicycle around, and to do a crawl with a volley ball. There was lots of water ballet in the pool class, lots of Esther Williams visuals, and slowly, as we played in the water, the women I didn't like in the beginning were beginning to be interesting to me. Like this one doctor who seemed so uptight when I walked into the Jacuzzi last night now seemed to be nice to me. I don't know whether that was because she was suffering as much pain as I was, but we were all sort of in it together, like kids at summer camp, if you know what I mean.

"By mid-afternoon on that first day, you start to feel your muscles cramp up. Just as you start to feel that crampy, uncomfortable feeling, they tell you that you're ready for an herbal wrap. Of course, I have no idea at this point what an herbal wrap is . . . but here's what happened.

"We all walk into the family bathhouse and a beautiful, blond, soft-spoken girl comes over to me and tells me to sit down on this hot massage table. Have you noticed how everybody here seems to be beautiful, blond and soft-spoken? Well, anyway, this beautiful blond girl then wraps me up (literally) like an Egyptian mummy. She uses linen wrappings that smell like tea bags or chamomile, and when I'm all covered, she puts a cold compress on my face and I'm so relaxed I have absolutely no memory of the next twenty minutes. The next thing I know, she's undoing me, and I really feel undone. That's when the first real layer of tension came off, I think—with that herbal wrap. I don't quite know how to explain it, but I guess you feel vulnerable then. You've got to be very careful here, because when you go into the slowdown part of the day, which has to do with the massage and the herbal wrap, strange things start to happen. You don't speak so clearly. You're kind of drunk, you know; like you can't get your thoughts collected easily. If there's a phone call for you in the afternoon, you get really crazy. I noticed that. Like, I went from my herbal wrap to my massage, and there was a phone call—and I absolutely couldn't take it because I was too numb.

"All I was ready for was a massage in my room. And that's what I got. Actually, I got Aiko (a little Japanese girl), who is with me the whole week. She watches to make sure everything is all right. She cautions me because I'm very tired the first day and tells me I should go to yoga class.

"Well, if there's anything I don't want to do at this point, it's take yoga. I've been up since five in the MORNING, after all, and I'm relaxed and I'm tired and the last thing I want to do with myself is get into yoga postures. But the woman who gave the class was marvelous, so I pack up my body and I take it to yoga.

"The first thing Eleanor (the really swell-looking blond woman who taught the class) did was tell us about how all the food we were eating was bad for us. Now I had a clue that the eggs I was getting from the local supermarket weren't all that they should be, but I never knew they had ARSENIC in them! So we started with that realization. Then Eleanor put us into deep relaxation. And I'd never had that experience before. It was just unbelievable. And just when I was really deeply into it, I started to cry, and I guess I had a breakdown. I don't know, I never cried anywhere else. I never cried on my trips to the Club Med, or on cruise ships ... but for some reason I was crying here. But it was a GOOD cry. It wasn't a depressing cry. It was a cry out of almost sheer exhaustion, and out of the insight that I'd never before, ever in my life, been in touch with my body on anything more than a surface level.

"When I stopped crying, I went back to my room for a bit, then headed to the dining room for dinner, which was a liquid gazpacho. It was beautifully served, but basically dinner was very quiet and low-key because we were all so tired. Everybody seemed to drift off to go to bed around eight thirty. You could go to the family bath if you wanted to, but I was so exhausted I just wanted to get back and be by myself. I'm tired and I hurt and I'm annoyed because I don't know for sure whether this is all worth the money, and the schedule seems like more of a work camp than a glamour spa ... and it's not fun, it's hard work ... and even though I know it's good for me, I don't feel good. In fact, the next morning when I wake up to go to the bathroom at four o'clock I can't move. And I think to myself, 'This is really AWFUL!'

"However ... the instructor told us that the second day WOULD be awful. They told us that we'd have a terrible blood-sugar drop. And they told us to just 'go with it.' They also told us to go on a 700-calories-a-day diet the second day and to start eating solid food. They even said that the crabbiness we were experiencing has to do with the speed at which we were cleaning out our systems.

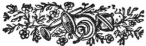

"So the next morning walk was not enjoyable. It hurt. But we're *all* hurting. We're all sharing our hurts, which seems to make it better. And I *loved* that. I loved everybody saying, 'Yes. I hurt.' Even the women who came here in jogging suits all limber from Beverly Hills were really aching, and I loved sharing that with them. I thought, 'Well, see, I'm not so bad.' We were all hurting. We were all hurting and talking about what parts of our bodies seemed to hurt most. Like it seemed to me to be LEGS. Most women hurt in their legs and their lower backs. And then some woman got started talking about her childbirth. And breathing. And we realized how important breathing was. And this woman shared her natural childbirth experience with us ... and suddenly it was an encounter. That morning walk became very important because we were sharing gut experiences. As we walked, we would let go and unwind. So suddenly I was closer to these women than I was with my friends at home. Yet I knew nothing about them. I knew (in the back of my mind) that even if we exchanged phone numbers, I would never see them again. On that level it reminded me of a cruise ship. But even on a cruise ship you never get this in touch with people's intimate, personal stuff.

"The body is really the ultimate personal thing, you know. Also, we didn't care about things that would seem awfully important to us at home. Like we didn't care about body odor or bad breath, because we were always so busy we couldn't constantly spritz under our arms with Ban or spray Binaca into our mouths every minute.

"We'd go back to our rooms after the walk and have that tiny moment of peace. And we were alone with that. In fact, it was after one morning walk as I sat there with my grapefruit juice that I started to see food as a ritual. A ceremony. Not just something you stuff in your mouth and abuse. There was a message in that beautiful little tray saying: Good morning ... drink me slowly. Think about me. That kind of thing.

"The classes were tough that third day. The pool class was the most soothing, because it was like water therapy for cripples. And the teachers went easy. I was kind of depressed and cranky with my body, because I hurt too much to push it very far, but even that was a lesson. And then the masseuse was very good, and the yoga class was marvelous that night. You really appreciated the place the yoga teacher was putting you in. You know, the drinking in of energy."

At this point Barbara got up, stretched and put on the tea kettle. "Another cup of broth?" she asked me. I accepted gratefully, because as she had been drinking in all that yoga energy I was riddled with envy. Broth before us, Barbara began again, slightly west of the place she'd left off.

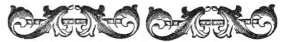

"I think I'm going to skip toward the end of the week now, because everything I've already explained sort of continued. The schedule was the same every day. The classes got easier. But basically everything just continued through Wednesday and Thursday. Toward the end of the week, during the facial, a woman broke down. Each woman, I noticed, had a breakdown there. It happened in two ways. Either you'd cry during your facial, or you'd cry during yoga, or you'd have a fit of the giggles at dinner. Having a breakdown at a spa, I realize, is a sign of letting go. And every woman by Thursday night had let go at least once. We were talking about very intimate details of our sex lives now, and it was quite wonderful. But more than that, everyone had dropped at least four pounds by Thursday. Feeling good was beginning to be the issue now, not weight loss. Feeling really, really good within yourself. Knowing that you could go to an exercise class when you got home—and be Advanced.

"Oh yes, and our skin was looking really good, too, because of all those facials we were having. And we had avocado oil in our hair all the time. I always thought I hated that. I always thought it was so awful to walk around with oily, greasy, yucky hair. But what it did to the texture of your hair was so beautiful I didn't care.

"By the end of the week the women suddenly looked very beautiful to me in their terry cloth robes. It seemed they looked better in terry cloth robes than in anything else they could possibly wear, no matter how expensive it was or which name designer had his tag in it. The evenings got a little longer because we could stay up later—we didn't need as much sleep. By Friday night we were going to bed at eleven and getting up at five with no problem. We were even looking forward to it. That morning walk was fabulous. We cried from the beauty of it.

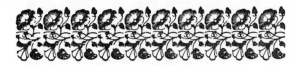

"The evenings were mostly spent in the bathhouse, although they did have a flower-arranging course we could take if we wanted to. But all that seemed too planned out, somehow. I didn't want to get back into anything that reminded me of the real world yet. Flower arranging! Fashion shows! It all seemed sort of silly. And besides, there were cliques forming. Certain twosomes and threesomes would eat together and everybody had found the one person she was most interested in talking to. We were all making friends, and it wasn't the horrible feeling I felt that first night when I thought all these women were together and I was alone.

"The spa felt like boarding school the first night, but by the end I felt like I belonged to this great sorority. At the end there was a betting pool. We put in two bucks apiece and bet how much the whole group had lost. There were twenty-five women. We'd lost about 120

pounds. The jewelry saleswoman from Beverly Hills had won and she couldn't have been happier.

"That last night they served us steak and potato shells for dinner. We couldn't even finish it. None of us could finish it. I didn't have the steak, myself . . . but none of us could finish the meal.

"Then Michel came out and gave us a cooking class. And we learned the value of paprika and parsley . . . and the meanings of good, empty tomato skin and potato skin. The amazing things you can do with Mayonette Gold Diet Mayonnaise! He was wonderful, Michel was. He told us all to get Adele Davis's *Let's Cook It Right,* and really drove home how important nutrition is. He showed us the miracles of the blender. The gazpacho we'd been drinking for a week wasn't even made out of gazpacho, it turns out. It was made out of every herb you could possibly imagine . . . with maybe a TOUCH of tomato. Those wonderful stuffed mushrooms on the hors d'oeuvre platters weren't stuffed with caviar . . . they were stuffed with other mushroom stems, chopped up. The class was amazing. We all sat there enthralled. Michel became a Wizard of Oz figure who whipped away the curtain and all of a sudden you could see how all the tricks were done. They were so beautiful and so obvious.

"We all got terribly carried away with ourselves then. We started ordering Cuisinart food mills on the phone. You get very inspired by the cooking course, because you see that you don't have to eat badly. I cried at Michel's cooking course, actually. I finally saw how well food can be prepared and how I abused food. There were high moments in the class, moments when he lectured us about using food as a friend. Which, of course, I always do. I'm always eating when I'm depressed or anxious or something. Anyway, Michel is up there in the dining room, saying, 'Don't use food as a friend. Find other friends. Find jogging. Find going shopping. Find something ELSE. Don't use food as a friend . . .' And I'm crying and the other women are ordering

Cuisinarts. It was really quite something. Then the bell rang and we all went off and sat in the family bath for the last time and cried because we realized we had to go out into the real world soon, and the real world doesn't serve you lovely fresh grapefruit halves with pretty little flowers on your bamboo tray in the morning. The real world doesn't give you a list of things you have to do for the day written out on a beautiful Japanese silk fan. The real world is going to be yourself.

"Here I had lost 12 inches and 7 pounds. And I was going out into the real world and I didn't want to ruin it, so I was crying.

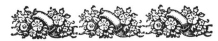

"But just at this moment I realized how important this vacation was. I realized that I'd had this moment in time that was all to do with myself. It was just me. When I got into that white station wagon to go to the airport, I wasn't crabby. I knew that I wouldn't have baggage-claim blues. I really felt like a new year had started. And, more important, I realized how ridiculous those vacations at the Club Med and in Las Vegas had been. How they had nothing to do with learning about me. And how learning about me was definitely something I owed myself. I've never been through analysis. I've never taken drugs. And yet I had all these very heavy experiences at this spa. That is the really miraculous thing. Finding out that my body was never taken on a vacation before. My MIND was always taken on a vacation, but this was the first time my body was allowed to let go. I didn't realize it before, but I just never took it to the shop. And it *craves* this. So what I took home with me was a new sense of self. I liked the way I looked when I left. I had no feelings about walking around naked. I walk around naked in my apartment now. I'm surprised I don't go to the supermarket naked.

"Also, I took home the idea of food being a celebration. So when I sit down at the table now,

I'm not going to wolf down my food. I'm going to think about it. Before I go to a restaurant, I'm not going to be ashamed to wonder, 'What should I eat?' I'm going to think about what I should eat, and the fact that I really don't need those four glasses of wine. I obviously didn't need it at the spa, even though I was working twice as hard and under four times as much body stress.

"So I came home with a new attitude about myself, and with a new attitude about food and with an overpowering desire to set up my life so I HAVE a beautiful tray in the morning. I want to be good to myself. I want to have a massage once a month and a facial every six weeks. There's no reason why I shouldn't do those things. I want to surround myself with teensy little reminders of what that whole spa number was like. I want to join a gym, and if I don't take the exercise classes I want to at least step into a whirlpool and close my eyes. I got a tape of my yoga teacher taking me into deep relaxation, and believe me, I intend to use it. And I even stole a pink T-shirt just to wear to bed so that I know I'm still mentally that person who went to the spa. That wasn't a different person who went through that—that was ME."

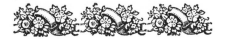

So that's the story my friend Barbara told me when she got back from her first brush with a glamour spa.

During the two years following her return, I heard many stories and read many articles about what it's like to go spa hopping. Still, Barbara's story sticks in my mind as the most graphic, the most detailed and the most honest.

Yet even after hearing Barbara's story, two questions began to bother me: Not being Barbara, how would I choose a glamour spa? And where, exactly, would I start? It became one of those bewildering problems, which began to look like it could be best solved at random—or, as my friend Dale once suggested, by sticking a pin into an open book.

On the surface, making this sort of a decision should be a snap. You know what you want out of your spa adventure. All you have to do is pick the spa that looks like it will deliver the goods. Easy, yes?

Well, yes . . . and, then again, no.

Unless you have eight or ten close friends who have personally taken themselves to the spa you're considering, you will have almost no trustworthy way of finding out what's going on there.

The magazine pieces you read about spas may actually be the author's way of paying off a free trip to the spas she's covering for that magazine. Besides, people always pamper writers, so depending on an author for your information isn't always reliable.

Of course, you *can* talk to someone you know who has a close connection to spa society. Like my cousin Betty, whose dentist's nephew is rumored to be the sauce chef at a top Southern society spa. But then I've never met my cousin's dentist's nephew. So how do I know I can trust him? Besides, once the information filters back to me (if it ever does), it will surely be worthless.

The biggest trouble with talking to people (even if they've been *personally* in touch with one spa or another, or several) is that THEIR taste is almost guaranteed not to match up with YOUR taste.

Take, for example, my neighbor Angie. She had a simply glorious time at a remote mountain spa offering little more than inspiration and shredded vegetables. It sounded like something out of *Watership Down*, but Angie was *wild* over it. She was rapturous about the sheer physicality of the place. She loved its rusticity. She was thrilled to live in jeans and work boots for seven whole days.

Okay for Angie. That's HER trip. If she prefers white-water canoeing down the Snake River to spending an equal amount of time at the Top of the Mark having her meals delivered by room service, that's fine.

I, however, would HATE that. In fact, I try never to get any closer to the Snake River than I absolutely have to. If I go to a spa, I want to be pampered and fanned by slaves. I don't even want to hear *stories* about roughing it. Which brings me to my next problem with Angie: Once I got her started talking about her spa vacation, it was almost impossible to get her to stop.

"So what's left?" I asked myself. "How can I make an intelligent decision? How can I choose a spa for myself with the least possible strain? Where can I go for accurate information?"

Believe it or not, I came up with a single word: BROCHURES.

You probably think brochures are simply blatant advertising ploys, right? You also probably think that the chance of there being an accurate representation of a spa in a brochure is about as slim as your last tax refund, right?

RIGHT! And so did I. I did, that is, until I talked with Bruce Becker, the author of a dynamite new book called: *Decisions! How and When to Make Them* (Grosset & Dunlap, $9.95).

It was Bruce who set me straight about brochures as they relate to deciding which spa you finally entrust with your body.

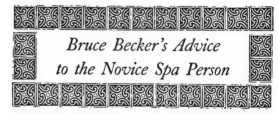

Bruce Becker's Advice to the Novice Spa Person

Actually, brochures *are* blatant advertising ploys and should be treated somewhat like you treat any other salesperson. Unquestionably, they have but one aim: your money. And, of course, they are biased. But, taking this into consideration, there is a lot of information you can get from brochures that can help you make a better decision as to where to go. And they even have one advantage over the salespeople: They are *written*, so later you can't be told that you misunderstood and no one ever said such a thing. There it is, in black and white—or, possibly, some glorious living color that pops off the page at you.

That's the first thing to look for: the way it's printed, the style of the brochure. Remember that this material is in fact the spa's own self-image: This is not only the picture they want you to get, it is also their own impression of what they are (or, at least, of what they'd like to be). For example, I have one in front of me that has not only a Botticelli reproduction on its parchment cover, it also has another from Michelangelo on the underlying cardboard second cover! Before I even opened that brochure I knew a lot about the place—which, in fact, was confirmed when I saw their rates. And, also, the aerial view of their grounds. This is a spa that smacks of wealth and high society; it also means all kinds of indulgent pampering in return for high tips. It is a far cry from the other end of the spectrum: a single photo-offset page that guarantees weight loss by "natural, fast and effective means." Which, of course, means very little equipment and lots of manual workouts. And it's probably very close to the old mom-and-pop candy store: not too many on the staff. Then somewhere in between is a very simple folder with a lot of single pages slipped in; this one offers "plenty of room to be yourself." And so you know that it is not fancy, not formal, and not nearly as expensive as the Roman Empire you first looked at.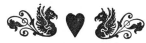

Now, with this initial information—that is, the style and price of the place—you can easily pick out from your bunch of brochures those that appeal and those that don't. In fact, you probably had some intuitive feelings about each of them as you removed them from the envelopes, and have already, in effect, done just this.

Then look at the pictures of the spas you have narrowed your choice down to. Here you not only can get an idea of their self-images, but you can get some clues as to what their *best* is. Remember, that's what they're showing you: their ultimate. They certainly are not going to show you their lesser sides, so what you see is the cream of what they have to offer. Therefore, you can now compare their best against that of the others you are considering. For example,

what's the age range of the guests? One brochure shows them going from seventeen to seventy; you *know* that's a fake! Are they old, run-down, dreary-looking—therefore assuring a staid but quiet week? Or are they younger, more active, more weekender types? And what does the dining room look like? Will you be comfortable in jeans (if you wear them)? Or is mink *de rigueur?* Is there a picture of a bedroom? If so, is it simple or fancy? Does it look cold and formal, or is it warm and inviting, conducive to your frame of mind and your own self-image? And what are their facilities like? For example, when you see a picture of a steam cabinet and no mention of other facilities, you know there is no sauna—which may or may not be important to you. Look carefully; even the use of a magnifying glass is not a bad idea: It may save you some time, money and grief.

Most important, don't assume. The fact that it's a "health spa" doesn't mean anything per se. Read between the lines carefully and cynically; to be "nearby" anything, for example, could mean half an hour away. And "all the facilities on the premises" is meaningless: What facilities? Look for the specifics; go for the facts.

What you must do is have an idea of what will please you and what you are looking for, and then read through these advertisements carefully to see which best satisfy your requirements and offer what you want.

But always remember that, if they do meet your needs, what you see is the best they have, and so you may have to accept something not quite the same as shown. However, what they have may be close to your desires and, hopefully, having some idea of what the spa is like before you make your choice, it should turn out to be worthy of your decision.

Good luck!

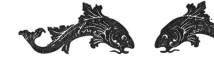

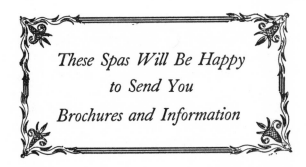

*These Spas Will Be Happy
to Send You
Brochures and Information*

RENAISSANCE REVITALIZATION CENTER (nonresident spa)
Cable Beach
P.O. Box 4854
Nassau, Bahamas

> Specializing in rejuvenation and antiaging processes, including hydro, cellular and chicken-embryo therapy.
> Approximate cost: $2,500 for 10 days of treatments.

MAINE CHANCE (women only)
Maine Chance Reservations Office
5830 East Jean Avenue
Phoenix, Arizona 85018

> Offers a return to an opulent, affluent, pampered childhood. Guests have included Clare Booth Luce, Cornelia Otis Skinner and Mrs. Dwight D. Eisenhower.
> Approximate cost: $1,000 per week.

THE GREENHOUSE (mostly women. Couples allowed twice a year)
Inn of the Six Flags
Arlington, Texas 76010

> Presidential wives and daughters have flocked here for major overhauls.
> Approximate cost: $1,200 per week

THE GOLDEN DOOR (women only)
2104 Hancock Street
San Diego, California 92110

> The smallest of all the major spas, The Golden Door builds a supportive climate while concentrating on the psychic benefits of redirecting your life toward health and exercise.
> Approximate cost: $1,500 per week

LA COSTA (the family spa)
Carlsbad, California 92008

> A full-service country-club resort with an international reputation for attracting millionaires, movie stars and first-rate mobsters.
> Approximate cost: $600 per week

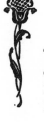

THE SPA AT PALM-AIRE (separate facilities for men and women)
2501 Palm-Aire Drive North
Pompano Beach, Florida 33065

> Billie Jean King, Sam Levenson, Hughes Rudd, Senator Jacob Javits and Jimmy Hoffa have all done time at Palm Aire.
> Approximate cost: $600 per week

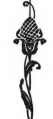

HARBOR ISLAND SPA (coed)
7900 Harbor Island
Miami Beach, Florida 33139

> Most of the guests here are merchant millionaire couples out for a good time. Regulars include the owners of BVD Underwear, Bazooka Bubble Gum and National Tea. The food is kosher and terrific.
> Approximate cost: $450 per week

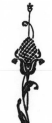

RANCHO LA PUERTA (coed/vegetarian)
Tecate, California 92080

> Rustic outpost popular with mellow youth, tightly budgeted school teachers, ex-nuns, virile bachelors, vacationing stewardesses and character actors.
> Approximate cost: $450 per week

MURIETTA HOT SPRINGS
Murietta Hot Springs Hotel
Murietta Hot Springs Road
Murietta, California 92362

The Temucula Indians bathed and healed themselves here. Now sports and resort facilities are available to everyone.

Approximate cost: $400 per week

THE GREENBRIER (coed)
White Sulphur Springs,
West Virginia 24986

Eighteen different United States presidents came to Greenbrier, which now specializes in water therapy and rejuvenation treatments.

Approximate cost: $300 per week

PAWLING HEALTH MANOR (coed/fasting)
Hyde Park, New York 12538

No gadgets, gimmicks, shortcuts or miracle treatments here. No smoking, either.

Approximate cost: $300 per week

BERMUDA INN (coed)
BERMUDA INN REDUCING RESORT
43019 Sierra
Lancaster, California 93534

In the words of its owner, George Alexander, the Bermuda Inn is "... a nuts and bolts fat farm which offers the best blubber bargain in America."

Approximate cost: $150 per week

NEW AGE HEALTH FARM (coed)
48 Haverstraw Road
Route 202
Suffern, New York 10901

Diets, fasts, natural foods plus lots of classes in astrology, I Ching, tarot and numerology.

Approximate cost: $150 per week

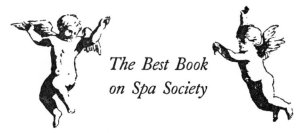

The Best Book on Spa Society

Before you do anything, before you even lift the phone to make a reservation, before you put the stamp on your letter asking for brochures and information ... go read Kitty Kelley's marvelous, gossipy, informative book, *The Glamour Spas.*

Find out exactly what goes on behind the gilt-edged gates of reducing shrines made famous by women like Ava Gardner, Zsa Zsa Gabor, Sophie Gimble and Dinah Shore—or men like Frank Sinatra, Bill Blass, Joshua Logan and Buddy Hackett.

Read about tipping and escort services. Get the servant's-eye view of famous patrons. It's all in *The Glamour Spas,* and it's the most intimate inside view of the billion-dollar-a-year fat-farm business you'll ever read.

In researching *The Glamour Spas* Kitty Kelley visited every beauty spa in the United States. She ate vegetarian food at Rancho La Puerta, soaked in mud baths at Murietta Hot Springs, baked in Hawaiian sands at the Royal Door. She was massaged, manicured, pedicured, pampered, preened, stretched, steamed, slimmed and pounded. She got into every program, asked terribly embarrassing questions of the employees and the guests and turned out one of the best (and dishiest) books that's ever been written on the subject.

THE GLAMOUR SPAS
by Kitty Kelley
Pocket Books (Paperback, $1.50)

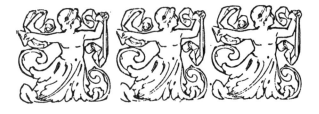

Smelling Marvelous

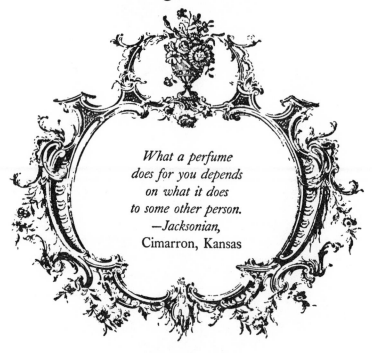

*What a perfume
does for you depends
on what it does
to some other person.
—Jacksonian,*
Cimarron, Kansas

*More Power
to the Perfumed Pulse!*

Basically, the more you know about perfume, the more you'll get out of it. An educated sniffer can spend an intoxicating afternoon (or a lifetime) expanding her emotional repertoire at the tester counter of any good department store. A whiff of oak moss can send her hurtling back to a rambling forest walk she's not thought about in years. Blue Grass may bring forth memories of her grandmother's scent, or of the first perfume she ever got tucked into her Christmas stocking. Mitsouko will remind her of her first love's laugh, Vent Vert of the day she became a career woman or got her first large raise.

Perfume is like a fine painting. It's full of emotion, meaning, color and texture. The more you open yourself up to the whole *experience* of scent, the richer it becomes for you.

Beyond the sheerly practical advantage of smelling wonderful, you'll find you can make friends with one certain fragrance—or a number of them. You might find that lavender calms you after a tough day, or that rosemary cologne is just the thing to wear on a long drive because it's stimulating enough to keep you from snoozing out behind the wheel.

As you begin to know about which fragrance does what (and to whom), you'll start enjoying the devastating effects of *specific* scents on the men of your choice ... and your friends, co-workers, the check-out kid at the A & P, cab drivers, neighbors, your children—just about everybody.

The best, most effective way to find out about fragrance is to experiment like crazy. You needn't *buy* anything; but you can and should work your way through the mysteries of the whole range of scents (from Abano to Zen). Almost every company makes testers or tiny samples available with its fragrance displays, so trying on for size can be an inexpensive as well as a delightful pastime.

Read this section for some of the legend and lore and basic vocabulary you'll need to experiment wisely. Then don't hesitate to try anything (and everything) that intrigues you.

Speaking of Power...

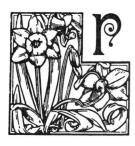

uth Revzen is a Chicago sorceress who puts "body spirits" into ¼-ounce Art Deco bottles. ENLIGHTENMENT and SUCCESS (two fragrances named for the qualities you want to call *into* your life) are to be rubbed on the back, from the base of your spine to the nape of your neck. They cost $14 each. LOVE ($22) and GOODNESS ($8), two other Revzen essences you might like to *radiate out* to those around you, are made to be put only on the front of your body and over your glands.

For more information on BODY SPIRITS (or to find out why LOVE is more expensive than GOODNESS), write:

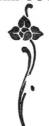

Ruth Revzen
BODY SPIRITS
221 East Clark
Box 1968
Chicago, Illinois 60601

The Nose Knows

Napoleon used sixty bottles of cologne a month.

One fourth of the people who lose their sense of smell also lose their desire for sexual relations.

Ruth Winter, science columnist for the Los Angeles *Times*, writes about our sense of smell and its irresistible subliminal messages in *The Smell Book.*

She writes about two men who earn their livings with their acute senses of smell: Smelly Kelly, who sniffed out gas leaks in the New York subway system for thirty-four years, and Albert Weber, food sniffer for the U.S. Food and Drug Administration, who smells up to four thousand raw shrimp a day, testing for freshness. There is a society matron who can match her guests to their coats by smell. Mrs. Winter says, "We could all equal them if we used our potential." The average person smelling a skunk is smelling 0.000,000,000,000,071 of an ounce of scent.

Smell is extremely important to doctors, because each disease has its own unique odor, which helps them make rapid diagnoses. Yellow fever smells like a butcher shop, typhoid fever like freshly baked bread, plague like apples, and measles like freshly plucked feathers.

Experiments have shown that if young boys have no sense of smell and their sex glands are underdeveloped, they will probably be sterile and should be placed on testosterone therapy at puberty. If they have some sense of smell, rather than none at all, they are probably normal and will eventually be fertile.

Hippocrates, the most famous physician of all time, advocated scented baths and recommended perfumes as medicine for certain diseases.

Bloodhounds can follow an individual's trail by its scent two weeks after the fact.

Freud considered repression of the sense of smell a major cause of mental illness.

Today it costs perfume manufacturers one million dollars to develop a new scent. The manufacturers have about five thousand raw materials to choose from, both natural and synthetic. There are vintage years for flowers and other natural raw materials just as there are for wines.

We are constantly being lured, without our conscious knowledge, into buying products because of the way they smell. Less than 20 percent of all fragrance presently employed is in toiletries and perfumes. Many marketing experts claim that how a product smells is more important than how well it works ... $500 million a year is spent making products smell pleasant. A new-car smell—a blend of oil, leather and metal scents—is sprayed on used cars to give the impression of newness. Plastic shoes are sprayed with the odor of leather.

Incredible as it seems, *The Smell Book* is the first book ever completely devoted to the sense of smell.

THE SMELL BOOK:
Scents, Sex, and Society
by Ruth Winter
J. B. Lippincott (Hardcover, $7.95)

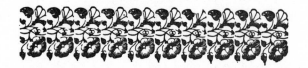

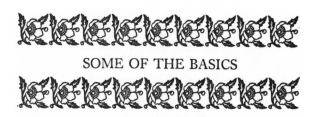

SOME OF THE BASICS

Scentual Terms
You'll Want to Know About

This may be a very personal bias, but I am enthralled by technical terminology. Give me five or six pithy phrases used by professionals and I find I can fake a certain amount of wisdom. Coupling this scant knowledge with a dollop of enigmatic smile has made me the recipient of enormous amounts of inside information. The rule I've found to apply is: People tell you things if you've got a bit of jargon and seem interested.

For the short course in instant fragrance expertise, you will need to get a handle on the following terms and definitions. They're not in alphabetical order because they're easier to understand chronologically. Armed with no more than these, you'll be able to talk intelligently to anyone in the fragrance business. And you might even understand them when they talk back.

Fragrance Dabbler's Dictionary

TOP NOTE. This is what you smell as the fragrance is applied to your skin. Never judge from a tentative sniff at an open bottle. The true bloom of a great scent NEVER shows up until you put it on your body.

A fine perfume should have a lovely lift and sparkle about it. The first hints of its character should impress you right away (within about thirty seconds after you put it on). Think of the TOP NOTE as the first impression you get of someone you've just met.

MIDDLE NOTE. This is what you smell in five to twenty minutes, when the fragrance dries on your skin and the essences come into play.

MIDDLE notes are like your second meeting with a new friend ... the second date where you share experiences and really get to know a little more about each other.

BOTTOM or BASE NOTE (also called DRY DOWN). What you smell hours after your first application, when the TOP and MIDDLE notes begin to fade. BOTTOM notes make the quality of the fixative apparent. It's like all the good, lasting things that cement a friendship or a love affair.

CHEMISTRY. Your body chemistry *does* affect the way a perfume smells on you. If you perspire heavily, you may have trouble keeping a perfume on the right note. If you try a perfume when you have your period, it may smell completely different to you when your cycle is over. (For some reason, menstruation alters the way your mind translates odor.) Body chemistry relates to scent in such a strictly personal way that one woman in a hundred will bring out *all* the notes and subtleties in an aroma. Fifty women will keep it at what it was at first smell; the rest either lose it entirely or alter its structure so that it smells different on them than it does on anybody else. CHEMISTRY has everything to do with why you may *love* a particular perfume on a neighbor. Unfortunately, chemistry can also cause that same perfume to smell like hair straightener when *you* wear it. The moral then, is: Test before you buy.

FIXATIVES. Fixatives are vital to the architecture of a fragrance—they hold the scent together. They equalize the evaporation rate of all the note-giving elements and make the perfume last. Although many fixatives come from mosses and resins, the ones we hear most about come from animals. Civet comes from wild jungle cats. Musk is gathered from the male musk deer, and ambergris (the most precious product, by weight, taken out of the sea) is merely a lovely name for whale vomit.

CHARACTER. This does not apply to the woman behind the counter who tries to sell you the stuff, but rather to the personality of the perfume itself. A fine fragrance should establish its character and identity at the TOP NOTE; maintain that presence through the BODY of the perfume (the MIDDLE NOTE) and remain through the DRY DOWN without going through any major, radical changes.

EFFUSIVENESS. Effusiveness is the ability of a fragrance to reach out from your skin and surround you with its aura. The best way to test if you're wearing an effusive perfume is to keep track of how many people ask you, "What are you wearing?" The more questions, the more effusive the scent.

VEHICLE. Vehicles are carriers for perfume oil. Most vehicles are alcohol or oil mixtures. Oil vehicles will tend to make a scent last longer, but can cut down on its effusiveness.

CONCENTRATION. The ratio of actual perfume oil to the VEHICLE gives you its concentration. By custom, perfumes have at least 20 percent perfume oil. Colognes have about 3 to 6 percent and toilet waters have between 5 and 8 percent.

In other words, perfume is the strongest, most concentrated and longest lasting of the forms. Next in strength is EDT (eau de toilette or toilet water), which carries the original essence in an expanded, more subtle form. Then comes cologne, which (these days) is followed by even lighter, more subtle categories like splashes and coolers and body lotions. On the other end of the scale, there are also super colognes (which have as much as 15 percent actual perfume oil in them) and essential oils, which are all perfume essence and seem to last forever.

Colognes, incidentally, are meant to be put on all over the body with a lavish hand. Perfumes (or perfume oils) get applied OVER colognes; at the pulse spots. The pulse spots (just in case you've forgotten) are wrists, backs of knees, throat, temples, just below each ear, the nape of your neck and anywhere else you can feel a heartbeat.

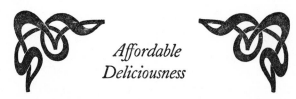

Affordable Deliciousness

No longer need you be as rich as Croesus to surround yourself in a sparkling veil of perfume. Don't let the prices of the perfume oils themselves put you off. It doesn't matter that a pound of pure jasmine petals costs three thousand dollars. For most of us, life is made bearable because fragrance comes in lots of beautifully *affordable* forms. So if the real stuff sells for $80 an ounce and you just want to get used to the feeling, the aura of it, start with two bars of hard-milled, scented soap instead. This does only about $6 worth of damage to your pocketbook. A bottle of soft cologne may cost $10 and a teeny, tiny, travel-sized cologne spray can be had for as little as $3.50.

If the scent is *really* lovely, you can work your way up to the real perfume slowly. Or you can put in an early Christmas request with your neighborhood Santa Claus ... or raid the grocery money ... or ask a friend to bring a bottle back from Paris ... or ... well, I'm sure you'll find a way to work it out.

While you're thinking, here's a brief recap of the many forms of fragrance you've got to choose from:

PERFUME—The real McCoy. Expensive. Luxurious. Meant not to be saved, but to be used often once it's opened.

PERFUME PACQUETTES—Towelettes moistened with scent, in little foil envelopes. Very much like pretty-smelling Wash & Dri. Great for traveling.

SOLID PERFUME—Scent suspended in a soft, beeswaxlike base. Solid perfumes are neat for traveling because they're (by definition) unbreakable, unspillable and all that. They also tend to come in nice jewelry cases that look very elegant when carried around in a handbag.

TOILET WATER—Lighter than perfume, but more concentrated than cologne. Should be used lavishly.

COLOGNE—Lighter than toilet water, perfect when used as an overall base fragrance. Add the real perfume to your pulse points for extra sparkle.

SOFT COLOGNE—An after-bath tingle. Some people keep huge bottles in the fridge just to heighten the experience.

PERFUMED BATHING OILS—Time was when one used to cheat by using bathing oils as perfume. (At least *I* used to cheat, until a master perfumer told me that bathing oils are meant to diffuse only in water. This means they don't release fragrance evenly if you put them directly on your skin.) My master-perfumer friend also mentioned that bath oil used as perfume sometimes goes rancid. I stopped cheating.

CREAM PERFUME—Sometimes called by other names, like perfumed body lustre or moisturizing creme perfume. A cream perfume is meant to be used like an allover moisturizer. Nice to slick on the backs of knees, legs, elbows—like I said, allover.

PERFUMED MILK BATH—Usually a powder, but sometimes a creamy liquid, milk bath softens, perfumes and extends the pleasure of an otherwise routine bath into a patent-leather luxury.

PERFUMED BATH POWDER—A sheer dusting of dry scent. Great in the shoes during the summer.

PERFUMED SOAP—Fragranced bars of bath soap leave you squeaky clean *and* smelling pretty. Not recommended for using on your face. But do feel free to use them liberally as company soap in the powder room.

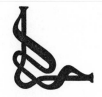

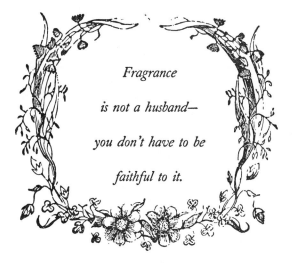

Fragrance

is not a husband—

you don't have to be

faithful to it.

—Francois De Roussy De Sales,
Christian Dior Perfumes

SHOPPING FOR PERFUME

Five Sure-Fire Ways to Shop for Scent

1. Whatever you do, DON'T stand there with your nose over the open bottle. A fragrance doesn't start to live until you put it on.
2. Spray (or dab) the perfume on the inside of your wrist. Wait two minutes. Then sniff for the top note.
3. Try to get involved with the character of the scent. Close your eyes. Smell Vetiver for dry wood (like cedar chests or the chips you line the gerbil cage with). Or try to pick up the traces of vanillin in Shalimar. Oddly enough, they smell just like chocolate. Citrus notes are easy to pick up because they smell lemony or limey. Florals may be a bit more elusive—try looking for the carnation in Norell, for example. If you find it, you've already got an educated nose.
4. About half an hour after you've sniffed your wrist for the TOP NOTE, smell it again for the middle tones. (I am assuming you've gone about your business and are not still standing at the counter chatting it up with the saleslady.) See if anybody notices that you've got a new perfume on. Ask a friend how he or she likes it.
5. Three or four hours after you've checked the MIDDLE notes, you'll be able to see what the BOTTOM note is like. Sniff again. If you're still pleasantly intrigued, then (and *only* then) consider buying.

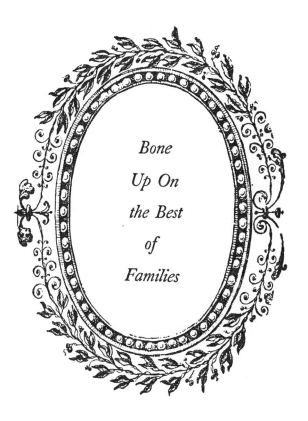

Bone

Up On

the Best

of

Families

Suzanne Grayson is the brains behind a marvelous place called The Face Factory. She's also a person who believes in making things easier for people. To that end, she's created a system of charting the family tree of the best-known scents of the century. The chart makes it superbly simple to find the thread that connects the scents you've always loved with the newer perfumes you'd like to try.

THE EVOLUTION of PERFUME

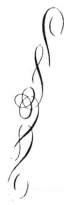

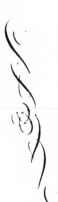

FLORAL

The fragrances of flowers gathered around the world. Some familiar. Others quite rare. Single florals...Or multi-florals blended into distinctive scents basically floral in character.

SINGLE FLORAL
One note...The essence of a single blossom, either floral, citrous or fruit "flavored."

FLORAL BOUQUET (BLEND)
A harmonious blend of several flowers. Sometimes one note predominates, but usually specific florals are not readily recognizable.

ORIENTAL-SEMI-ORIENTAL

Very rich and full-bodied. Woody. Sometimes sweet or smoky with amber or musk. Modern or semi-orientals are softer blends, highlighted by floral, green or spicy notes.

> Perfume. A magical, mystical word that conjures up all the romance of life. It has been thus since the dawn of history.
>
> Because of their exquisitely elusive nature, fragrances cannot be totally confined to a precise "type" or "class." THE EVOLUTION OF PERFUME attempts instead to place each of the world's great perfumes in the category most representative of its particular type. (Some fragrances in the same "family" will be similar, others will be quite different. But each one has its own soul.)
>
> And for each of the classic categories, I have lovingly created one beautiful new perfume. Each a totally new interpretation of the category. Each one a treasure.
>
> *Suzanne Grayson*

FLORAL (by year)

- **1975:** ONCE UPON A SUNRISE / *Suzanne Grayson*; FLEUR de VIE / *Suzanne Grayson*; JONTUE / *Revlon*; CHLOE / *Lagerfeld*; A ROSE IS A ROSE / *Houbigant*; BIGARADE / *Ricci*
- **1970:** LOVE'S LEMON; FRACAS / *Piguet*
- **1960:** ECCO / *Borghese*; CAPRICCI / *Ricci*; PLAISIR / *Raphael*; DIORISSIMO / *Dior*
- **1955:** WINDSONG / *Matchabelli*
- **1950:** L'AIR du TEMPS / *Ricci*; JUNGLE GARDENIA / *Tuvaché*; JEAN NATÉ
- **1945:** LAVENDER / *Yardley*; MUGUET de BOIS / *Coty*
- **1940:** WHITE SHOULDERS / *Evyan*; FLEURS de ROCAILLE / *Caron*; JOY / *Patou*
- **Pre-1935:** CHANEL 22 (1926); MY SIN / *Lanvin* (1924); JE REVIENS / *Worth* (1932); QUELQUES FLEURS / *Houbigant* (1912); JEAN MARIE FARINA / *Roger & Gallet* (1806); 4711 (1792)

ORIENTAL-SEMI-ORIENTAL

Herbal/Spicy:
- BAKIR / *Monteil*
- ULTIMA / *Charles Revson*
- HERBESSENCE / *Rubinstein*
- TUVARA / *Tuvaché*
- ROYAL SECRET / *Monteil*
- YOUTH DEW / *Lauder*

Woody/Mossy:
- VIA / *Lanvin*
- CHAMADE / *Guerlain*

Classic:
- KHUSHI / *Suzanne Grayson*
- TIGRESS / *Faberge*
- CHANTILLY / *Houbigant*
- SHALIMAR / *Guerlain* (1925)
- JICKY / *Guerlain* (1898)

Floral:
- CIARA / *Charles Revson*
- PRIVATE COLLECTION / *Lauder*
- ZADIG / *Pucci*
- WEIL de WEIL
- BAL A VERSAILLE / *Desprez*
- TABU / *Dana*
- EMERAUDE / *Coty* (1921)
- L'HEURE BLEUE / *Guerlain* (1913)

Musk and its variations:
- MUSK / *Jovan*

Time scale (left axis): 1975, 1970, 1965, 1960, 1955, 1950, 1945, 1940, Pre-1935

MODERN BLENDS

Aromatic blends, often *creations* rather than duplications of products of nature. Predominantly in sub-categories of all nature's fragrance sources. Characterized by brilliant top notes and full body. Many contain notes from several fragrance categories, so it is their *major* notes which place them in their appropriate family.

MODERN FLORAL
Sparkling floral. with specific flower notes not easily identifiable.

MODERN GREEN OR WOODY FLORAL
Fresh, grassy, drier (less sweet) blends than florals. but not as dry as true greens.

MODERN GREEN
Noticeably green in character. Crisp. Fresh. Dry. With grassy or flower-stem notes.

MODERN MOSSY/LEAFY/WOODY/FRUITY AND HERBAL OR SPICY BLENDS
From light and airy to rich and resinous. Difficult to categorize because of their sophisticated harmony and complex structure. but more beautiful because of it.

MODERN FLORAL
- 1975 — I AM-HE IS-WE ARE / *Suzanne Grayson*
- GEOFFREY BEENE
- NUANCE / *Coty*
- DAISY L. / *Love*
- GUCCI
- CERISSA / *Charles Revson*
- FAROUCHE / *Ricci*
- INFINI / *Caron*
- RITZ
- CLIMÂT / *Lancôme*
- GERMAINE / *Monteil*
- CALANDRE / *Rabanne*
- ZEN / *Shiseido*
- L'INTERDIT / *Givenchy*
- HYPNOTIQUE / *Max Factor*
- CASAQUE / *D'Albret*
- MADAME ROCHAS
- MAGIE / *Lancôme*
- LE DIX / *Balenciaga*
- ECUSSON / *D'Albret*
- SORTILEGE / *Le Galion*
- L'AIMANT / *Coty (1927)*
- CHANEL 5 / *(1924)*
- ARPEGE / *(Lanvin 1927)*

MODERN GREEN OR WOODY FLORAL
- FILLY / *Suzanne Grayson*
- LAUGHTER / *Tuvaché*
- CHARLIE / *Revlon*
- NORELL
- FIDJI / *Laroche*
- DETCHEMA / *Revillon*

MODERN GREEN
- CHANEL 19
- ALIAGE / *Lauder*
- VENT VERT / *Balmain*

Floral/Mossy
- S ∞ / *Suzanne Grayson*
- MADAME JOVAN / *Jovan*
- AVIANCE / *Matchabelli*
- ANBHAMO / *Borghese*
- RIVE GAUCHE / *St. Laurent*
- IMPREVU / *Coty*
- LE DE / *Givenchy*
- MAJA / *Myrurgia*
- ANTELOPE / *Weil*
- REPLIQUE / *Rafael*
- UN AIR EMBAUMÉ / *Rigaud (1913)*

Woody/Mossy
- STEPHAN B. / *Max Factor*
- HALSTON
- VIVRE / *Molyneux*
- ELAN / *Coty*
- VIVARA / *Pucci*
- Y / *St. Laurent*
- CHANT D'AROME / *Guerlain*
- CHYPRE 53 / *Guerlain*
- MA GRIFFE / *Carven*
- APHRODISIA / *Faberge*
- CRÊPE de CHINE / *Millot (1925)*
- CHYPRE / *Coty (1917)*

Mossy/Fruity
- VERVE / *Suzanne Grayson*
- COURANT / *Rubinstein*
- AUDACE / *Rochas*
- GIVENCHY III
- CACHET / *Matchabelli*
- EAU DE LOVE
- FIAMMA / *Borghese*
- CALECHE / *Hermes*
- IMITIMATE / *Revlon*
- QUADRILLE / *Balenciaga*
- JOLIE MADAME / *Balmain*
- MISS DIOR
- FEMME / *Rochas*
- MITSOUKO / *Guerlain (1921)*
- RUMEUR / *Lanvin (1924)*

Mossy/Spicy/Herbal
- PRIMA CLASSE / *Suzanne Grayson*
- EMPREINTE / *Courreyes*
- DIORELLA
- SUPER MOON DROPS / *Revlon*
- ESTÉE / *Lauder*
- AZURÉ / *Lauder*
- MISS BALMAIN
- CABOCHARD / *Grès*
- AMBUSH / *Dana*
- ROBE D'UN SOIR / *Carven*
- BANDIT / *Piguet*
- HEAVEN SENT / *Rubinstein*
- BLUE GRASS / *Arden*
- MOMENT SUPREME / *Patou (1933)*

Years (chart axis): 1975 · 1970 · 1965 · 1960 · 1955 · 1950 · 1945 · 1940 · Pre-1935

Men Test the Perfumes You Wear— Here's One Man's True Story

"Every day during the testing of Ciara, we would wear it on each arm, reporting every hour or so about how the notes were holding up, how they were changing and so on. As you know, it's a heavy, rich, pervasive fragrance, so I usually washed it off after work. One night, however, I forgot and left the office, and took a cab home to 83rd and Park.

"So there I am in the cab and the driver started asking me questions like, 'Where are you going? Do you like baseball? Are you married? Do you have children? Where do you hang around at night?'—very strange questions for a New York cabby. I guess by the time we'd gotten to my apartment, he'd determined that I wasn't gay. But he still wasn't totally sure, since I'd filled the whole cab up with Ciara.

"When I was paying him, he said, 'Are you going upstairs? Is your wife home?' And as he was giving me my change, he asked if I minded him telling me something. I said no, and he said, 'I can still smell the other broad on you.' So I gave him a big tip and destroyed all his illusions by telling him I worked for Revlon."

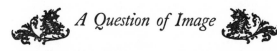

A Question of Image

You wouldn't believe how much the fragrance makers know about you. They know how old you are, if you're married or single, what you do for a living, what you do with your time off, how much money you make and (in all probability) what you eat for breakfast.

Scads of people in the industry are employed to find out everything they can about you, your fantasies and the image you have of yourself.

Once they know you as well (or better) than you know yourself, they can gear a perfume to fit your life-style or play on your deepest, most secret dreams. That's why when you look at any fragrance counter, you'll find all sorts of different perfumes, each geared to a particular image.

There are the liberated fragrances, the ladylike fragrances, the designer fragrances, the cosmetic house fragrances, the naturals, the fragrances that become part of you, the ones that insist they stay true to themselves; there's one if you're sports-minded and a few that'll keep you locked up in the bedroom for the rest of your life.

In fact, there are so many things that attract us to perfume, it's hard to know just where to start. Sometimes it's a crystal bottle that catches us, or the brief whiff of a new scent on a beautiful woman as she crosses the room. Sometimes it's a romantic or interesting story about how the perfume came to be—or even an attachment we form to a picture in an ad or an item in the evening paper.

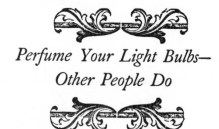

Perfume Your Light Bulbs— Other People Do

Dr. Schiller, a venerable pharmacist (who was seventy-five at the time, if he was a minute), told me that ladies of questionable reputation once perfumed their light bulbs with Patchouli oil. No longer need you be engaged in the ancient art of hooking to perfume your light bulbs. Today, in fact, light-bulb perfumery is merely a very nice way to fill a room with scent. There is even a special little gadget made for light-bulb perfuming called The Perfume Vaporizer. What it is, is an asbestos disk. You put a few drops of essence on it, allow several seconds for the perfume to absorb, put it on your light bulb, turn the light on and *voilà:* perfumed room.

Perfume Vaporizers (in Jasmine, Roman Hyacinth, Stephanotis, Sandalwood, Ormonde and Tantivy) are available from:

FLORIS OF LONDON
702 Madison Avenue
New York, New York 10021
Vaporizer $7.50
Scent $6.00 (15 cc); $11.50 (34 cc)

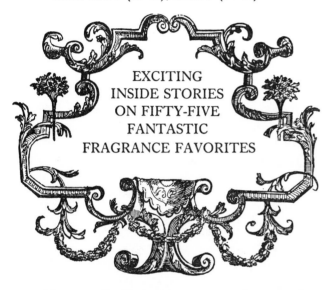

EXCITING
INSIDE STORIES
ON FIFTY-FIVE
FANTASTIC
FRAGRANCE FAVORITES

The more I talked with master perfumers and marketers, the more images came into play. Each time we talked about fragrance, we talked about *the women who wore the scents* and the men and women who created them. We talked about history and literature and princes and pilots and designers and debutantes. We talked in terms of image and life-style and got ourselves all tangled up in the intangible things that link the power of perfume to the mind.

The more we talked (the perfumers and I), the more I wanted to set down once and for all the images associated with all my favorite perfumes. Also, because I am a practical person as well as a double-dipped romantic, I wanted to set those images against all the vital information anyone would need if she wanted to try the scent herself. That meant "How much do they cost?" and "How DO you pronounce those names, anyway?" The result, which you'll get to in a minute, is meant to be sampled at leisure. You might want to leave it around the house (with appropriate pencilings) as a subtle hint to someone who'd be happy to buy you perfume, if only he knew what you'd really like.

NOTE: *Prices listed here range from the least expensive product on the line to the largest, most expensive size available. Prices (as always) are subject to change without notice.*

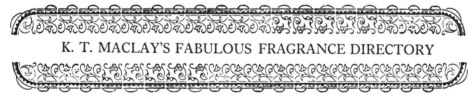

K. T. MACLAY'S FABULOUS FRAGRANCE DIRECTORY

1. AMBUSH (pronounced AM′-BOOSH) by Dana, $2.50–$25.00. A pretty bunny named Wendy who works at the Playboy Club in Ocho Rios, Jamaica, told me she loved Ambush because it was so perfect for the tropics. The perfumers who make it call it "unconfined and unconventional. A pretty floral with just a hint of musk to make it animal." Oddly enough, the surveys show that more teenage girls wear Ambush than almost any other cologne.

2. APHRODISIA (pronounced AF-ROW-DEESE′-YA) by Fabergé, $1.50–$40.00. Chief jeweler to the last two czars of Russia, Peter Carl Fabergé's finest creations were the small gold enameled and jeweled Easter eggs commissioned each year by the Russian imperial family and their friends.

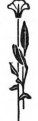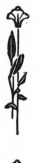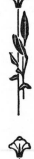

When the glittering era of the czars ended, Peter Carl retired to Switzerland, leaving his two sons to reopen The House of Fabergé in Paris. It was there in 1937 that Aphrodisia was born.

Named for Aphrodite (the Greek goddess of love), it's a regal scent; light enough to wear to lunch with an old beau, mysterious enough to wear for the most special man in your life.

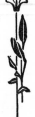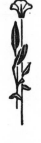

3. ARPEGE (pronounced AR-PEJ') by Lanvin, $5–$55. The name comes from *arpeggio,* which my Webster's Dictionary defines as "a non-simultaneous but swift sounding of the notes in a chord, as in the playing of a harp." The scent celebrates its fiftieth birthday this year. For those of us who have long known and loved it, it's a dressy, special fragrance that's just too beautiful to be taken lightly.

4. A ROSE IS A ROSE IS A ROSE by Houbigant, $2.50–$33.00. The name is inspired by a line in Gertrude Stein's famous poem, "Sacred Emily." The feeling is pure romance. Imagine all the velvet textures and sunlit colors of one perfect, full yellow rose. The woman who wears this clear, subtle fragrance truly regrets that parasols have gone out of style.

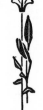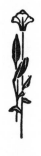

5. AVIANCE (pronounced AH-VEE-AHNCE') by Prince Matchabelli, $4–$10. Aviance is the aura of the "other woman" inside each of us, that very sensuous, very private other woman who knows nothing of Hamburger Extender and PTA Meetings. She's lush, perfumed, beautiful and totally feminine.

6. BAL A VERSAILLES (pronounced BAHL'-AH-VAIHR-SIGH') by Jean Desprez, $8–$285. Monsieur Jean Desprez developed BAL A VERSAILLES because he wanted to create THE great, classic French perfume. The name means "Ball at Versailles" and M. Desprez was so convinced that the Versailles Palace epitomized all French romanticism and elegance that the Bal A Versailles package, with its crystal cap, gold cord, and silk brocade, and its colors (gold and white) was taken directly from the Palace of Versailles. The label itself is a reproduction of a Fragonard painting called "Coupe des Sens" ("The Senses"), which is the only part of the design not taken from the palace, but included because it was a tribute (perhaps even *the* tribute) to sensuality. Bal A Versailles, then, was created to be the *most* romantic, classic French perfume you could possibly find.

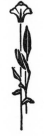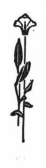

7. BELLE DE JOVAN (pronounced BELL'-D'JOE-VAN') by Jovan, $10. According to legend, BELLE DE JOVAN was created for a prince whose wealth was beyond imagination. It was to be his tribute to the woman he cherished beyond all others. It's the sort of scent given by every man who has ever cherished a woman—and worn by every woman who wants to be cherished.

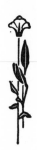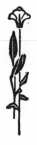

8. BLUE GRASS by Elizabeth Arden, $3–$30. "Gladys (Elizabeth Arden's sister) was discovering a wonderful new perfume that had been concocted by a

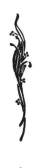

chemist in Grasse, in the south of France. She leased it in the name of the Arden company and dispatched a flagon to Elizabeth, along with a list of possible romantic-sounding French names for the fragrance. Elizabeth took one whiff and said it would be called Blue Grass in honor of her horses. One of her managers complained, 'You'll never sell it with that name. It'll remind people of manure.'

"He was wrong. Blue Grass was a winner, the largest-selling perfume she ever manufactured." *

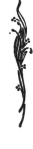

9. CABOCHARD (pronounced KAB'-OH-SHAR) by Gres, $3.50–$120.00. In Paris patois, *cabochard* means "stubborn." It's the fragrance of the hard-headed, the irresistibly willful, the captivatingly persistent woman. *Vogue* once called it "dazzle by the drop."

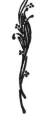

10. CACHET (pronounced KA-SHAY') by Prince Matchabelli, $2.50–$35.00. Cachet's woman prides herself on her individuality. She's sure of herself; sure of what she stands for. She wouldn't be caught dead looking (or smelling) like the girl next door. The story on Cachet is that it's designed to work with your own body chemistry to create a totally unique scent that's as individual as you are.

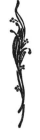

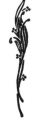

11. CALANDRE (pronounced KA-LAHN'-DRAH) by Paco Rabanne, $9–$72. The Calandre woman has a crisp, cool sparkle. She's the sleek creature who zooms through life with the grace of a gazelle. Calandre matches the pace she sets and sets the pace she makes. By the way, the word *calandre* is French for the perfectly tooled grille of a racy sports car. It also applies to the perfectly balanced perfume of a racy woman.

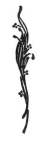

12. CALECHE (pronounced KAL-ESCH') by Hermes, $18.50–$200.00. The House of Hermes began in 1837 by making the finest, most fabulous saddles in Paris. That's right, I said *saddles*. They also made leather harnesses and sporting accessories for kings and noblemen and toilet accessories and tea caddies for queens and courtesans. The Hermes workmanship was painstakingly thorough, the materials the finest, the designs faultless ... and the prices high. Today, only a small percentage of Hermes's products are concerned with horses, and the only connection with carriages is the carriage trade clientele that still flocks to the famous House of Hermes on Rue du Faubourg, St. Honore, in Paris.

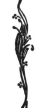

In 1961 (shortly after they introduced the illustrious Hermes signature scarves, which women still collect like jewels), the House of Hermes created a beautiful perfume called Caleche, which was named after the most elegant and beautiful carriage. Caleche is floral without being flowery; sultry without phoniness, sunny without being *naïve*. If this sounds paradoxical, it is. And perhaps that explains its universal appeal. The other nice thing about Caleche is that its personality is submissive—meant to let your own character shine through.

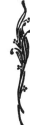

13. CHAMADE (pronounced SHA-MAHD') by Guerlain, $10–$60. Antoine

* From *Miss Elizabeth Arden*, by Alfred Allan Lewis & Constance Woodworth (Pinnacle, $1.50).

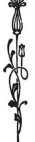
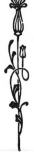

meets Lucille at a fashionable dinner party. Nothing for either of them is ever quite the same again. The next time they meet, they are alone. Antoine takes Lucille's hand.

Françoise Sagan describes the moment in her story "La Chamade," whence comes the inspiration for this perfume: " 'Now come,' thought Lucille, 'he's holding my hand as we cross the park. It's Spring, no need to worry, I'm not sixteen anymore.' But her heart thumped wildly. She felt the blood drain from her face and her hands rush to her throat . . ."

In France today, *chamade* quite simply means "the heart beating wildly." But for the woman who wears Chamade, a word of warning: *Chamade* also means "the beating of a drum to signal the moment of final surrender." Don't say you haven't been warned.

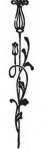

14. CHANEL NO. 5 (pronounced SHA-NELL′ #5) by Chanel, $5–$400. Rumor has it that Chanel No. 5 was a mistake. As the story goes, Coco Chanel was looking for a fragrance that had the same flawlessly tailored freedom her other designs (the Chanel suit, the jersey dress, the turtleneck sweater, the blazer jacket, the pantsuit and the "little black dress") did. She was getting samples of everything from the Paris perfumers, who were at the time playing around with a new synthetic ingredient called an aldehyde. In one of the test bottles they submitted for Mlle. Chanel's consideration (the bottle marked No. 5), they had *by mistake* put in about ten times as much aldehyde as they wanted to. Mistake or not, it was *beautiful.* So Mlle. Chanel chose it, named it after the number on the test bottle and started a whole new (aldehydic) trend in fragrances.

15. CHANEL NO. 19 (pronounced SHA-NELL′ #19) by Chanel, $6.50–$100.00. Chanel No. 19 comes in the same celebrated bottle, whose classic design is on permanent display at the Museum of Modern Art. It's the first new fragrance from Chanel in forty years. Originally Mlle. Chanel created Chanel No. 19 for herself. She kept it in private stock, giving it only to special friends and select couture customers, because it was said to embody the very essence of Chanel herself. It's named both for her birth date (August 19) and for nineteen of her most obvious good qualities. A confidante recounted her attributes this way: "You will always be young no matter what age you reach. And truly elegant in your manner and life-style. Intensely female. Graceful. Casually understated. Contemporary. Brilliant. Witty. Fascinating. Generous. Honest. Courageous. Outspoken. Supremely confident and completely independent as few women are or ever hope to be. You are logical. A perfectionist. Unforgettable and way ahead of your time."

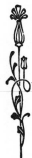
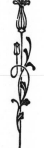

16. CHARLIE by Revlon, $3.50–$8.50. Charlie was the first American fragrance to turn the perfume industry around and set it on its ear. It was, for instance, the first woman's perfume with a man's name. It was fresh, not terribly expensive, clean and (and this was the new part) it was aimed at a new kind of woman—the Charlie person. She is fun and serious and dynamic and God knows

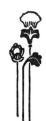
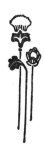

what all else. She is a get-around-town girl who is just as comfortable barefoot in the country. She'd fly a kite on Sunday and a 747 on Monday morning. She is an eager extrovert who gets shy sometimes and can still blush. She pretty much speaks for all of us.

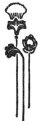

17. CHLOE (pronounced CLOW′-EE) by Parfums Lagerfeld, $12.50–$100.00. Chloé is a designer fragrance created by Karl Lagerfeld, who thinks of perfume as another kind of "body dressing." The woman who wears Chloé doesn't have to *prove* anything. She has her own personal mythology, her own muses, her own friends. She loves the drawings of Aubrey Beardsley, the sculpture of Brancusi, she likes Colette, Isadora Duncan, Marlene Dietrich, Andy Warhol and David Bowie. She's a one-of-a-kind who, in the words of Lagerfeld himself, "does not just *put on* my fragrance; she *enters* it."

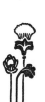
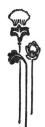

18. CIARA (pronounced SEE-AHR′-AH) by Revlon, $8–$45. There was one year at Revlon when all the fragrances seemed to have something to do with the name Charles Revson. The first, of course, was Charlie. Next came Ciara (a poetic arrangement of Mr. Revson's initials), then Cerissa (another play on the initials CR). In contrast to the very liberated, fun feeling of Charlie, Ciara was made for the woman who is both gentle *and* strong—warm, willing and exuberantly alive. The warm bosom, tender kiss, silken curtain of hair sort of woman who will fight to the death to protect and care for what is hers.

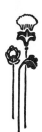
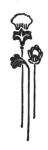

19. DAISY L by Love, $3.50–$6.50. Daisy L goes with sexy black dresses or ancient bluejeans; romantic ruffles or cool classics; hiking boots or dancing shoes. It's as marvelous at a candlelit dinner for two as it is sharing a peanut butter sandwich on the road. It goes to the opera or off-off-Broadway and smells just as great on a yacht as it does on a Sunfish.

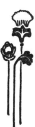

20. EAU DE LOVE (pronounced OH-D'LOVE′) by Love, $1.50–$8.00. For the woman who's successful enough to have a full-fledged career under control, but romantic enough to walk in the woods at dawn, love her very own husband and want lots of babies when the time's right. The Eau De Love woman lives in a man's world, but never forgets for an instant that she's a woman.

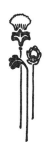

21. EMERAUDE (pronounced EM-EHR-AWED′) by Coty, $2.75–$30.00. The people of Persia kept emerald jewels in their temples and believed that mysterious powers were hidden within their depths. Fascinated by the Persian reverence for this precious stone, François Coty wanted to capture the intrigue of the land and the beauty of the stone in a perfume. In 1923 he created Emeraude—earthy, provocative, mysterious as the emerald for which it was named.

22. FRANKINCENSE & MYRRH (pronounced FRANK-INCENSE and MURR) by Jovan, $5–$10. The Wise Men brought frankincense and myrrh (two of the most precious aromatic oils in the history of the world) as gifts for

the Christ Child. These precious oils have been blended into a sultry, almost smoky, deeply provocative fragrance.

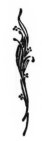

23. HALSTON (pronounced HALL'-STON) by Halston Fragrances, $10–$100. Halston by Halston is the major fragrance designed by the very same man who created Jackie Kennedy's internationally famous pillbox hat. A pretty, intricate, *interesting* fragrance, it comes in a revolutionary asymmetrical bottle designed by Halston and Elsa Peretti (the noted jewelry designer for Tiffany). For the woman who buys Halston, quality is merely the beginning.

24. HOPE by Frances Denney, $3.75–$15.00. Made for the romantic snow queen with tinsel in her hair, Hope wafts on free and winsome—before caroling, while wassailing, at brunch, unwrapping presents beneath the tree on a sparkling Christmas morning. A winter fragrance. Innocent? But of course! *Naive?* Never!

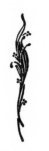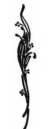

25. IMPERIALE (pronounced IM'-PERI-AL) by Guerlain, $9–$35. Napoleon III adored women, but until he met Eugénie de Montijo, he had never adored one woman for very long. Eugénie was startlingly beautiful, with blue eyes, red hair and alabaster shoulders. She transformed the Royal Palace of the Tuileries into a glittering spectacle of crinolined ladies and elegantly bedecked gentlemen, thrilling to masked evenings of dance and endless games of charades. In 1860 Pierre François Guerlain created an eau de cologne of such outstanding purity and distinction that the Empress Eugénie allowed him to name it after her: Eau de Cologne Imperiale. To wear Imperiale today is to recall the splendor of France's Second Empire and the story of one, very beautiful woman.

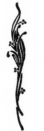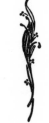

26. IMPREVU (pronounced OHM-PRAY-VOO') by Coty, $3.50–$30.00. Imprevu was made modern for the woman who dared to be daring; the woman who delighted in being different; the woman of whim who'd rather be herself than anyone else in the world.

27. INTERLUDE by Frances Denney, $3.75–$17.50. Think fantasies of the great indoors … emerald earrings and satin sheets. Think of a mood to bathe in, sipping brandy before a roaring fire, dancing beneath a tinkling crystal chandelier, driving home snug beneath a silver fox lap robe. Mysterious. Magnetic. All those things.

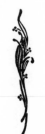

28. INTIMATE by Revlon, $1.85–$7.50. A marvelous old standby for women who liked boys at twelve and thoroughly appreciated men by the time they were twenty-one. The woman who wears Intimate leaves coyness to the also-rans and thinks cute is something kittens are.

29. JEAN NATE (pronounced JHUN-NAH-TAY') by Lanvin–Charles of the Ritz, $1.75–$25.00. Treats are part of the Jean Naté life-style; little treats like

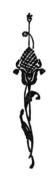

buying jonquils in February or playing hookey from the office to see a lunchtime movie. You can get 128 ounces of Jean Naté Friction Pour le Bain for $25 and still have enough money left over to place a $2 bet at the race track.

30. JICKY (pronounced GHEE´-KEY) by Guerlain, $6–$35. From Truman Capote's book *Answered Prayers:* "The room smelled of her perfume (at some point I asked what it was, and Colette said: 'Jicky. The Empress Eugénie always wore it. I like it because it's an old-fashioned scent with an elegant history, and because it's witty without being coarse—like the better conversationalists. Proust wore it. Or so Cocteau tells me. But then he is not *too* reliable.')."

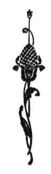

31. JONTUE (pronounced JOHN-TOO´) by Revlon, $3.75–$6.75. This is another one of those Revlon fragrances that was named for a member of the Revson family—in this case, for John Revson, son of Charles and vice president of Revlon's Fine Fragrance division. It's an unabashedly pretty perfume with a gentle feeling. It's meant for the woman who secretly wants to live like Jacqueline Onassis and look like Cybil Shepard; the sexy woman who (even though she's absorbed by consumerism) would still rather be loved by Robert Redford than by Ralph Nader.

32. JOVAN MUSK OIL by Jovan, $1.50–$12.50. Jovan Musk Oil is dedicated to the proposition. Need I say more?

33. JUNGLE GARDENIA by Tuvache, $4–$25. A very Victorian young woman I once knew wore Jungle Gardenia in the winter. She'd move gracefully through the snow, surrounded by the aroma of tropical midnights, cloaked in the romance of a pale jungle moon. It would be silly to add that she had a tremendous effect on ski instructors that season, but there's the fact of it.

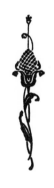

34. L'HEURE BLEUE by Guerlain (pronounced L'ERR BLUEH´) $9.50–$40.00. A man pauses to reflect on his way home. It's another gloriously warm summer evening. The sky is cloudless. The deep blue of the sky grows darker and stars begin to appear in the east. For a brief moment it is as if all the elements are conspiring to say something tender. Guerlain legend has it that Jacques Guerlain's inspiration and appreciation of that particularly soft evening were heightened by some unrealized premonition of a war that would soon devour Europe. True or not, the woman who puts L'Heure Bleue to her pulse points will be caught up in an unforgettable spell. What happens then is another story.

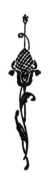

35. LOVE'S FRESH LEMON by Love Cosmetics, $1.25–$4.00. Created for the girl who gets straight A's without really trying. Young in spirit and spirited in everything, the Love lady founded her campus jump-rope league, plays a mean game of Scrabble and can occasionally be found giggling in the bushes with an interested friend.

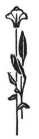
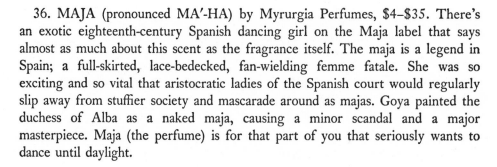
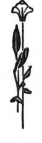

36. MAJA (pronounced MA´-HA) by Myrurgia Perfumes, $4–$35. There's an exotic eighteenth-century Spanish dancing girl on the Maja label that says almost as much about this scent as the fragrance itself. The maja is a legend in Spain; a full-skirted, lace-bedecked, fan-wielding femme fatale. She was so exciting and so vital that aristocratic ladies of the Spanish court would regularly slip away from stuffier society and mascarade around as majas. Goya painted the duchess of Alba as a naked maja, causing a minor scandal and a major masterpiece. Maja (the perfume) is for that part of you that seriously wants to dance until daylight.

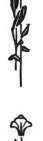

37. MITSOUKO (pronounced MITTS-SOO´-KOH) by Guerlain, $9.50–$40.00. A young British naval attaché is aboard the Japanese flagship . . . so is the admiral's wife. Her name is Mitsouko. Her beauty is unequaled. The impossible happens. History does not record the affair, but Claude Farrere's love story *(La Battille)* inspired this marvelous Guerlain perfume.

38. MUGES DE BOIS (pronounced MOO-JHAY D'BOWAH´) by Coty, $2.75–$4.50. The legend says that a young man was walking through the woods near Paris on the first day of May. He picked a sprig of lily of the valley *(muges de bois)* to take home to his lover. She gave him a kiss in return (it was a *long time ago,* you have to remember). Anyhow, it's still the custom in France to offer *muges de bois* to a loved one on May Day. Every woman who accepts this offering is honor-bound to respond with a kiss.

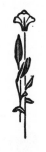

39. MUSK by Houbigant, $3.50–$15.00. Consider the harem builder who mixed musk oil into his construction materials . . . or the Empress Josephine, who used musk in her bedroom (where you can still smell it today). Then clear your calendar and prepare for a change in your life—for the power is yours. But remember to use Houbigant's musk with caution, because while you may not be aware of its potent qualities, others fall under the spell almost instantly.

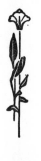

40. MUSK by R. H. Cosmetics, $3–$9. Science hasn't proved yet that musk is an aphrodisiac. *Vogue* magazine, however, proudly says that its animal odor probably does "prod our subconscious into erogenous reaction by suggesting sex, pleasure, warm skin and the contact of bodies." In other words, musk is a turn-on. R. H.'s Musk Oil is milder than most, and meant to be used as a base that makes your own favorite fragrance last longer.

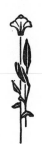

41. MY SIN by Lanvin, $5–$55. A very young-in-heart fragrance that's sensuous in a *provocative* way. Sensuous the way life was in the 1920s and 30s. It's just not a blunt-up-front kind of perfume. It's a vamp scent. A fun, *teasing* kind of fragrance. You get the feeling that the woman who wears it knows it's sexier to wear something dangerously revealing than to wear nothing at all. More than anything, My Sin is (like the ads say) "a most provocative fragrance."

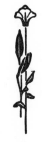

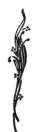
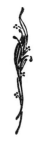

42. NORELL by Norell Perfumes, Inc., $6–$80. Norell is a regal, enormously self-assured scent that has the happy quality of smelling lovely on almost anybody. Designed by Norman Norell (who also gave us the sequined mermaid evening dress Lynn Revson wore everywhere), Norell perfume almost single-handedly opened up the great American fragrance boom. Before Norell appeared on the scene, everyone thought great perfumes were FRENCH perfumes—by definition. Norell changed all that by being the first great perfume born in America.

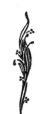
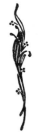

43. NUANCE (pronounced NOO-AHNCE') by Coty, $4.50–$40.00. As soft and provocative as a whisper in his ear, Nuance is the sort of fragrance that speaks softly, but carries a big stick.

44. OLD ENGLISH LAVENDER by Yardley, $1.75–$5.00. Forget about lavender being the fragrance little old blue-haired ladies use. What this fragrance was all about during the eighteenth century was S-E-X. Lavender was the how-to-turn-a-man-on fragrance of the 1760s. Oh yes, Cary Grant used it, too.

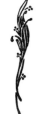
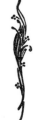

45. PARURE (pronounced PEAR-ROO') by Guerlain, $12–$120. *Parure* is hard to translate. About the closest you can come is to say that it means "ornament," but only in the sense of a jeweled tiara. It also means "adornment," but in the sense of an aura, a presence that is *felt* more than seen. The scent is by turns innocent, angelic, disarming, defiant and proud.

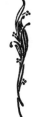
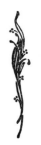

46. QUELQUES FLEURS (pronounced KELL'-KIH FLEWR) by Houbigant, $2.50–$33.00. Houbigant's royal clientele included such stellar personalities as Marie Antoinette, Napoleon, Queen Victoria and the Empress Eugénie of France. You can join this titled assemblage with QUELQUES FLEURS—*the* fragrance of the 20s and 30s—now staging a nostalgic comeback. QUELQUES FLEURS is one of those classics that is said to mark "the beginning of a beautiful past." (I have no idea what that means either.)

47. REPLIQUE (pronounced RAY-PLEEK') by Raphael, $4.25–$70.00. A full-blooded aristocrat, Replique is sultry, sophisticated and just a touch exotic. Blended to bring out a bit of gentled wildness in the woman who wears it, Replique calls up images of sharing champagne cocktails with an amorous leopard.

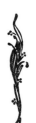

48. RIVE GAUCHE (pronounced REEVE GOASH) by Yves Saint Laurent, $3.50–$12.50. One of the most striking women I know says she'd be lost without her little $3.50 bottle of Rive Gauche Cologne. Maybe that's because designer Yves Saint Laurent (pronounced EEVES SAN LAW-ROHN') has packed this young, contemporary perfume full of the adventurous madness of Paris's Left Bank, for which the scent was named.

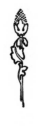
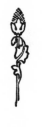

49. ROSEMARY COLOGNE by Weleda, $2.50. More relevant than a cup of coffee, the clean, herby smell of rosemary is a definite stimulant. If you use it in cooking (the herb, not the perfume), it will wake up your digestive juices. If you dab the cologne behind your ears and under your nose, it will keep you alert. Rosemary Cologne is just one of several nice natural fragrances put out by Weleda. They also make Lavender, Orange Blossom and Pine Scents. They require a minimum $3 order, though, so send for their catalog:

WELEDA
30 South Main Street
Spring Valley, New York 10977

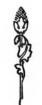

50. SHALIMAR (pronounced SHALL' IH MAHR) by Guerlain, $10–$100. "Shah Jehan (the third mogul emperor of India) had many wives. But he adored only one. Her name was Mumtaz Mahal. Some say he loved her unto madness, that she was not his wife, but his fever. Victories, empires, riches were as dull as dust compared to her. Jehan created a series of gardens at Lahore for Mumtaz. He called them the Gardens of Shalimar and brought to them the most fragrant, delicate blossoms. Deep pools were built and crystal fountains with marble-paved terraces. The rarest birds sang here and lighted lanterns rivaled the brightness of stars. It was here, in the gardens of Shalimar, that Jehan and Mumtaz were truly happy."

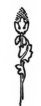

This story was told by a maharaja to Pierre and Jacques Guerlain in Paris in 1925. They were so moved by it they created a perfume called Shalimar, which (they say) has "been the beginning of a never-ending tale."

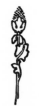

51. STEPHEN B by Stephen Burrows Fragrances, $4.75–$40.00. Two-time Coty Award–winning fashion designer Stephen Burrows was already famous for embellishing his ensembles with lettuce edging and zigzag red stitches. Then he created Stephen B, an adventurous, exuberant young fragrance about which he says: "When a woman wears my fragrance, she will feel alluring, adventurous and alive. She will be happy with today and ready for tomorrow."

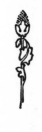

52. TATIANA (pronounced TAH-T'YA'-NAH) by Diane Von Furstenberg, $10–$14. Tatiana was the first fragrance pleasure-tested on New York cab drivers. What happened was that Diane Von Furstenberg takes a lot of taxis. And while she was testing the fragrance, she was almost subconsciously waiting until the cabbies turned around and asked: "Mmmmmmm . . . what IS that you're wearing?" So by the time she developed what she thought was a good fragrance, she had as many as ten cab drivers a day turning around to ask what perfume she had on. Now that I think of it, Tatiana may be the reason traffic is always so messed up in New York.

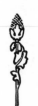

53. TWEED by Yardley, $4.00–$8.50. Rumored to be one of the first underground unisex fragrances, Tweed was used by men and women during the Second World War, long before anybody thought anything about unisex. The women used it because it was beautiful. The men used it as an aftershave because they liked the way it smelled and because they were secure enough about their own masculinity not to worry about smelling good.

54. VOL DE NUIT (pronounced VOL D'NOO-EE) by Guerlain, $9.50–$40.00. Vol de Nuit expresses a very personal view of courage and compassion. The name comes from *Vol de Nuit* (Night Flight), the famous story by French poet/aviator Antoine de Saint-Exupéry.

An airplane carrying mail to Buenos Aires loses radio contact. There are storms over the entire Patagonian plateau. At Bahia Blanca a message is received: "Commencing descent. Entering clouds..." Two final words are picked up at Trelew: "...see nothing..." The pilot Fabien has been married only six weeks. His wife waits in the flight-operations office listening to the seconds tick by. Each second carries something of Fabien away...

Saint-Exupéry (himself a wing commander in the French Air Force) disappeared during a mission over occupied France in 1944. Now, every year, the French Air Force College orders bottles of Vol de Nuit, specially emblazoned with French wings, to be given by its Air Force cadets during official visits abroad.

55. ZEN by Shiseido, $4–$30. Zen is the most indefinable form of self-discovery. It's a special technique of teaching without words. Zen is also a fragrance created with many similarities to the philosophy for which it's named. Zen confuses; it dazzles, yet quiets. It's sensual, yet still ... innocent, yet worldly; youthful, yet sophisticated. Zen is made for the woman to whom the art of BEING is more important than the art of being busy.

 ## GETTING THE PERFUME TO THE PULSE POINT

THE BEST WAY TO PUT ON PERFUME is to spray it on. This means you'll need an atomizer.

CASWELL-MASSEY (the oldest apothecary in the United States) carries marvelous atomizers. Prices range from $39.00 for a cranberry-glass sphere with frosted glass flowers and a natural pump spray device to $13.50 for a clear glass, ribbed pyramid that looks as if it were snatched from a vanity table in 1929 or so. Both these atomizers hold about two to three ounces of scent. They're also a great deal of fun to use.

By the way, if you're going to have an atomizer, you're going to need to fill it. Those of us with unsteady hands have learned to depend on small plastic funnels for filling large atomizers. For the smaller (purse size) sprays, there's a little bulb-syringe device that works wonders.

Plastic Funnel $1.00
Moulin Rouge Perfume Spray Filler $1.50

Atomizers and accessories can be ordered from:

CASWELL-MASSEY, LTD.
320 West 13th Street
New York, New York 10014

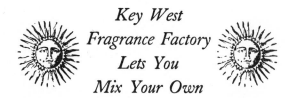

Key West Fragrance Factory Lets You Mix Your Own

You can visit the famous Florida factory and watch the perfume laboratory at work. You'll be able to test your nose at the Make Your Own counter, where you can choose from over sixty different fragrant oils and make perfumes and colognes to your heart's delight. You can also get elegant, *finished* perfumes and colognes in beautiful packages. Everything is made in small batches, so you can be sure they're absolutely fresh. For catalog, send a self-addressed, stamped envelope to:

KEY WEST FRAGRANCE FACTORY
P.O. Box 1643
528 Front Street
Key West, Florida 33040
Phone: (305)294-6661
Open 9:30–5:30 daily except Sunday
Credit Cards Honored

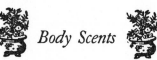

Body Scents

Miriam Nunberg and Paul Lindenbaum run a dear little shop in Woodstock, New York, where they dispense essential luxury oils. Their stock covers all sorts of good smells from almond to wisteria. Tiny ¼-ounce bottles ($3), if you order them by mail, come shipped in lovely little rattan baskets for which I seem to have found thousands of uses. One is at the moment holding paper clips; another, sachet; and the one in the kitchen keeps laundry change. For a Body Scents price list, send Miriam a self-addressed, stamped envelope. She likes getting mail.

BODY SCENTS
P.O. Box 266
Woodstock, New York 12498

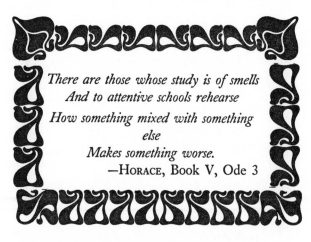

There are those whose study is of smells
And to attentive schools rehearse
How something mixed with something else
Makes something worse.
—HORACE, Book V, Ode 3

HOW I DIDN'T BECOME A MASTER PERFUMER

by K. T. Maclay

Somewhere on my list of favorite fantasies, cuddled in between owning a white Silver Cloud Rolls Royce and being stranded on a desert island with Robert Redford, down on page two somewhere, there's a little note that says: "Make perfume."

Not that I hadn't been warned about this. The same people who'd nod indulgently when I told them I wanted to be chauffeured around in an elegant car or spend some time weaving hibiscus into Robert Redford's hair would become furious about my wanting to dabble in the fragrant arts.

Ed Blaumeiser, manager of fragrance planning and evaluation for AVON, smiled indulgently. *Then* he went on to tell me that anything I could possibly whip up in my kitchen would be a drastic oversimplification, doomed to failure. Like making a photocopy of a great work of art.

Well, I thought. Avon is a big company. The biggest fragrance producer in the world. They have thirty active lines and make about 150 pure fragrance products. They take anywhere from sixteen months to two years to develop a single scent. I was certainly not foolish enough to go after anything THAT complicated. No. What I wanted was perhaps an unpretentious toilet water. A blend of four or five beautiful aromas. Something that was simple, but essentially *me*. So when Peter De Marfy (president of Continental Perfumes, Inc.) invited me to his laboratory to create my own scent, I was thrilled. I was flattered. I had no way to know he was kidding.

Being invited by a real perfumer to make your own perfume is like being invited by Mozart to come in to knock off a fugue. Or having Picasso ask you if you'd like to play with his brushes.

My first disappointment was with the laboratory itself. After all, I'd envisioned fragrant vats of spice and herbs, a rococo clutter of petals and vials, mahogany panels and a crystal chandelier. Perfume was romance and romance (in my fantasy) demanded a romantic setting.

Was I ever *wrong*. Mr. De Marfy's lab looked more like a shipping room than an artist's studio. Actually, it looked like a cross between a shipping room and a NASA space station. Immense cannisters of raw materials side-by-next delicate scientific equipment. Aluminum casks of nutmeg and cumin-seed oil weighing 250 pounds sharing space with a serious-looking machine that measured specific weight and gravity of each raw material before creation even began. A Xerox-like machine hummed softly in the corner, quietly vaporizing Linalool at one end and producing a Linalool "fingerprint" read-out at the other.

"Where's the romance? Where's the mystery? Where's Peter De Marfy?" I wondered. But he was behind me, struggling with the cap on a small cannister of ambergris. "Ambergris!" he said as he proudly held the open jar to my nose.

"Nothing!" I said, after inhaling deeply. "This stuff smells awful." "Right you are!" said De Marfy (in a really attractive, soft, French accent). Then he went on to explain that that's where the romance came in. "It's the curve of pleasure," he said. "The point at which an unpleasant odor like ambergris or musk or civet becomes pleasant." In pure concentration most animal products smell *ghastly*. It takes the perfumer/artist to know how to modify them, dilute them, distill them and combine them to make them beautiful.

So, Lesson #1 seemed to be that (in perfume) things are not always what they seem. Take lavender, for example. "Okay," you say. "Lavender is lavender." But the truth of the matter is that the lavender I sampled next was the product of some fifty ingredients, all working together to simulate one aspect of lavender. The amazing thing was that that delicious lavender was only one of the thousands of products a good perfumer has at his fingertips. So where in heaven's name do you start?

For purposes of illustration, WE started at Mr. De Marfy's perfumer's organ. (I *know* that sounds dirty, but hang on for a minute and I'll explain.) A perfumer's organ looks just like a pipe organ. It's a U-shaped series of stepped shelves that starts at the perfumer's workbench and works its way up to a point where he can easily reach the top shelf. The shelves themselves are lined with little brown bottles full of all the raw materials the perfumer needs to make his perfume: natural oils, aromatic chemicals, synthetic chemicals, solvents, extracts and like that.

Have you ever seen someone play a pipe organ, sitting in the middle of it, reaching with his left hand to play some notes, reaching with his right hand to play others or working at the center keyboard to orchestrate a melodic run? Well, that's exactly what a perfumer does. And to get back to my story, Mr. De Marfy, who was by this time seated before his perfumer's organ looking very sage and wise, dipping blotter strips into small brown bottles, told me that there were no shortcuts to making perfume.

A good perfumer starts sniffing blotters of contrasting scents. He begins with lemon, say, then moves on to sandalwood, cloves, anise and jasmine. Contrasts are easy to learn because each one is strikingly different from the other. As his nose gets more experienced, he can move on to similar scents. Which is a much more difficult task. The apprentice nose must tell the difference between lemon, bergamot, tangerine, sweet orange, bitter orange, orange from California, Florida orange, Italian orange and oranges from Portugal and Guinea. And that is just a tiny part of a single fragrance family. Once you have the citrus notes committed to memory, you can move into woods, spices or florals—then synthetics.

This fragrance thing was more complex than I'd imagined. (And I *knew* it was complicated.) Could I spend two or three years committing to memory the distinct odors of some three thousand different raw materials? Could I remember my name in the morning, or where I'd left my housekeys? It looked unlikely that I'd be able to keep all these different things in my head, no less master the intricate technique of writing them down. And believe it or not, writing it down is important. No perfumer sits at his workbench indiscriminately ladling oils and powders into a beaker hoping for the best. He starts with a formula, the way Mozart might have started with notes on a page. And even before he puts pencil to paper, he starts (according to Mr. De Marfy), "with a melody in his mind."

"You decide in general terms . . ." he told me. "Then you work backward from there. It's like hearing a song sung softly in your ear. So you start with chords, not single notes. Each chord is orchestrated. If you have a clarinet and an oboe and a violin and a piano all playing the same note at the same time, each instrument will develop that note differently. And that's what you try to do with fragrance. You're trying to harmonize a jasmine, a rose, a wood and a musk, for example. You try to get a nice, round, velvety sound to it; you're constantly trying to smooth out jagged edges, to make the colors of the scent blend beautifully—like a Renoir painting."

So scent has color as well as sound? Mr. De Marfy told me to close my eyes and sniff. Yes. Of course, scent has color! Naturally, color is a highly personal thing, but with my eyes closed, resins were definitely brown, jasmine and roses were red, mimosa was yellow with a blue background (very springlike), woody notes were the color of autumn leaves in Vermont, lavender, not surprisingly, was purple (like a mountaintop at sunset), galbanum was a sharp spinach-green while lentisc seemed creamy green (like asparagus soup).

While I was smelling for color, something else was happening, too. Because each odor seemed to have its own "depth," my scentual experience became like looking into clear water or listening to the violin score in a symphony, then ignoring the violins and listening only to the bass.

The more complicated each raw material became for me, the more I marveled that perfumers were able to break each note into its component parts, then smell one part and know instantly how it would work with other components. The process is like a composer inventing a new instrument to go nicely with oboes and flutes.

Here was the creative part, the romantic part, the part of perfumery I could relate to. It took Mr. De Marfy to break in on my reverie. And what he said convinced me that I'd never, ever make a go of it in perfume. It went above and beyond mere simple questions like, "Does the muguet still smell the same with synthetic hydroxycitronellal" and "Does the rose still have the lift and life it had before geraniol became synthetic?" It got right to my heart and right to my major weakness: tidiness and thrift.

There are four hundred raw materials and compounds on a small perfumer's organ. Each is very clearly marked. Alphabetically arranged. Its name, the date it was poured into its bottle—

everything is organized and clear. Each blotter is marked not only with the name of the ingredient being considered, but with the time it was wet with scent. (They do this so they can check how quickly a component evaporates.) Every minute detail must be weighed and noted, because each ingredient matures at different times in different ways. Every experiment is cataloged with monklike devotion, for the good perfumer must be accurate to one part in ten thousand. Or, as Mr. De Marfy was quick to point out, "There's nothing more frustrating than creating a fantastic fragrance and not being able to reproduce it." This way lies madness (for me at least).

No. Clearly I am not tidy enough to be a perfumer, nor scientific enough. Nor am I wealthy enough. Oh, maybe I can afford a little bitty mistake ... throwing a $2 mixture of essential oils down the sink would not seriously unhinge me. But when you talk about toilet water that costs $25 a pound and gets mixed in thirty thousand pound batches—you are definitely out of my league.

And so it was that I decided not to become a master perfumer. To bid *adieu* to Mr. De Marfy and his sunlit laboratory, and make my way back to the perfume counter to revel in a new appreciation of classic scents created by REAL masters.

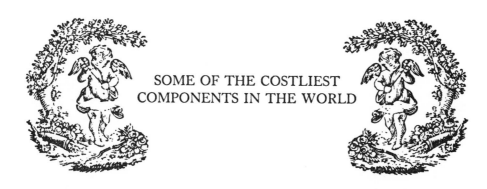

SOME OF THE COSTLIEST COMPONENTS IN THE WORLD

Amber	40 pounds average per whale yields 2 pounds musk	$1,100
Civet	2 pounds yield from 100 cats makes 2 pounds musk	$2,000
Orange Flowers	11,000 flowers, gathered from 2 acres equals 2,200 pounds, which yields 2 pounds orange flower essence	$2,000
Jasmine	11 pounds to 2 acres; 19 pounds of jasmine yields 2 pounds of essence	$6,200
Rose	55,000 pounds to 2 acres; 9,000 pounds yield 2 pounds of essence	$5,500
Sandalwood	900 pounds yield 2 pounds of essence	$200
Musk	(Deer) 2 pounds from 33 musk deer yield 2 pounds musk	$10,800

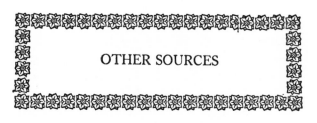

OTHER SOURCES

Not Kidding Around

My spies tell me that kids in California are wearing *food extracts*. The kind you cook with. This may seem like just a step away from dabbing garlic salt behind your ears, but as far as initial investment is concerned, it's hard to beat. Ehler's extracts cost 49¢ per 1-ounce bottle. They're carried in supermarkets everywhere and come in the following fragrant flavors: vanilla, chocolate, lemon, almond, anise, banana, orange and peppermint.

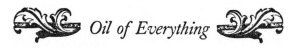

Oil of Everything

If extracts don't do a thing for you, but you DO like pure, fragrant essential oils, you can MAIL ORDER them from two wonderful suppliers.

First there's the Indiana Botanic Gardens, who'll send you a charming almanac ABSO-LUTELY FREE when you ask for their price list.

Then, there's Aphrodisia, a tiny shop that's been the haunting grounds of New York fragrance and herb enthusiasts for years. Their catalog will cost you $1. Here's where to write:

INDIANA BOTANIC GARDENS
P.O. Box 5
Hammond, Indiana 46325
APHRODISIA PRODUCTS
28 Carmine Street
New York, New York 10014
NOTE: Perfume oils can be quite expensive—from $.50 a half-ounce to $20 and up, so be sure to check the price lists before placing your order.

What the Elves Hid In the Perfumer's Workshop

I imagine that if Saint Theresa of Avila showed up in your living room, she'd flood it with the delicious odor of tea rose, the fragrance is that heavenly.

In the middle of summer 1975 the scent and odor of New York City changed dramatically from musk to tea rose. Personally, I hold the Perfumer's Workshop directly responsible. You couldn't get into an elevator here without being gently tossed into a rosy summer garden. It was magnetic. It was haunting. It was enough to make me stop someone on the street and ask her where she got it. She told me . . . so naturally I went to see for myself, and personally tested sixty-four delicious essential oils.

And I found out a secret. Hidden in with the simple single florals and the key notes and the animal tones are four glamorous, absolutely exquisite perfumes that were famous in the 20s and 30s. They were hidden in the Perfumer's Workshop collection by one of the gentlemen who founded the firm because he was still captivated by these specific nostalgic scents.

If you'd like to test the acuity of your nose or take a trip back in time, I heartily suggest you look into Bergamote, Oakmoss, Marguerite and Wisteria from the Perfumer's Workshop. They have branches all over the country, but should you rather order by mail, write:

PERFUMER'S WORKSHOP
1 East 57th Street
New York, New York 10022
Enclose $1.50 (over and above purchase price to cover postage and handling.)

GIVING BIRTH TO CHARLIE

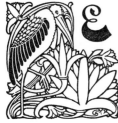 ver wonder how a huge company creates a great fragrance? Red-headed Carol Allen, one of the people who was there when Revlon's famous CHARLIE was created tells ALL:

"First came the CHARLIE image, a 1972 dream of sassy New York chic. Charles (Revson) code-named it COSMO—and then we all went to work. We went to our offices, alerted our staffs, our suppliers, our agencies and our research firms. We called our husbands and wives and told them we were going to be late for dinner . . . for the next year . . . and we settled in.

"From the initial decision to go ahead, we decided on a target market—a woman we thought would be *our* woman—and we set out to describe her: CHARLIE was aimed at a twenty-eight-year-old woman, but she was bigger than all that. And there was a chunk of everybody at Revlon in her. The CHARLIE user didn't have to be twenty-eight. She could be sixty-eight or forty-eight or eighteen or twelve and a half—or anywhere in between. She was probably unmarried, probably in the creative arts kind of business, interested in improving her mind, her body, her career . . . interested in doing her own thing. The more we got to know her, the more life we pumped into the product, the more CHARLIE began to live.

"Developing the fragrance itself took a terribly long time. From the initial submissions of scent (which come from fragrance houses like Flora/Synth), we tested and modified and refined and reformulated until we got a fragrance that gave us what we wanted. A familiar top note. A great lasting quality. Bright. Spirited. Freewheeling. A green floral. The floral being the romantic base note. The green giving us a clean, light, spirited touch plus a certain prettiness.

"The top perfumers in the world were at our disposal; and we told them what we wanted and they came back with their submissions. Then we'd work with the submissions till they were right. We'd say things like, 'It's too harsh on top. Make it less sweet. Make it greener. Make it more herbal. Make it brighter. Make it more floral. Increase this note. Decrease that note.' Until we came to a place where we were happy enough to send the submission on to a test panel. Everything gets tested. CHARLIE had over five hundred different submissions that were fine-tuned and modified until eighteen months later we had *the* scent.

"But the scent isn't the only important thing we had to think about. There was Research & Development, too. As *we* tested for scent, *they* were testing for things like compatibility, sensitivity, microbiology, color . . . does it last? . . . does it break down under adverse conditions? . . . It takes three months just to find out if a product is stable. We spent hundreds of thousands of dollars just to be sure all these problems were solved. And they have to be solved before any product gets out into the marketplace.

"The marketers, the perfumers and the scientists at work on the project were all excited, but there were other people involved in it, too. And other problems to be solved. Like what kind of bottle would do? We wanted it to be classical as far as shape was concerned. But we didn't want to be cute, or to be out of style in a year, so we put our designers to work and they submitted maybe twenty to thirty final designs and lucite molds from which we narrowed down a final decision. There are so many considerations even in something as simple as a bottle. Things like what is the perfume going to look like in here? Will there be a pocket of air at the top of the bottle that'll distort its shape? Can we technically blow the glass? How does it look in the different proportions (1 ounce, 2 ounces, half an ounce)?

Can we get a cap for it? What's the outer package going to look like? And what are we going to call it?

"The code name for CHARLIE just happened. We were talking about how Helen Gurley Brown and *Cosmopolitan* magazine had turned around the whole image of sex. So the code name COSMO just evolved. But as for the real name—we saw five hundred of them written by just about everybody in the company until we came up with CHARLIE.

"Selling fragrance is fantasy. And selling fantasy has its own special mystique. It's not like selling some detergent that's going to get your laundry white. With CHARLIE we were faced with selling the CHARLIE fantasy to 10,000 independent drugstores; 3,500 chain drugstores; and 3,200 department stores. Hundreds of thousands of women spent $14 million for CHARLIE in the first year. It gave women more than most products did. It fulfilled all its promises. It was interesting to wear, made you feel good, and was (and continues to be) exciting. And it took the dedicated work of ad people, marketing people, packaging people, legal people, fragrance people, public relations people, salespeople, testers, panel people, chemists, dermatologists, writers, artists, designers, printers, noses, secretaries and most of all Charles Revson to get it that way."

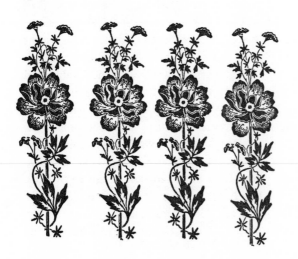

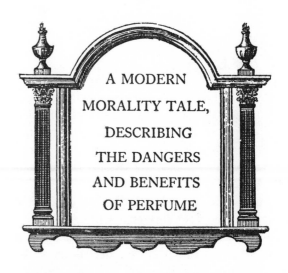

A MODERN MORALITY TALE, DESCRIBING THE DANGERS AND BENEFITS OF PERFUME

(with thanks to Ken Meeker, vice president of marketing, Lanvin)

"Once upon a time, not very long ago, there was a man whose wife loved a particular fragrance. The man loved his wife, and to demonstrate his devotion he would mark each birthday, each anniversary, each joyous event in their lives with a beautiful bottle of this characteristic scent.

"Time went on, and the man in question met another woman whom he also loved. Her perfume intoxicated him. They dined and danced and made merry until one fatal evening when our amorous hero met his mistress and discovered she was wearing that very scent he associated only with his wife.

"Although his mistress had changed nothing (save trading her usual perfume for one that came disastrously close to all our hero's vital emotions), he suddenly felt so incredibly guilty and so totally uncomfortable in her presence that he went home immediately and lived happily (and faithfully) ever after."

THE MORAL: Your fragrance says so much about you, you must be *very* careful how you use it.

TAKING CARE

OF YOUR SKIN,

FEET AND

FINGERNAILS

Wrinkles. There's no way to avoid them.
You're going to get them anyway.
My own approach is to learn to enjoy them as early as possible.

—NANCY ABRAHMS,
author of *Wrinkles: Coping with the Inevitable*

Take care of your skin and it will take care of you. Ignore it and you'll be miserable. Your skin, if you haven't thought much about it lately, does not just sit there. You are literally all wrapped up in it. It's the largest organ in your body (or rather, on your body) and it has all sorts of important work to do. You breathe through it. You get messages of heat, cold, pain and pleasure through it. It regulates your body temperature. If you're a normal-sized person, you've got some twenty square feet of skin to maintain, which accounts for 6 percent of your body weight, and if you don't take care of it, it will eventually look dreadful.

K. T. Maclay's Philosophical Approach to Skin Care

Good, effective, basic skin care depends on four baby-simple operations: Cleansing. Toning. Masqueing. Moisturizing. In addition to these basics, application and narcissism play hefty roles. The woman who spends two hours a day lovingly applying creams and lotions to her skin and reminding herself that she is (and always has been, and always will be) beautiful is going to get better results than the woman who slaps it on, dashes it off and hopes for the best.

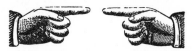

This is the most intricately constructed, uniquely designed, least expensive and simplest application device ever invented: The human finger. Use it with care.

Almost every company that makes treatment products has a basic cleanser, toner, moisturizer and masque as the cornerstones of its treatment line. The large companies may have anywhere from three to seven different lines under one large corporate umbrella. Each individual line has a full range of products geared to take care of almost every skin type. The main difference between the lines is how much they cost, or where they're sold, or who (or how old or how affluent) their projected customer is. The Ultima II customer is a bit older and a bit wealthier than the woman who buys Moon Drops, for example. And the Moon Drops woman may be slightly more mature than her younger sister at Natural Wonder, but all three lines have products that do good things for almost every type of skin.

Taking good care of your skin depends on your age and your skin type. Contrary to popular belief, not every teenager has oily skin, nor does every woman over thirty have a dryness problem. Your skin does, however, change as you get older. Your sebaceous glands don't work double-time anymore to produce oil. Your cells hold less moisture. Your skin becomes less elastic and you may need more help to keep it soft and supple. You'll know when you've gone through a major skin change, because the methods you've been using just won't work anymore. That's the moment to recheck your skin type. Naturally, a woman whose skin is a personal solution to the international oil crisis is going to

be using different products than the one who feels drier than the Magna Carta. People with excess-oil problems need oil-free (or oil blotting) products that deliver *moisture* but blot up the bad stuff. People with dry or sensitive or mature skin may need moisturizers which sit on top to keep the wetness inside, or lubricating creams to go to work beneath the surface, plumping up from the underside, as it were.

When in doubt, ask the woman behind the counter. Erase from your mind all thoughts of cosmetics harridans placed behind counters for the sole purpose of prying as much money as possible from your purse. These days, the woman behind the treatment counter is a highly trained technician who's there not only to push the product but to answer your questions. More important, she's your link to the product itself. She'll help you test it, help you figure out if it's the right product with which to treat your specific problem and, should you decide not to buy then and there, I promise you she will not open her veins in the bathtub. So relax, and depend on her.

Once you've settled on your own private method of treating your skin like a loved one, your expectations play a bigger part in the success or failure of any new product you might be trying than any other single factor.

Compared to the product you're using now, is the new product less or more expensive? If it's less expensive, will you be happy with it because you're getting a bargain? Or will you feel like you're shortchanging your skin every time you smooth it on? This is important. And so is packaging. Do you feel more exquisite using a fluffy pink cream that comes in an ornamentally flowered package than you do using a colorless cream that's wrapped up in brown paper and string? Are you more secure using a product that's fragrance-free? Or do you miss that lift you get when you use an orange-and-honey-scented nourisher that smells good enough to eat? The more you match your expectations to the way your treatment method looks and feels—

and how much it costs—the happier you will be with it, the more faithfully you'll use it—and the more successful it'll be for you.

Before you run out to get yourself a whole new clutch of treatment goodies, here are some things you should know about your skin and the things that are made to keep it beautiful.

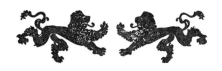

MACLAY'S SIMPLIFIED GUIDE TO SKIN TYPE

Perfect Skin

Smooth, blemish-free, almost translucent skin that never flakes, peels, roughs up or gets sunburned instead of tropically tanned can be listed as practically perfect skin. Most of us (45.9 percent), while we are not completely perfect, have close to perfect skin. Most people call it normal. (Given the option, I'd rather call it perfect—makes me feel better.)

Oily Skin

If you're on the oily side of perfect, and 28.19 percent of us are, you're probably too busy worrying about its drawbacks to congratulate yourself for having skin that will stay younger looking and wrinkle-free longer than any other type of skin. You look in the mirror and the first thing you see looking back at you is SHINE. You tan beautifully, cope very nicely with the cold, but have a maddening tendency to blemish.

Dry Skin

If you're on the dry side of perfect, your skin probably has that uncomfortable size-too-small, fragile feeling. You're the first one at the ski house to chap during the winter, and the first one on the beach to get burned. Your skin can go red in blotches for no apparent reason, or start to flake off like pie crust when the humidity gets low.

Before we get down to specifics, let's have a look at who's doing what in the industry, and how they might be helping you solve your problems.

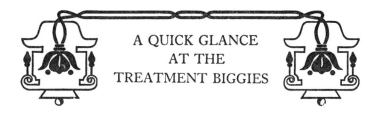

A QUICK GLANCE AT THE TREATMENT BIGGIES

Adrien Arpel

For quickie lunchtime facials at department stores everywhere, Adrien Arpel is hard to beat. The Arpel line is based on treatment, so specially trained operators will not only analyze your skin, but prescribe for it, vacuum it and apply the special cleansers, toners, masques and moisturizers you need right there on the spot. There are Adrien Arpel minisalons at fine department stores all over the country. The prices vary, but figure on $13–$30.

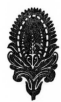
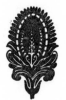

*We always say that Lauder is the Lincoln, Ultima is the Cadillac and de
Markoff is the Rolls Royce of the cosmetics industry.*
—UNIDENTIFIED SOURCE AT ALEXANDRA DE MARKOFF

Alexandra de Markoff

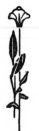
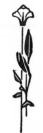

A luxury line at luxury prices ($7.50–$55.00), de Markoff products are made
specially to be used with Countess Isserlyne makeup. This is because of the
unique anhydrous (without water) formula of the countess's products. Since
they're made without water, they're extremely long-wearing and consequently
very difficult to take off. Other than the special compatibility of de Markoff
treatment products with the Countess Isserlyne makeups (especially in cleansing),
de Markoff concentrates on the woman who thinks enough of herself to go out
and spend the kind of money it takes to take advantage of the de Markoff line.

Almay

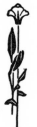
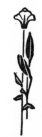

For the last forty years Almay's been developing pure products at sensible
prices. Both product lines (Almay for Normal/Oily Skin and Deep Mist for
Normal/Dry Complexions) are fragrance-free, recommended by dermatologists
and distributed in drugstores everywhere. Prices range between $2.25 and $7.50.

Avon

Yay! Treatment products you can buy at home. Avon has at present three
different treatment lines (Moisture Secret, Delicate Beauty and Perfect Balance).
It's the personal service that counts here. Not only can you buy Avon at home or
at your office, you can earn extra money selling it. Avon advertises for
representatives in most local newspapers. Or look them up in the White Pages of
your phone book.

Biokosma

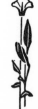
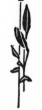

One of the oldest Swiss natural cosmetics companies, Biokosma's products are
made from pure plant substances, with no mineral oils or animal fats or synthetic
fragrances. They're very economical and pleasant, sell for $1.50 to $5.00 and can
be gotten at your local health food store or by writing to Weleda, Inc., 30 South
Main Street, Spring Valley, New York 10977.

Bonne Bell

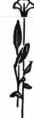
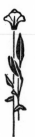

There really IS a Bonnie Bell. She was named for the heroine in a syndicated
newspaper series her parents were reading shortly before she was expected. She's
also a corporate executive in the Bonne Bell company.

The Bonne Bell customer skis, sails, swims, jogs, mountain climbs and involves
herself. So do the people who run the company. The president's wife (Julia Bell)

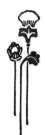
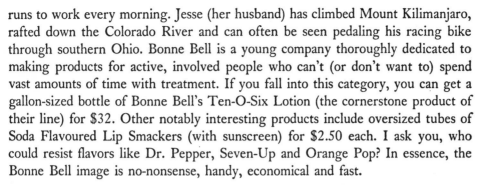
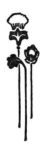

runs to work every morning. Jesse (her husband) has climbed Mount Kilimanjaro, rafted down the Colorado River and can often be seen pedaling his racing bike through southern Ohio. Bonne Bell is a young company thoroughly dedicated to making products for active, involved people who can't (or don't want to) spend vast amounts of time with treatment. If you fall into this category, you can get a gallon-sized bottle of Bonne Bell's Ten-O-Six Lotion (the cornerstone product of their line) for $32. Other notably interesting products include oversized tubes of Soda Flavoured Lip Smackers (with sunscreen) for $2.50 each. I ask you, who could resist flavors like Dr. Pepper, Seven-Up and Orange Pop? In essence, the Bonne Bell image is no-nonsense, handy, economical and fast.

Caswell-Massey

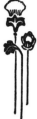

Superb for imported products across the board, Caswell-Massey will be happy to mail you such wonderful items as: French Anti-Wrinkle Petals (60 little pieces of paper imbued with wrinkle-banishing solution), $8.75; or Creme Simone, a 115-year-old face cream that's been moisturizing continental complexions since 1860 and still comes in its own antique jar (4.5 oz., $8.50). Caswell-Massey also has Cosmetic Toilet Vinegar (wonderful for toning and normalizing) and a large selection of natural mitts, sponges and brushes which you'll be reading about presently.

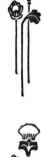

Christian Dior

European women knew about and depended on beauty treatments (not just makeups) long before their American sisters caught on and began to catch up with them. This means that European-based or European-oriented companies like Dior have a special attitude about beauty treatment. They cater to women who think that any time spent caring for their skin is the best investment they could possibly make. Their treatments (Dior's, that is) tend to be moderately expensive and exquisitely packaged.

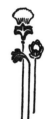

Coty

The phrase from Coty is: "You shouldn't do less for your skin, and you shouldn't pay more." Equasion (the Coty treatment handle) is coordinated for every skin type, mass distributed and available in drug and department stores everywhere. It sells for anywhere between $2.75 and $6.00.

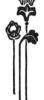
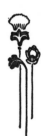

Dorothy Gray

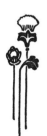
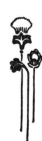

Dorothy Gray was one of the original big three turn-of-the-century cosmetics pioneers. While not as invitingly interesting as either Elizabeth Arden or Helena Rubinstein, she did (at one point) have her hands insured for $100,000 by Lloyds of London, so she must have been doing something right. Skin care is still a big thing with the Dorothy Gray company. But, unlike a cute little walrus-fur cosmetic case that sold for $125 in the 1920s, the line is now medium-priced, with most beauty treatments selling in the neighborhood of $5.

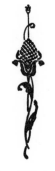

Elizabeth Arden

The Arden image has changed recently from a firm which catered mainly to chic little old ladies to a young, with-it company that cares very much about *treating* skin and treating it right. Miss Arden herself was a passionate devotee of treatment products. So much so that she used to rub her creams and lotions into the flanks of her thoroughbred race horses; the stable boys used to call her Miss Mud Pack. But those days are long gone, and today, the Arden philosophy is best explained by their vice president of research and development, Dr. John A. Cella:

> At Elizabeth Arden, we believe that beauty begins with good skin. Our first goal, as a company, is to do the most we can to help women take care of their skin. To this end, the major thrust of our research and development effort is aimed at the study and understanding of the factors that contribute to skin quality and proper care. From this research we seek to develop efficacious products with proven performance profiles.

Arden beauty treatments cost anywhere between $2.75 and $25.00.

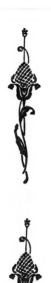

Estée Lauder

A recent entry into the field, Mrs. Lauder is the sole surviving queen of the cosmetics industry. Her company is responsible for products that are as beautifully conceived and executed as they are prettily packaged and presented. People at rival companies still call her The Blue Lady. There are two stories on this. One source says the sobriquette refers to her blue packaging. Another insists there's a tinge of blue in all the products. Neither story is substantiated. Prices range from $5 for a toner to $125 for a golden jar of Re-Nutriv Creme.

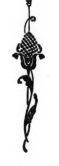

Etherea

Another unsubstantiated but wonderful story is the one about how Etherea came about. It goes like this: Charles Revson wanted to test the mettle of an up-and-coming young vice president, so he gave him an impossible task. "Go," he said, "and create an ultrapure cosmetic line. Gear it to skin type, and make it both exciting and different. You've got two months."

Thus the up-and-coming executive, clutching his Maalox, commissioned his trusty staff to get the lead out and eight weeks later was hand-filling the bottles at the plant and personally delivering the stock for the opening day of sales at Bonwit Teller. I don't know if this story is true. I DO know that Etherea is NOW fragrance-free, tested by dermatologists, and sealed up for last-ditch assurance of freshness and purity. All Etherea programs are formulated for specific skin types, but the mainstay of their treatment line (Maximum Moisturizer, 2 oz., $8) is good for every kind and class of skin. The Etherea price range for beauty treatments: $6–$15.

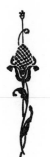

Evelyn Marshall

This woman began her career in the 1930s in show business. She was a makeup artist for film stars. She loved it and hated it (because her film work

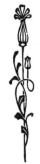
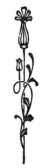

became static), so she finally decided to devote her time and energy to skin care and makeup for civilians rather than starlets. Fashion models flocked to her small New York studio, and soon she began to invent and market her own products. "Need," says Ms. Marshall, "was the mother of invention." And so, it seems, was artistic inspiration.

"I was at the Prado Museum," Ms. Marshall says, "looking at a painting by Renoir of 'Girl At Piano.' She had beautiful contouring under her cheekbones and a luminous blue-white look in her eyes. I thought if Renoir can shape like that on canvas, the very same colors would be great on the face. I went to a chemical house and bought a complete sample set of color additives and, with the cooperation of the Prado Museum, stayed in Madrid until I'd developed the colors for my Shading Rouge, and the Blue Eyeliner to use on the lower rim of the eye." Then and there Evelyn Marshall promised herself that she'd one day own a Renoir painting. She now owns "Dancing in the Garden," which constantly reminds her of the inspiration for her two revolutionary products.

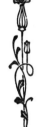
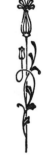

But enough of makeup—what does Evelyn Marshall do about skin care? My friend Susan, who gladly volunteered her face as a testing ground for the Evelyn Marshall program, reports as follows:

"When I grew up in San Antonio, it was an extremely social activity to have an Evelyn Marshall facial and complete makeup for your social debut. Things haven't changed. A visit to the New York salon for a free consultation is a pleasure. She started by dragging me into the bathroom and teaching me how to wash my face. Odd, I thought, but then I realized that I'd be doing the same procedure in my own bathroom, so why not learn in situ? During the rest of the hour and a half we spent together, Ms. Marshall devoted all her energies to teaching me how to look my best. And it was so easy I carried the information home and put it into practice on a daily basis with no trouble. Besides, an assistant takes detailed notes all through the session, so at the end you have a complete and accurate record of what was going on. The Marshall salon also keeps a record on file (just in case you lose yours). Consultation starts with cleansing and follows through to the final, finishing touches, and while it's billed as FREE, you do have to agree to buy $25 worth of products. You WILL need them. In fact, if you really buy everything you need and want, it'll run you closer to about $60. You can, however, make an appointment for a Special Occasion Makeup for $10."

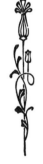
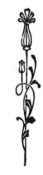

Susan also told me that she "felt quite ravishing" after her appointment and supplied me with a complete list of Evelyn Marshall Salons throughout the country. (Evelyn Marshall-affiliated salons use Evelyn Marshall products and the services of specially trained operators.)

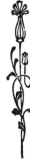
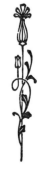

Dallas:
Betty Myers Faces
c/o Lou Latimore
4320 Lovers Lane
Dallas, Tex. 75225

Fort Worth:
Joanne Moritz
5817 Boca Raton
Fort Worth, Tex. 76112

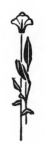
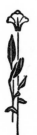

El Paso:
The Gazebo
9616 Sims Drive
Morningside Mall
El Paso, Tex. 79925

Houston:
The Smart Shop
2411 S. Post Oak
Houston, Tex. 77027

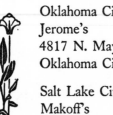

Oklahoma City:
Jerome's
4817 N. May Avenue
Oklahoma City, Okla. 73112

Salt Lake City:
Makoff's
2nd East & S. Temple
Salt Lake City, Utah 84111

West Bloomfield:
Marlene's Faces
6575 Orchard Lake Road
West Bloomfield, Mich. 48033

Shreveport:
Jammy Willingham
501 Ratcliff Street
Shreveport, La. 71104

Beverly Hills:
The Salon of Beverly Hills
301 N. Robertson Boulevard
Beverly Hills, Calif. 90211

David Fausone
c/o George Deming's Salon
461 North Beverly Drive
Beverly Hills, Calif. 90210

Los Angeles:
Jim Daniels
10323 Santa Monica Boulevard
Los Angeles, Calif. 90025

In addition, EM products are carried in selected high-fashion department stores such as Henri Bendel in New York.

Frances Denney

Mrs. Denney came to the United States from Ireland in 1893 to open a very chi-chi beauty salon off Rittenhouse Square in Philadelphia. Her grandson, Bob Denney, who literally grew up in the business, told me she ran her operation with an iron hand. He was quick to add that "it was always a well-moisturized iron hand"—but that's the way cosmetics people talk.

One day Mrs. Wannamaker, long a happy participant in the afternoon teas Mrs. Denney held in her salon, told John Wannamaker (in no uncertain terms) that he should carry Mrs. Denney's creams in his Philadelphia department store. That's how the ball got rolling. Currently, the Denney company considers itself a dark horse in the industry, a medium-sized company moving quickly on a track where all things are possible. .

The Denney treatment products are carried in fine department stores and can be had for anywhere between $4 (for Spot Remover—a blemish stick, not a cleaning fluid) to $32 for 4 ounces of Source of Beauty Cream.

Helena Rubinstein

The people at Rubinstein pride themselves on their treatment products. They're very quick to pick up on new trends and seem to come up with a new line just about every season. The regular Helena Rubinstein line (Skin Dew) is aimed at anyone from teenage to mid-twenties ($1.50–$12.50), but there are two other main product groupings under the HR umbrella: Ultra Feminine ($5.00–$18.50) and Skin Life ($5–$40). Both are geared to more mature skin.

Lancome

A very sophisticated, mature and enlightened French-oriented company. Their packaging is pretty but not superfluous, and there seems to be a serious reason for each of the four to five items specifically prescribed for your skin type. Prices are upwardly mobile, from moderate to middling expensive. You can get your hands on a Lancome Tonique Douceur (freshener) for about $5.50 and work your way right up to Lancomia Night Cream (2 oz., $40). You might also want to look into Lancome's Hydrix hydrating cream, made with a patented "water trap" process to keep the moisture in and fend off aging lines and wrinkles (⅞ oz., $7.50; 1¾ oz., $12.50).

Max Factor

Lines within lines here run the gamut from drugstore goodies to ultraluscious, expensive treats in the Geminesse Collection. Factor started as a theatrical makeup and just grew like Topsy into a company that really does have a little something for virtually everyone.

All skins need help. I've never heard of a skin that doesn't need anything to keep beautiful.
—SUSAN WINER,
Special Correspondent, *Town & Country*

Orlane

Jackie Onassis uses Orlane. Orlane is in all probability the most expensive treatment line in the world and is aimed at the "woman whose skin is over 21." That's not to say that the woman herself is over 21, but her skin definitely is. To help solve some of the problems of a skin that's past its second decade, Orlane has things like their B-21 line, which has five products working together to rejuvenate and replace lost moisture (Creme B-21, 2.5 oz., $85; B-21 Creme Fluide for Body and Bust, 7 oz., $45; and their best-selling Super Hydratante B-21, 1.76 oz., is yours for another $45 in check, money order or coin of the realm). Although most Orlane products *are* geared to normal to dry skin, their new Ligne Integrale is a special program for dehydrated skin that's also *sensitive* . . . and they make a soap, a cleansing milk and a normalizing base for blotting and moisturizing oily skin that doesn't need extra oil.

Payot of Paris

In addition to making superb treatment products for every known type of skin, Payot of Paris also has facial salons everywhere. They are thoroughly dedicated to doing the job and doing it well.

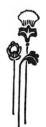
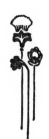

The whole thing started around 1917, when Dr. Nadine Payot met Anna Pavlova (the famous ballerina) in New York and was so impressed with her lasting beauty and well-toned skin that the good doctor decided to use her medical training to help other women look as good. She (Dr. Payot) developed the "Method of Physical Culture for the Face and Neck," which was based on exercising the facial muscles, massage and a selection of facial products based on natural ingredients like extracts of plants, herbs and flowers. A Payot massage includes some forty-six different movements and takes a full fifteen minutes. But that's just the beginning, because the Payot estheticians then go on to classify your skin (from among some twenty different skin types) and clean, tone, mask and moisturize it during a full hour-long treatment session. All this for approximately $25. You can also avail yourself of some sumptuous Payot treatment products for anywhere from $2.50 for a hand cream to $35.00 for a 3.66-ounce night cream. If you'd like the name of a salon offering Payot services in an area near you, write:

> Ron Klass
> Payot of Paris
> 320 Park Avenue
> New York, New York 10022

Princess Marcella Borghese

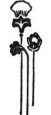

Superrich and superbeautiful are two collections of words that come to mind when you think of Borghese treatments. There actually IS a Princess Borghese, by the way, who now lives in Italy and is rumored to be breathtaking. It was she who inspired the line, but the company itself is now wholly United States-based and -operated. Devout skin-care enthusiasts, the Borghese company started as a program for the mature woman, but has in the last ten years extended the line to cover younger, more oil-prone skin. Price range for Borghese products settles between $7 and $70.

Revlon

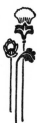
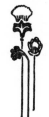

Chronologically, Revlon's empire runs all the way from Natural Wonder (which is geared and priced for teenagers and more mature women with strict budgets and oily skin problems) through Charlie (a brilliantly conceived, easy to use, gel-formula line based on noncomplicated, no-muss no-fuss treatment that delivers what it promises and gets you out the door in a hurry) all the way to Moon Drops (which is made for the woman whose skin is over thirty and who wants to spend time and money getting it to look gorgeous). Prices vary accordingly. Natural Wonder, $1.50–$4.00; Charlie, $3.00–$6.50; Moon Drops, $3.75–$7.00.

Shiseido

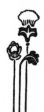
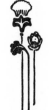

Have you ever known a Japanese woman with rotten skin? I haven't. And therefore I have nothing but respect for the Japanese influence on the American treatment market. Shiseido products all seem to combine good beauty-treatment sense with technical expertise. The three lines (Shiseido, Assimila and Benefique)

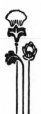

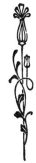

are fairly expensive ($6–$30), but I expect miniaturization helps make them economical. In other words, a little product goes an awfully long way.

Ultima II

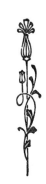

Expensive, exciting, beautifully packaged and somewhat sexy. The Ultima II philosophy as regards the woman who buys and uses it was best defined by Ultima II's director of marketing when he said:

> I like to think our Ultima II customer is every young girl after she finishes her acne period. Once her skin has normalized, we offer her products that will help keep her skin good-looking for life. She's a little like Lauren Hutton: active, bright, fun, successful. Most of our beauty-treatment products are well within the range of the working woman, although we do have a C.H.R. night cream that sells for about $17.50 an ounce. But we feel the best treatment should be in the range where any woman can afford to buy it.

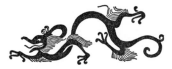

Lines, lines, go away, go and visit Doris Day.

—LUPE, the World's Oldest Beauty Expert
(a Lily Tomlin character)

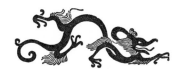

ADVENTURES AMONG THE SKIN PEOPLE

by Gillian Eltinge

How the *Guinness Book of World Records* missed me, I'll never know, because surely I've held the American Lightweight Facial Care Championship for the last twenty years (at least!). To put it simply: Since my very childhood, I have been steamed, ozoned, masqued, massaged and vacuumed by the best estheticians in the country.

I have walked in the wake of the incomparably dramatic Aida Grey in her Beverly Hills Institut de Beauté. I have been tutored by Aida Thibiant (whose other clients include some of the most perfect glamour-puss faces in American filmdom. I have been vacuumed by Christine Valmy and steeped with fragrant herbal concoctions by Georgette Klinger. What's more, I have healthy, glowing, beautiful skin to show for it.

Ordinarily, I would keep the secrets of the facialists' trade to myself. But an impassioned petition by my friends and relatives (who threatened to have me locked up in a dark, dry room) has convinced me to set down this very personal gazetteer.*

The Eltinge Guide to Elegant Esthetics

Georgette Klinger

I started with this blond Czeck bombshell when I was twelve. That was at the beginning. Way before the Klinger salon was crowded with working women bent on more beautiful complexions. Years before Miss Klinger opened her second-floor headquarters for men.

On my first visit Miss Klinger took me right in hand. She examined my face with a magnifying glass, grimaced slightly, then her uniformed assistant proceeded with a relaxing massage of my shoulders and neck. When I was thoroughly

---

* As in diet and exercise some skin care methods are controversial and should be evaluated by the consumer with care.

relaxed, the assistant steamed my skin with a fragrant herbal tea, cleaned my pores (by hand), applied three different types of masques (which smelled strongly of camphor and other good stuff) and sent me out into the world feeling (and looking) 200 percent better.

I was twelve, but I knew a good thing when I saw it. In fact, I have a yellowing letter, right here on my desk, that I wrote to Georgette Klinger after my tenth facial. It reads:

> Dear Miss Klinger:
>
> I just wanted to let you know that I am coming along just fine with my face. I still have a couple of bumps, but it's improved considerably from before. I'm sure it will get even better as I continue to use the products.
>
> My mom told me to switch to something else because I can't afford them . . . But, if they're really helping, I guess the cost shouldn't really matter. . . .

Things haven't changed much since I was twelve. The bumps are gone, of course—but both the products and the procedures remain top-notch and have contributed not only to the way MY skin looks, but to Miss Klinger's country-wide reputation as a skin-care authority.

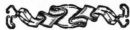

Prices and Other Vital Information

GEORGETTE KLINGER has salons in New York, Beverly Hills, Chicago and Bal Harbor, Florida

Facials	$19–$25
Surface Peeling	$10 extra
Series of 6 Facials	$99.50
Skin Examination and 5-Product Starter Kit	$8.25

Georgette Klinger products are available by mail. For information, write:

GEORGETTE KLINGER
501 Madison Avenue
New York, New York 10022

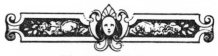

Christine Valmy

Christine Valmy comes from Rumania, where she trained long and hard until she'd mastered the ins and outs of facial esthetics. Like Miss Klinger, Miss Valmy came to the States to build an empire. *Unlike* Miss Klinger, (who does virtually everything by hand), Christine Valmy believes in the beneficial qualities and powers of machinery. In fact, she has probably done more for the vacuum than Hoover. Miss Valmy does not, however, beat as she sweeps as she cleans. The Valmy facial vacuuming technique is meant solely to clean your skin and unplug your pores.

Outspoken and direct, Miss V believes that one of the best all-time skin-perkers is a professional facial. At one time she even went so far as to offer a *free* facial to those men and women who lived in the vicinity of a Valmy salon yet had never before been tempted to have a salon face treatment. The offer is *still* good at her 57th Street branch in New York City.

I myself am most partial to her national network of salons. Just knowing that there are nine hundred of them gives me the freedom and security of knowing I can zip in for a lunchtime facial just about anywhere in the country. So if you're a novice at this facial game, or if you travel a lot (the way I do) and you'd like to have a *handy list of all the Valmy salons* everywhere (or even just the name of one closest to you), all you have to do is write to Christine Valmy, Inc., 767 Fifth Avenue, New York, New York 10022.

CHRISTINE VALMY has salons everywhere

Facials	$25
Ultra Biogenic Facial	$50

Personally worded, beautifully hand-written gift certificates available in any denomination. Products are available by mail. Write:

CHRISTINE VALMY, INC.
Change Bridge Road
Pine Brook, New Jersey 07058

Mario Badescu

I had a brief fling with Mario Badescu in the early 1960s. I always look at it as my organic, flower-grown-up period. Anyway, he was quite the fashionable item then ... quite the man to see. He used to be Georgette Klinger's chemist (or something) until he went out on his own. Someone told me they'd had a nasty lawsuit ... but at the time I was more intrigued with his organic products and the fact that he mixed the fruits and the jams and the jellies into face creams and tonics and lotions right there before your eyes and whipped them into the fridge for you, than I was with court battles. You'd have to use the products instantly (of course) or they'd have a tendency to "go funny," but that, too, was part of their charm.

Though Mr. Badescu now restricts his activities to supervision and analysis, his blender and his unique health-food approach to beauty are still alive and well and busy.

Prices and Other Vital Information

Facial	$20

FREE Consultation

Products available by mail. For questionnaire, write:

MARIO BADESCU
320 East 52nd Street
New York, New York 10022

Aida Thibiant

I was in Los Angeles last year having a somewhat rowdy lunch at the Brown Derby when Sophie (star-struck childhood chum that she is) convinced me that I had to meet Aida Thibiant. Sophie *swears* by her, as do Cher Bono, Ali McGraw, Candice Bergen and just about every other raging Hollywood glamourpuss.

Philosophically, Miss Thibiant falls somewhere between Klinger and Valmy, because about fifty percent of her treatments are done by hand, the remainder by machine. She doesn't believe in either method all by itself. She also doesn't believe in letting her clients become completely dependent on her. Being from Paris, Miss Thibiant is the first to admit that, unlike the French, Americans such as myself don't know Schrafft's from Shinola about skin care. So she spends a lot of time training her people how to do for themselves. This can involve working up to a basic vocabulary of as many as fifteen or sixteen different special creams (exclusive of moisturizers and masques), so believe me, learning how to take care of your skin here gets pretty complicated.

One more thing Aida Thibiant doesn't believe in is hot water. She says it's too much of a shock for your skin and forbids you to use facial saunas, steam or any other variety of heavily heated H_2O on your face. Miss Thibiant took exceptional care of me that afternoon with her exclusive *hydradermie* deep-cleaning and deep-moisturizing procedures. The only depressing part of the hour and a half I spent in her chair that afternoon was that I didn't see Candice Bergen, I didn't see Ali McGraw and Aida Thibiant refused, denied and flat-out wouldn't tell me whether Cher Bono ever had pimples!

Prices and Other Vital Information

Facials	$25–$30
Basic Skin Care	$50–$60

Products available at salon only.

AIDA THIBIANT SKIN AND BODY CARE CENTER
353 North Canon Drive
Beverly Hills, California 90213

Aida Grey

Just across the street from Aida Thibiant's tranquil facial palace is the bustling chaos of Aida Grey's Institut de Beauté. Well, it's actually *not* just across the street, but in Hollywood everyone allows themselves a healthy dose of theatrical license.

My ex-husband gave me a $100 gift certificate to the Institut because he knew I'd enjoy basking in the glow of Miss Grey's utterly unbelievable charisma. So I went in, and thirty seconds later Miss Grey had personally plucked out most of my eyebrows: "They control 40% of your facial expression . . . and you don't want to look like an animal, do you?" she said. Then she told me to change my frames: "They make you look sad! You deserve to wear HAPPY glasses . . . so much better for your disposition." When this was done, she led me away to a facial-treatment room, where I was summarily thrummed and steamed and cleaned and buttered with natural-based Aida Grey products whose names were so tasty, they sounded like rich, fattening desserts. (I mean, wouldn't you rather have Peau d'Ange smeared under your eyes than plain old wrinkle eye cream?)

My ex-husband had been right. Miss Grey treated me like a concerned Jewish mother. And I have to admit I loved every second of it. She also stood over me and helped me fill out a long questionnaire about my skin and promised to mail me anything I ever needed to take care of it. What could be easier?

Prices and Other Vital Information

Cleansing Facial $20
Exfoliation Facial $30
For gift certificates and products by mail, write:

AIDA GREY Institut de Beauté
9549 Wilshire Boulevard
Beverly Hills, California 90212

    Erno Lazlo

Erno Lazlo died in 1970. He came originally from Rumania, where he was an up and coming medical doctor. The story on how he got into the skin business starts with a young member of the Rumanian royal family, a girl who had terrible, terrible skin problems.

Now in those days, girls who had skin problems lived in closets. They disappeared. They just didn't have anything they could do about it. Their skin was too bad . . . and that was that. Anyway, Dr. Lazlo was called in to counsel this one acne-plagued princess . . . and he came up with all these lotions and things, and they proved to be extraordinarily good, and they cleared up the princess's skin, and that's how the Lazlo Institute started.

Pretty soon Dr. Lazlo had an international reputation, so it was a short hop from that position into being convinced to come to America to make the big time.

Years ago, when you went to Dr. Lazlo in New York, it was a procedure. It was dramatic. It was an event. You went into a consultation room and it was black. Black! You spoke to an esthetician, or a nurse, and she was dressed in black. For a facial salon it had the atmosphere of Forest Lawn. Dr. Lazlo gave you two hours of intense examination, told you what your problems were and exactly how to fix them. You took whatever you needed home, followed his program religiously and in six weeks or so your skin looked better.

The premise of the Lazlo program was (and still is) that you must wash your face with soap and water sixty times a day. That's thirty times in the morning and thirty times at night. With Lazlo's soap and the same rinse water. Why do you use the same old yucky rinse water over and over again? Because the soap takes a certain amount of oil out of your skin, part of which is restored in the rinses. See?

Now, if the thought of washing your face in dirty water makes you cringe, I can tell you the story of my friend Marge, who (on being told what she had to do) exclaimed: "Brown soap? Dirty water? Who *needs* all this stuff in my life?" Well, six weeks later (when all this nonsense was working for her) Marge became a convert. She thought the soap and water stuff was so fantastic she became an absolute bore on the subject.

Now that Dr. Lazlo is no longer with us, the

Institute still functions as the most exclusive beauty club in America. Other members include such notable beauties as the duchess of Windsor, Gloria Vanderbilt Cooper, Audrey Hepburn and the Rothschild family. Be warned, however, that membership does not come cheap. To have your skin analyzed and pick up your initial complement of products (at any fine store in the country carrying the Lazlo method) will cost you $75. Upkeep can (and usually *does*) run between $250 and $300 a year. The Lazlo Institute will be happy to send you a list of stores through which you can become more personally involved in the Lazlo way of life.

Prices and Other Vital Information

Initial analysis and program $75
Yearly upkeep and replacements, $250–$300
For information on the Lazlo program, write:

LAZLO INSTITUTE
10 East 53rd Street
New York, New York 10022

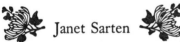 Janet Sarten

Janet Sarten has a hypnotic voice, a Svengali attitude toward restoration, a special skin-care routine (which may have been influenced by the nine years she spent working for Dr. Erno Lazlo) and a restorative machine you just wouldn't believe. The machine is what makes Miss Sarten different. She won't tell you exactly how it works (of course), but one beauty editor I know told me that it was sort of like the old Relaxaciser. My editor chum also said the machine exercised the facial muscles and was mildly uncomfortable. Miss Sarten, however, insists her machine is the next best thing to having personally discovered the fountain of youth. She also avers that the machine treatments are much better for you than having your skin peeled or indulging in anything so permanent and irreversible as plastic surgery.

I, myself, am particularly intrigued with Miss Sarten's strangely syrupy voice. This means that I'll nip in for a treatment just to hear her *talk.* My face does look swell, but sometimes I think it's merely some subtle form of hypnosis.

Prices and Other Vital Information

By personal appointment only
Series of 6 restorative treatments $450
For mail order facial care products, write:

JANET SARTEN COSMETICS
480 Park Avenue
New York, New York 10022

 Catherine Hinds

I was standing in the Catherine Hinds Salon in Boston early one evening when a very stylish eighty-five-year-old English woman stepped bouncily up to the receptionist and bought out the store. She settled the bill for her complete facial, picked up an entire collection of makeup and then went on to assemble an enormous bagfull of skin-care products. She was just about to spin out the door with her sack of goodies when she remembered something, stopped, then came back to the cosmetic counter and asked for a night cream for her mother. When Miss Hinds could find her voice, she stood very straight and (as tactfully as she could) asked just how old the woman's mother was.

The English woman adjusted her cape and told us (very proudly) that her mum had just turned 103, that she was (at that very moment) back at the Ritz-Carlton washing her hair, and that she "wouldn't dream of going to bed without creaming her skin." So there are OTHER people who never give up!

I go to Catherine Hinds for plain old garden variety cleansing facials, but the real specialty of the house is peeling and placenta. Miss H believes that the peeling removes tiny wrinkles and the placenta (which was used as burn therapy during the Second World War) helps skin cells rebuild themselves. Her method is based on three salon treatments in quick succession, followed by using placenta-based products on the home front.

Prices and Other Vital Information

Skin analysis, treatment and *complimentary* makeup $25

For mail-order makeup and beauty treatment products, write:

CATHERINE HINDS, INC.
692 Madison Avenue
New York, New York 10021

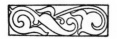 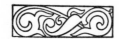

Other Beauty Biggies
You Might Want to Investigate

Atlanta
Jamison & Don
1375 Peachtree Street
Atlanta, Georgia 30301
Great for deep cleaning and massage.

Chicago
The Face Place
102 East Oak Street
Chicago, Illinois 60601
European facials plus intensive instruction in at-home care.

Cincinnati
Face Biz Cosmetics
2710 Erie Avenue ·
Cincinnati, Ohio 45201
Facials and a COMPLIMENTARY makeup.

Cleveland
Makeup Center
5885 Mayfield Road
Cleveland, Ohio 44101
Facials with a heavy emphasis on massage.

Dallas
Mister Lee
Fairmont Hotel
Dallas, Texas 75201
Fabulous for dealing with Texan tans.

Denver
Ilona of Hungary
361 South Colorado Boulevard
Denver, Colorado 80201
Fully equipped to clean, analyse and cope with almost any skin problem.

Detroit
Aesthetics of Mira Linder
29563 Northwestern Highway
Detroit, Michigan 48201
Have every part of your face treated differently here.

Honolulu
The Royal Door Health and Beauty Spa
The Royal Hawaiian Hotel
2259 Kalakaua Avenue
Honolulu, Hawaii 96801
Spend a magic morning being facialed in this exquisite spa.

Houston
Neiman-Marcus
2600 South Post Oak Road
Houston, Texas 77001
Experts at biocellular and minifacials.

Kansas City
La Secret
1410 West 47th Street
Kansas City, Missouri 64101
Machines and enzyme-layering a specialty.

Miami
J. Baldi
330 Miracle Mile
Coral Gables, Florida 33134
Fantastic facial stimulation, aeration and nutrition.

New Orleans
Godchaux's Beauty Salon
828 Canal Street
New Orleans, Louisiana 70101
Nip in here for a lunchtime minifacial.

Philadelphia
Adolf Biecker at Nan Duskin
1739 Walnut Street
Philadelphia, Pennsylvania 19101
The newest, niftiest machines are used here to clean and stimulate.

Pittsburgh
Beti Weitzner Salon
Carlton House
Pittsburgh, Pennsylvania 15201
 European facials in a large, full-service salon.

Saint Louis
Judy Bean, Ltd.
9918 Clayton Road
Ladue, Missouri 64758
 Facials done with machines and a full range of European products.

San Francisco
Fabulous Faces
305 Grand Avenue
San Francisco, California 94101
 Biological facial peeling and aroma therapy are specialties of the house.

Washington, D.C.
Saks Fifth Avenue
5555 Wisconsin Avenue
Chevy Chase, Maryland 20015
 Adrien Arpel's Skin Spa at Saks offers you both full and minifacials for a leisurely or an instant perker-upper.

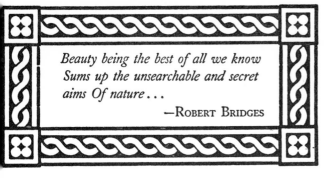

Beauty being the best of all we know Sums up the unsearchable and secret aims Of nature . . .
—ROBERT BRIDGES

ON THE SUBJECT OF YOUNGNESS: BOOKS BY A DOWN-TO-EARTH DOCTOR

When Bedford Shelmire's book *(The Art of Looking Younger)* came out in 1973, it was greeted by scores of gasping women who hadn't even opened the cover. What caused the violent reaction was the dust jacket, which proudly displayed a white-haired, seventy-year-old, naked woman.

"Awful!" you're saying. But wait . . . If you looked more closely, you saw that the cover illustration was really a seventy-year-old *head*, photographically attached to a *twenty*-year-old naked body.

Dr. Shelmire was making a point here, the first of many points tucked beneath that astounding dust jacket.

The Art of Looking Younger is a downright wonderful book on corrective and preventive skin care. Shelmire names names, does away with scientific mumbo jumbo and tells us good, basic, useful facts. Like the fact that the skin on your face probably looks twenty years older than the skin on your bottom (for example) or that Crisco is a terrific moisturizer. *The Art of Looking Younger* also has great chapters on hair, hands, nails, makeup and tanning.

Dr. Shelmire's *second* book, *The Art of Being Beautiful,* picks up where *The Art of Looking Younger* left off by recommending specific products and giving us reams of beauty advice based on AGE. "Your skin's age," says Shelmire, "is not always the same as your chronological age." To find out how old your skin is, you can take his personal skin-index test, then flip to the appropriate section for help. The doctor also covers problems affecting every age group from infant to senior citizen. He tells why and when to consult a dermatologist, cosmetologist or plastic surgeon. He also gives us an inside look at the beauty business, its products and practitioners . . . and lets us sit in with him while he speculates. It's a charming book, full of good sense. One gets the feeling it was written to help those of us who sometimes worry that (like the woman on the cover of his first book) we too will end up with twenty-year-old bodies and seventy-year-old heads.

THE ART OF LOOKING YOUNGER
by J. Bedford Shelmire, Jr., M.D.
St. Martin's Press (Hardcover, $6.95)
Dell (Paperback, $1.25)
THE ART OF BEING BEAUTIFUL
AT ANY AGE
by J. Bedford Shelmire, Jr., M.D.
St. Martin's Press (Hardcover, $7.95)

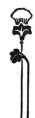 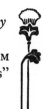

Most Women are not so young as they are painted.
—Sir Max Beerbohm
"A Defence of Cosmetics"

 SKIN CARE

Sand Rash? Windburn? Chapped Lips? Tennis Toe?

Do you have super skin? Well, neither do I. And even though Dr. Jonathan Zizmor and John Foreman (coauthors of a wonderful book called *Super Skin: The Doctor's Guide to a Beautiful, Healthy Complexion*) won't give you a point-by-point program to get you into that condition, what they WILL do is tell you how to cope when something goes wrong.

"Good-looking skin is not difficult to come by," they say, "if only we understand how our skin functions and its reactions to various natural and chemical elements."

My favorite part of *Super Skin* is that it gives the lie to a lot of myths I'd carried around with me since heaven knows when. For example, they say that it's OK to squeeze pimples. (What a relief!) The good doctor also goes on to say that candy bars don't cause pimples and dandruff isn't catching (no matter what your mother told you to the contrary) and that you CAN get venereal disease from a toilet seat. See what I mean about myth destruction!

Super Skin is also chock full of advice about commercial products, so if you've got the heartbreak of a periodic case of pimples, you can run to the store without having to search the shelves for a generic item like tincture of greensalve. With book in hand, you can march right up to the counter and ask (in a loud, clear voice) for Zit Away (or whatever).

Unfortunately, *Super Skin* doesn't read with the ease of a two-penny novel, but as a source

book, or a reference guide, or a book to turn to when something goes wrong, *Super Skin* is hard to beat.

> SUPER SKIN: The Doctor's Guide to a Beautiful, Healthy Complexion
> by Jonathan Zizmor, M.D., and John Foreman
> Crowell (Hardcover, $7.95)
> Berkley (Paperback, $1.50)

Interesting Ways to Get Your Skin Clean

(and a Couple of Things You Might Not Have Known About Cleansing)

Getting your skin clean is not a complicated process, but there *are* some things you should know about the stuff you use to come clean with.

• Bath soaps and toiletry bars aren't made to clean your face with, and can leave you feeling taut, dry or, worse yet, itchy.

• The main difference between lotion cleansers and soaps is that cleansers supply their own water, are usually soapless, and are used to dissolve dirt that then gets rinsed or tissued away.

• Cleansing grains are little granules imbedded in soaps or creams, or used alone, to improve circulation and manually remove dead surface cells.

• Toners are lotions you use after you wash your face. You need them because every time you wash your face, you change the acid balance on your skin. Toners help get your skin back to a normal, healthy balance. They also get rid of any soap residue you may have missed in rinsing, and they tighten up your pores. Toners, by the way, are especially good for people with normal to oily skin.

• Refreshers serve the same function toners do, but with less alcohol. The difference between a refresher and a toner is that toners are more stimulating and more astringent, and refreshers are gentler and better suited to dry or sensitive skin.

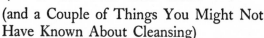

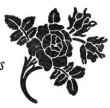

Luxury List:
The Most Expensive Cleansers
and Toners on the Market

Cleansers

Orlane	Lacta Creme, 17 oz.	$18.50
Stendahl	Fluid Demaquillage, 16 oz.	$18.00
Germaine Monteil	Super Moist Beauty Emulsion (Natural), 4¼ oz.	$15.00
Lancaster	Specific Cleanser, 5.4 oz.	$13.00
Etherea	Complete Cleansing Cream, 16 oz.	$12.50
Borghese	Clean Skin Treatment Soap, 6-oz. bar	$7.50

Toners

Germaine Monteil	Skin Freshener, 32 oz.	$16.00
House of Miriam	Apricot Toner, 8 oz.	$13.00
Ilona of Hungary	Overture I Complexion Freshener for Oily Skin, 16 oz.	$14.00

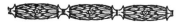

Cleansing your face and caring for your face is a laborious, time-consuming, ultimately boring process which never ends. What the beauty companies do, is try and capture your imagination with new ways of involving you in a regime. Just the way you think of new toys for children. Essentially, it's all a variation on soap and water, astringent and moisturizing. With makeup there's an immediate result and an immediate reward. You face the world and you get a reaction or you don't get a reaction. Treatment, on the other hand, is like belief in the Hereafter: it takes a while to pay off.
—TONI KOSOVER, *author of*
Diary of a New York Career Girl

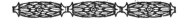

Some Very Special
Face and Body Soaps

Neutrogena: The Nifty Soap Found in the Very Best Hotels

If you travel a lot perhaps you've run into a little amber-colored bar of Neutrogena in the Fairmont in San Francisco, or tucked next to the spigot in the Ritz-Carlton in Boston. Maybe you've even picked it up and looked through it ... it's clear enough to see through. But you probably know all that. Here are some things you might *not* know about that cute little soap bar. Did you ever consider, for example, that one Dr. Edmond Fromont worked for seven long-suffering years in his Brussels lab to develop a soap formula that worked for all skin types? Did you know that Neutrogena SWEATS? That's right, it sweats because its rich in glycerine, and glycerine attracts moisture, which causes little beads to form on the bar. Did you know that you can brush your teeth with Neutrogena because there's no free alkali in it so it can't nip at your tongue? You can find out all about Neutrogena without ever leaving home.

NEUTROGENA REGULAR and NEUTROGENA UNSCENTED SOAP, 3.5-oz. bar, $1.25

   Oil Slick?

According to a national study, 97.6 percent of all teenagers report having skin problems. Here's the bad news ... so do a significant number of adult women who used to think pimples were only little kids' stuff. Neutrogena has a soap made specifically to cope with oily-skin problems. Special degreasing and drying things which take out excess oil and leave only clean, film-free skin behind ...

NEUTROGENA ACNE-CLEANSING BAR, 3.5-oz. bar, $1.50

   Homemade Soap

Merv Griffin's wife used to make her own soap. So did my grandmother. Ann Bramson's book *(Soap)* tells all about making soap in your kitchen the way our foremothers did. The difference is a new ease of equipment and materials, and embellishments our relatives hadn't even heard of. There are four basic toilet-soap recipes in the book: castile, copra-olive, palma-christi and vegetable. They're easy and fun. In the words of Michigan fifth-grader Craig Miller, who made soap in school recently, "If anyone said they weren't I'll sock 'em."

Homemade soap, like homemade bread, has little to do with the store-bought version. As Ann Bramson herself says: "Homemade soap has character. It charms." So does the book.

SOAP
by Ann Bramson
Workman Publishing Company, Inc. (Paperback, $2.75)

*The Most Incredible
Piece of Literature Ever Printed
On a Six-by-Six Piece of Paper:
The Dr. Bronner
Peppermint Soap Label*

I can't swear to this, but I have the feeling that if you wanted an answer to the question What is the meaning of life? you could probably find it on a Dr. Bronner label.

James Simon Kunen described it best (in an article he wrote for *Esquire*) as: "...a politico-religious fantasy tract comprising material drawn from Thomas Paine, Marx, Jesus, Khrushchev, Mark Spitz, swallows, God, popular music, and other sources featuring between four and thirteen moral absolutes, depending on the size of the bottle."

Dr. Bronner himself, a wiry man with the nervous energy of a sack full of hummingbirds, comes from a long line of soap makers. His father and his grandfather were making soap in Europe 150 years ago. When Hitler came to power, Dr. Bronner was disturbed. "The Nazis and the Commies were using soap," he says, "but their minds and their souls were still dirty." It was then and there that he decided to become a soap maker who cleaned not only the outside of the body, but the mind and the soul and the spirit. And that's how the label got to be a personal manifesto.

True, the label was the first thing about Dr. Bronner's Soap that fascinated me ... but then I got involved with the soap itself and I was *really* hooked. It's one of those products you can do everything with. You can shave with it, wash your hair with it, use it as a deodorant. You can brush your teeth with it or use it for mouthwash. You can wash out your underwear in it, use it for a hot-towel massage, rinse fresh fruit and vegetables in it or use it to kill the little white bugs that are taking over your aspidistra. Besides all that, it sometimes makes your crotch tingle.

DR. BRONNER'S PEPPERMINT SOAP is available at most drug and health food stores.

4 oz., $1.00; 1 pt., $3.00; ½ gallon, $9.50; 8 oz., $1.75; 1 qt., $5.00; 1 gallon, $18.00.

Bonne Bell Wants You to Know

Curious to see how cosmetics are really made? Call Bonne Bell. They'll take you through their plant and show you how Ten-O-Six lotion is created, you can visit the lab and talk to the chemists and see how they develop different formulas, you can browse through their shops, have a touch of wine and cheese and get answers to any questions you might have about their company.

BONNE BELL
18519 Detroit Avenue
Lakewood, Ohio 44107

You might also be interested in this: They have a toll-free consumer line. You can call up and get beauty advice, information about any of their products and a friendly contact with someone in the beauty business.

BONNE BELL
TOLL-FREE PHONE
(800)321-9985
Ohio residents call collect: (216)221-9191

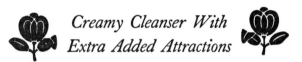

Creamy Cleanser With Extra Added Attractions

George Avery Bunting, the man who invented Noxema, raised ten-foot sunflowers and wrote awful poetry. In 1914 he went to the back of his pharmacy; cooked up a mixture of oil of cloves, menthol, camphor and vanishing cream; poured it into jars and quickly labeled it Dr. Bunting's Sunburn Remedy. When a satisfied customer told Bunting that the remedy worked wonders for his flourishing case of eczema, the original name bit the dust and Noxema was born.

That first satisfied customer was only one of thousands who found interesting (though sometimes odd) uses for the contents of that little blue Noxema jar. Mothers used it on babies. Teenagers used it to get rid of blemishes, men used it as an after-shave. Richard E. Byrd took a case to the South Pole to unchap the hands of his crew members. People used it as shampoo. They put it on cows and horses. Some doctored ailing tree limbs with it. Salesmen proved Noxema was pure by tasting it. Then, for a bit of sheer showmanship, they'd rub it on their suit jackets to prove it was greaseless. In 1950 a Noxell employee with sensitive skin used Noxema to wash her face. It was this brave woman who can be thanked for unintentionally introducing the washable cream cleanser to the American consumer. You can still buy Noxema for as little as 16¢ an ounce.

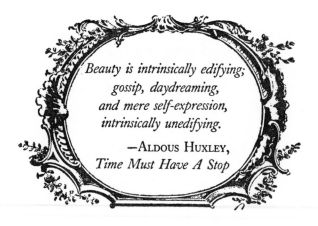

*Beauty is intrinsically edifying;
gossip, daydreaming,
and mere self-expression,
intrinsically unedifying.*

—ALDOUS HUXLEY,
Time Must Have A Stop

FREE FACIAL EXERCISES

The folks who make that cute yellow coco-butter moisturizing bar (TONE) have come up with a system of exercises called TONE-O-METRICS.

For those of us who've grown tired of trying to say *auk* and *ick* very quickly to tone our facial muscles—Tone-O-Metrics is an interesting alternative.

Your Tone-O-Metrics booklet may be gotten by writing:

TONE-O-METRICS
P.O. Box 20542
Phoenix, Arizona 85036

  Buff It Off

Pores your friends can see a mile away? Oil enough to fry eggs in? There's a handy new cleansing sponge made to buff the old, dull outer layer and excess oil away and uncover the fresher, moister, more translucent you that lurks underneath your problem skin. It's the BUF-PUF—a nonmedicated sponge made of inert polyester fibers and clinically tested by leading dermatologists on some fifteen hundred men and women (not the puff *you're* going to use, of course—you'll get a NEW one).

The Buf-Puf is round and white, rinses clean under water and should last you about two months if you use it regularly. You can get one for about $1.98 in the skin care section of your drugstore. If you have REALLY oily skin or acne problems, you might want to look into the Buf-Kit, which, in addition to giving you a Buf-Puf, includes a special soap-free cleansing bar that takes off excess oil without leaving a film behind. The Buf-Kit for acne comes with its own tidy, reusable tray, and an informative booklet that tells you more than you've ever wanted to know about acne. You can get your Buf-Kit for about $3.96 at drugstores everywhere.

  Newfangled Facial Care

For those of us who stumble around in the morning unable to deal with vigorous activity of any sort, Clairol has invented THE SKIN MACHINE. A first of its kind, it's an automatic skin-care system with a gentle hum guaranteed not to jangle the nerves.

The Skin Machine is a battery-powered, soft-bristled brush that automatically gets at the grime, gets rid of the extra oil and really gets your skin clean. Its rotating bristles respond to a battery-powered motor which slows down or stops if you get too aggressive about cleansing. Along with your Skin Machine you get a bar of dermatologist-recognized Fostex, a medicated skin cleanser, and a ventilated case to keep in your bathroom.

The Skin Machine by Clairol can be had for approximately $16.49 at drug, cosmetic and appliance stores everywhere.

Horrifyingly Expensive H$_2$O

Skin fresheners are mostly water with a bit of alcohol or a touch of scent and perhaps a tad of moisturizer added to them. The most expensive, most whimsical freshener I've ever seen is EVIAN MINERAL WATER. It comes in an unprepossessing 5-ounce spray can and sells for $5 (American). Amazing!

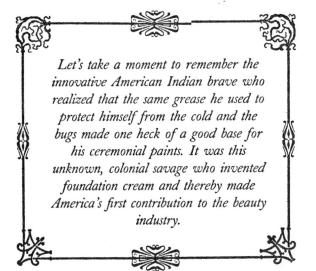

Let's take a moment to remember the innovative American Indian brave who realized that the same grease he used to protect himself from the cold and the bugs made one heck of a good base for his ceremonial paints. It was this unknown, colonial savage who invented foundation cream and thereby made America's first contribution to the beauty industry.

 ## The Marvels of Masqueing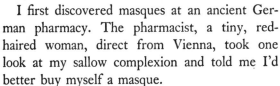

I first discovered masques at an ancient German pharmacy. The pharmacist, a tiny, red-haired woman, direct from Vienna, took one look at my sallow complexion and told me I'd better buy myself a masque.

I misunderstood her and asked if it wouldn't be cheaper just to wear a brown paper bag over my head till summer, when I could hide my miserable coloring under a fresh coat of tan. But she would have none of it. She dragged me to a long, low counter, sat me down and gave me a full-fledged introductory course on the marvels of masqueing.

"Masques," she said, "come in all kinds of shapes, sizes, types and varieties. They're good for extraspecial cleaning and to soup up your circulation. Besides, they're fun to play with, and I think you're going to love them." She then sold me a fresh batch of clay masque that had been made only that morning.

She was right on all counts. It cleaned like a white tornado. I had apples in my cheeks for the first time in years . . . and the masque WAS fun to play with—sort of like making fudge—there was one magic moment when the clay hardened. Unlike fudge, however, I was inside it and unable to move my mouth. Or anything else. It was an adventure to answer the phone in this condition. (The phone, by the way, will ALWAYS ring just as a masque hardens, so it's best to hide it in the sock drawer before putting the stuff on your face.) Anyway, I could tell I was well on my way to becoming a masque maniac. In the several years since my first masque experience, I've worked my way through the following categories with the following results:

Oil Blotting Clay Masques

Well, you pretty much know about these. They dry to a rock-hard consistency, soak up extra oil, get rinsed off and leave you pink, clean and glowing.

Moisture Masques for Dry Skin

Almost the direct opposite of clay, moisture masques never harden. They're rich, soft and creamy and meant to saturate your skin with moisture. Moisture masques are also wonderfully cool, refreshing and luxurious.

Masques that Dry to a Film (for any skin type)

These film-type masques have astringents added to them, so they firm and tighten your pores while they soften. They're wonderful for quick, pick-me-up beauty treatments.

Peel-Off Masques

Just the thing for facial muscles that need a bit of exercise. Peel-offs are made with a latex-type film-former that tightens up the skin and grabs onto imbedded grime, blemishes and other unattractive solids and literally pulls them off. The exercise part comes in when your facial muscles react to the peeling process. (Think of peeling off an adhesive bandage—it's very much the same feeling.)

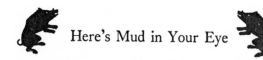 Here's Mud in Your Eye

I'm not the only one on my block who's nuts about masqueing. Pete (my garbage man) would be lost without his Sunday mudpack. I'm not kidding. I mean, he works in a dirty business and likes to save Sundays for little luxuries. His skin, by the way, is BEAUTIFUL; clean, sleek—truly healthy. He says he owes it all to mud. And why not?

Mud has a long, elegant history. Africans dye their hair with it. Resorts along the Black Sea plaster paying guests with it. The Egyptians used it fresh from the banks of the Nile. Just any old mud won't do, of course, and Pete's mudpack of choice is a special combination of natural earth clays carefully cultivated in England and Texas. The clays are aged in Chattanooga, Tennessee, then batch-tested for their ability to crumple up a special piece of test paper. The point is, if the mud is strong enough to crumple paper as it dries, it's strong enough to do a job on your skin. Pete says that MUDD (which is the name of the stuff he's using every Sunday) is especially good for keeping oil-rich skin in nice condition and at $2.79 for a 5.2-ounce jar ranks as one of his less-expensive indulgences.

Luxury List: Monied Masques

Alexandra de Markoff Peel-Off Facial Treatment Kit	$20.00
Eve of Roma Divine Mask	$12.50
Rose Ross Masque D'Elixir	$15.00

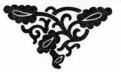

Moisturizers are the girdles of the face.
—Statement attributed to Estée Lauder

Ever Wonder How a Prune Got to Look That Way?

Water is the answer. Lack of water is what does it to prunes. Soak a prune overnight and it will look plump, moist and healthy. Keep the moisture in your skin and it, too, will look beautiful. Better than prunes, I assure you.

A good moisturizer used on clean skin will help protect you from the ravages of sun, wind, cold, air conditioning, high altitude, low humidity or any of the other moisture-robbing villains that human flesh is heir to.

Good moisturizers are made up of two basic ingredients: *emollients* (oils that soften and lubricate) and *humectants* (to absorb moisture from the air and keep the product from drying out).

Moisturizers either sit on top of your skin to keep the good stuff in and the bad stuff out, or they vanish into your skin to do their job. Vanishing creams are usually emulsions of oil in water. They feel cool when they're put on, and leave very little greasy aftermath. Moisturizers that sit on the surface of your skin are emulsions of water in oil. They're rich, protective and nourishing.

There's a SIMPLE TEST you can do if you want to find out whether your favorite cream is oil-in-water (or water-in-oil) based.

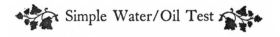 Simple Water/Oil Test

Dab a small bit of your moisturizing cream on a butter knife. Add a drop or two of water. Then try to work the water into the cream. If they mix together easily the product you're using is an oil-in-water emulsion.

If the water droplet beads up and refuses to mix with the cream, your product is water-in-oil. Finding out what kind of emulsion your moisturizer is helps fit the treatment to the need. While you're testing, here are two more professional tests for any cream or lotion.

Two More Professional Tests

Beauty people use the word *slip* as a noun, not a verb. They test a cream by how it feels when it goes on the skin. Is it waxy? Is it tacky? Is it dry? Sticky? Stiff? In other words, does it slide on easily or not.

Another measure of good creams is how they change once you put them on. Does your cream feel cool at first, then seem to sink in? Is it thick enough to stay put (like moisturizer)? Or thin enough to spread around (like body lotion)? What's the initial feel? The middle feel? The end feel?

The more aware you are about how your products work, the more you'll get out of them.

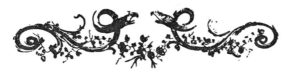

Luxury List: Madcap Moisturizers

Estée Lauder	Liquid Re-Nutritiv	16 oz.	$120
Orlane	Super Hydratante B-21	1.76 oz.	$45
Christian Dior	Hydra-Dior Equalizing Moisture Cream	2 oz.	$25
Elizabeth Arden	Cream Extraordinaire	8 oz.	$25
Germaine Monteil	Bio Miracle Cream	4.5 oz.	$50
Irma Shorell	Contour/35	7.5 oz.	$50
Borghese	Crema Concentra	3.5 oz.	$65

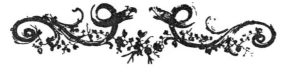

Fascinating Formula 405

My mother-in-law remembers when you had to have a prescription to get Formula 405 Moisturizer. She tells me she used to hoard it and that she'd never found a product that made her skin look and feel better.

Formula 405 is not a fluffy, romantic product line because it didn't grow out of a fluffy, romantic concept. It's the brainchild of Dr. Frank Panzarella, the biochemist president of Doak Pharmacal Company, who believes we should all know a couple of facts about our skin before we do anything disastrous to it.

"Your skin," he says, "everybody's skin, in fact, has three parts to it: the epidermis, the dermis, and a subcutaneous layer of fatty tissue.

It's all well and good to talk about skin generally, but when you talk about the way your skin LOOKS, you should know that you're ONLY talking about that terrifically thin little outer part of your epidermis: the stratum corneum.

"It's only about 1/1000 of an inch thick, but you've got to remember it's the *only* part of your skin anybody ever actually sees. Besides being highly visible, your stratum corneum spends most of its time as a natural barrier, keeping everything inside from getting out and anything outside from getting in.

"Naturally, your stratum corneum can't do all this work alone. In fact, since it's made up of cells which start down between the dermis and the epidermis and work their way up, if it weren't for the other layers, the stratum corneum wouldn't exist at all.

"These living cells in the other layers of your skin are very much like salmon swimming upstream. They keep moving up through the layers till they get to the top. It's a tough trip, so by the time they make it, many of them are literally quite dead and need to get washed off or sloughed away. Others of them desperately need a drink.

"The younger you are, the more your cells drink easily and naturally. They plump up your skin's outer layer so it looks firm, smooth and lovely. As you get older (and this is the bad news), it's harder for your thirsty little cells to hold in the water they drink up."

Knowing all this, Dr. Panzarella developed Formula 405 Cream to bring deep-action moisture down into the cells of your stratum corneum. He packed it full of water-loving ingredients to help fill out little lines caused by parched cells. The result: new freshness and pliability. Nice, yes?

Dr. Panzarella (who's also interested in clean, healthy—as well as moist—skin) says superficial cleaning doesn't go far enough. "There's no reason for a woman to look older than she has to," he tells us, and goes on to explain the benefit of his Formula 405 Cleansing Pac.

"The pac combines soapless pink cleansing and moisturizing lotions and two textured polyurethane sponges to whisk away pore-clogging junk that makes for rough or dull skin."

One of the best things about the 405 Cleansing Pac is you can use it all over your body as well as on your face.

> Formula 405
> Deep-Action Moisturizing Cream 2 oz., $5
> Formula 405 Facial Cleansing Pac (including 4 oz. of Deep-Action Cleansing Lotion and face and body size applicator sponges)
> $10

Baby Yourself—Free Booklets From Johnson & Johnson

Here's a company who believes in babying grown-ups. Especially grownups who are old enough to use makeup, shave their legs, or get a little dry all over. That's why they've put together three nice little booklets.

The first, called "Beauty Basics," gives tips on how to use baby oil for everything from tweezing your eyebrows to making your tan last longer.

The next, "You're Beautiful," is specially written for teenage girls who want to know more about skin and hair care.

Then, there's "Baby Yourself," which lists all the ingenious (and inexpensive) ways you can use baby products to take care of your skin.

If you'd like a copy of any or all of these booklets, or if you're a teacher and would like to know about the excellent educational materials the Johnson & Johnson Baby Products Company makes available to you, just scratch off a note and a self-addressed #10 envelope to:

JOHNSON & JOHNSON
BABY PRODUCTS COMPANY
Consumer Services Department
New Brunswick, N.J. 08903

Vonderful, Versatile, Vaseline

"Rod wax," said the workman at the oil refinery, as he crankily cleaned the stuff off the oil-pump rods for the third time that day. "Biggest nuisance in the fields," he told the visitor. Little did he know he was talking to Robert A. Chesebrough, a man who would turn that pesky rod wax into a product that now sells 69 million jars a year and has a thousand different uses.

Chesebrough was a struggling twenty-two-year-old chemist before that hot afternoon in 1859, when he decided to turn a nasty, waxlike residue into Vaseline.

Let's forget the fact that Vaseline's an excellent moisture-protective film, a superb lip gloss, a terrific way to take off your makeup. Let's forget that it's soothing and healing to minor cuts and burns. Let's forget all that for a moment and concentrate on some of the more arcane uses people have found for Vaseline over the years.

Peary took Vaseline to the Arctic because it

didn't freeze at 40 below zero. Indian natives buttered their bread with it. Chesebrough himself, in his ninety-sixth year (he died in 1933), ate a spoonful of Vaseline every day of his life. Africans use Vaseline like money. The *Gemini V* astronauts put it up their noses (to keep them moist in outer space). Long-distance swimmers grease their bodies with it. Movie stars use it to simulate tears.

You can shine your Mary Janes with Vaseline, or waterproof your riding boots or darken your eyelashes.

Photographers smear it on negatives to get rid of scratches. Motorists smear it on windshields to keep them from frosting over. Blind people keep their fingertips soft enough to read Braille with, with (you guessed it) Vaseline. And at least one major razor-blade manufacturer uses it to coat billions of blades so they don't rust. GIs used Vaseline for (among other things) shaving. A band of enterprising Chesebrough-Ponds employees stuck Q-Tips in jars of Vaseline, lit them, and created torches with which to light their way during New York City's 1965 blackout. Svetlana Alliluyeva left a jar of Vaseline on her dresser when she fled the USSR. It was immediately confiscated by Soviet authorities as evidence of her decadence. Charles Dickens used Vaseline ... and if that isn't enough ... a fisherman friend of mine named Henry tells me that small blobs of Vaseline Petroleum Jelly make fabulous trout bait.

VPJ comes in various sizes, from handy tote-it-around tubes to a jar that's almost too heavy to lift.

VASELINE PETROLEUM JELLY
by CHESEBROUGH-PONDS   49¢–$1.49

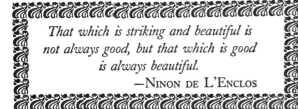

That which is striking and beautiful is not always good, but that which is good is always beautiful.
—NINON DE L'ENCLOS

GETTING TOTALED

I don't know about you, but there are days when (for me) getting totaled is the only answer.

The works. Manicure, haircut. Facial. Everything.

Recently my beauty-crazed friend C. B. Abbott had one of those days, and graciously volunteered to check out the full-service facilities at Saks Fifth Avenue. The following is her first-person report on what it was, and what it was like.

 Getting Totaled at Saks

by C. B. Abbott

No one had to tell me that my days of beauty neglect were just about over. The signs were all too obvious—hair out of control; skin a little dull and sallow from a carbohydrate binge; hands disgraced by fringed cuticles and multilength nails. In need of repair and wanting glamour, I immediately phoned the beauty salon at Saks Fifth Avenue for an afternoon make-over.

The salon is chatty, informal, bustling, and—the nice surprise—prompt about appointment times. I began with Annamaria, an expert manicurist who surveyed my digital damage with consoling words and practical advice on hand care. (Use creams, wear rubber gloves when scrubbing tubs, move hands gracefully and don't slam into objects, etc.) For instant glamour, I agreed to have Patti Nails applied.

To make a Patti Nail, a lengthy silver form is placed under your nail; a pink acrylic powder and liquid is mixed on your nail, then quickly brushed over both your nail and the extending silver form. *Voila!* You've got a pale pink nail (not unlike Cher's) that's harder than your own and "grown" before your eyes. When they are thoroughly dry, the Patti Nails are smoothed down and filed, in my case, to a manageable length. A minimanicure to clean up messy cuticles followed. Annamaria finished with a double coat of Revlon's Misty Lilac, then sealed the polish with a clear top coat. Gorgeous!

Next, to Ilona for an Adrien Arpel Bio-Cellular facial. Ilona noted my T-zone oiliness and proceeded with the fifteen-minute deep-cleaning and light-massage procedure to correct it. First, a soap-substitute foam cleanser to remove makeup and surface dirt, then a heavenly mist of Lemon & Lime Freshener to cleanse further and close the pores. Third, a much-needed peeling done with a gently abrasive cream to slough away dry and dead skin. The cream removal's done with a rotating pumice stone (this step is nonirritating). Any moisture loss is replaced by an application of Vital Velvet Moisturizer. A warm paraffin mask is then brushed on, left for a moment, then pressed to the skin by Ilona's skin iron (warmed for dry skin, iced for oily skin). Imbedded impurities are lifted out as the mask is lifted off. Finally, Adrien Arpel's Bio-Cellular cream is smoothed on to plump up cell tissues and replenish moisture. (This fifteen-minute facial is great not only for sybaritic relaxation and total deep cleaning, but *convenient*, too.)

Spirit restored, skin cleansed, wishing I'd owned a large cabochon ruby to wear with my new-look hands, I lazed back while my hair was shampooed and conditioned. I settled into Nicole's station for a cut and blow-dry. Though she was the last major step in my pampered afternoon, Nicole proved to be a talented stylist worth waiting for. I was given the *best* cut ever.

Before leaving, I stopped at the Adrien Arpel cosmetic counter to see Ilona for my complimentary makeup application (this is included in the price of the facial). I was skillfully moisturized, blushed-on, mascaraed, color-emphasized with dark lipstick, gray-green eye shadow—which gave me a *frisson*, being a look I hadn't considered (being the understated type). But I *loved* it.

For more information about the service, prices and locations of Saks beauty salons, see the following:

Saks Fifth Avenue—Nationwide Locations
(alphabetized by city)

Main Branch
Fifth Avenue and 50th Street
New York, N.Y. 10022

Peachtree at Lenox Road
Atlanta, Ga. 30326

Cityline Avenue at Decker Square
Bala Cynwyd, Pa. 19004

9600 Wilshire Blvd.
Beverly Hills, Calif. 90212

Prudential Center
Boston, Mass. 02199

5555 Wisconsin Avenue
Chevy Chase, Md. 20015

669 N. Michigan Avenue
Chicago, Ill. 60611

308 Fischer Building
Detroit, Mich. 48202

Sunrise Shopping Center
Fort Lauderdale, Fla. 33304

1300 Franklin Avenue
Garden City, N.Y. 11530

1800 S. Post Oaks Road
Houston, Tex. 77027

Milburn & Short Hills Avenue
Springfield, N.J. 07081

1 Plaza Frontenac
St. Louis, Mo. 63131

2901 E. Big Beaver Rd.
Troy, Mich. 48084

Bloomingdale Rd. & Maple Avenue
White Plains, N.Y. 10605

30 Woodland Promenade
Woodland Hills, Calif. 91364

Saks Fifth Avenue Service Price List for the New York Store
(prices may vary according to locations, but not a heck of a lot)

Haircuts:
   Cut: $15.00 and up
   Trim: $12.50

Hair services:
   Permanent: $50.00
   Straightening: $50.00 and up
   Blow-dry: $7.50 min.

Set: $8.00
Commercial conditioning: $5.00–$8.00

"Bone Marrow" treatment: •$15.00 (this treatment was originated by Sotiris Skrekas. Herbs, bone marrow and five natural oils are whipped together until creamy, then applied to the scalp and hair. Sotiris then bakes the conditioning in—hair is piled under a heatcap for half an hour. Three shampoos are necessary to rinse the formula out. Saks claims (Chris Fields does, anyway) that the treatment promotes the growth of hair while conditioning scalp and hair.

Coloring:
  One-process: $17.50 and up
  Two-process: $25.00 and up
Streaking:
  half-head: $25.00 and up
  full head: $50.00 and up
Hair-You-Don't-Want Services:
Arm waxing:
  half-arm: $8.00
  full arm: $12.00
Leg waxing:
  half-leg: $15.00
  full leg: $25.00
Facial waxing:
  lip: $4.50
  eyebrow arch: $4.00
  chin: $4.50
  face: $5.00
  neck: $5.00
Body waxing:
  bikini waxing: $5.00
Electrolysis:
  15 minutes: $9.50
  30 minutes: $18.00
  45 minutes: $27.00
  one hour: $35.00
Manicuring Services:
Manicure: $5.00
  ($4.50 with another service)

Nail wrapping: $15.00
Patti Nails:
  Full set: $35.00
  Single nails: $3.50
  Fill-ins: $2.50
Pedicures:
  Both feet: $12.50
Facials:
  European full facial: $30.00
  Adrien Arpel Mini-facial: $10.00
  Adrien Arpel Bio-Cellular facial: $12.50
Makeup:
  Adrien Arpel: $10.00
Lash and Brow:
  Eyelash dye: $5.00
  Eyebrow dye: $5.00

HAVE YOU THOUGHT ABOUT YOUR HANDS LATELY?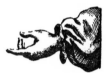

Beautiful Hands Are Happy Hands

"Nobody knows more about doing your nails than Cutex," or so they say. So when it comes time to give yourself a perfect manicure and you find you're all thumbs, all you have to do is write the Cutex Nail Care Clinic and they'll send you a FREE copy of the Cutex Nail Care Guide. It's a nifty little booklet that tells you exactly how to do it, and with what. Write:

THE CUTEX NAIL CARE CLINIC
415 Madison Avenue
New York, New York 10017

What a Palmist Sees
When He Looks at Your Nails

RIDGES show your nervous disposition. The more and the deeper the ridges, the more nervous you've been.

WHITE SPOTS show years' worth of trauma. Each white spot is a new one. If your spots show up near your cuticles, the trouble peaked recently. The farther the spot is toward the tip of the nail, the older the trauma.

SHORT, FLAT NAILS are critical nails.

POINTED NAILS belong to people who live in fantasy.

ROUNDED NAILS are realistic nails.

NATURALLY CURVED NAILS are artistic.

SQUARE NAILS belong to activists.

BROAD NAILS indicate muscular and physical endurance.

LONG, NARROW NAILS lack energy.

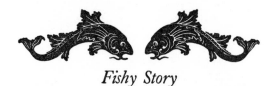

Fishy Story

That really IS pearl in your frosted nail enamel—but it doesn't come from an oyster, it comes from a herring, whose shiny scales (which the chemists call *guanine)* make your fingertips glisten.

The No-Polish Polisher

Buffers, nail buffers, are an old-fashioned invention with a newfangled knack for improving circulation and spiffing up a shine. Buffers actually smoothe away one of the major causes of cracking and chipping, while conditioning your nails and leaving them lustrous, strong, resilient and healthy looking. All this without any polish.

The JOVAN NAIL CONDITIONING AND POLISHING KIT has everything you'll need to buff your nails beautifully. There's a smoother to erase unsightly ridges in the nail surface—it's a very light abrasive on an especially easy-to-hold base—and there's Conditioning Cream and a padded chamois buffer that can turn problem nails into beautiful nails in minutes.

JOVAN NAIL CONDITIONING AND POLISHING KIT: $8.50

One Woman's True Story

Did you ever wonder about the women behind the luscious hands you see in all those diamond-ring ads? Did you ever wish your hands could look a little more like theirs do? If so, you'll probably want to read this fascinating story of a woman whose hands are (quite literally) her fortune.

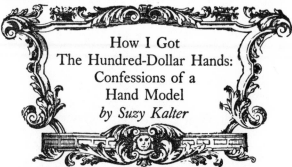

How I Got
The Hundred-Dollar Hands:
Confessions of a
Hand Model
by Suzy Kalter

My definition of a *lady* is someone with long, red fingernails. It's that simple. Real ladies have long, red nails; hence you can always tell a lady by her hands. I was *dying* to have long, red fingernails.

There was nothing wrong with my nails, mind you. I didn't bite them or anything. They grew out to a respectable length known as nice, and then they broke. It was cyclical; they just couldn't get beyond a certain point.

Then I met Him. He was rich (okay, *very* rich), social (yes, *very* social) quite hung up on his mother, but he was mine. Well, after he was his mother's, anyway. After two dates I could see I was moving in for a long affair, and I was in trouble. Could this millionaire *bon vivant* dream man of my childhood and bachelor of my mother's dreams find out the truth about me? Never! I would become a lady. Immediately. Before he found out otherwise.

A friend recommended René (Cilo of Milano, 9 East 53rd Street, New York, New York) and her famous Patti Nails. René could make me a lady in three hours and no one would ever know my secret.

I told Mr. Money I was having some dental work done and would be under the weather all

Saturday, so he should run on without me for the weekend ... there is nothing tackier than a woman admitting she'd spend the day at the beauty parlor, I always say.

I faced René as excited as a child facing Christmas. This was one of those cultural rituals Margaret Mead never mentioned. When I had my first menstrual period, Mother told me, "Today, you are a woman." But she never said anything about being a lady.

René explained that Patti Nails were invented by a dentist (whose wife's name was Patti), and that the nails are made from a material similar to the one used in temporary fillings. After a hand treatment of soaking, massaging and cuticle bending, René crowned each finger with a silver foil semicircle. The silver form fit exactly around my own nails as René expertly bent them into perfection with the tip of her trusty paintbrush. Out came two tiny jars: one filled with pink dust; the other holding a strong-smelling liquid René poured fresh from a larger bottle.

She filed each of my nails coarsely across the top, for adhesion, then dipped her magic paintbrush into the liquid, then into the powder. The tip of the paintbrush is about the size of a fingernail, so the liquid pulls up the powder and forms a nailish shape which René then applies to each fingertip; actually painting on a nail that stretches from the base of your own nail up onto the silver form.

It was painstaking work and took almost an hour, plus another half-hour to dry. I sat dreamily thinking of Ellen Ross. Ellen Ross was sort of my best friend when we were sixteen—we roomed together in college and I was in her wedding, but we were hardly speaking then. Anyway, at the age of sixteen, when I still had acne and an irregular period, Ellen Ross was perfect—and she had long, manicured fingernails. I hated her. She had them done every week, with Naked Pink polish, and she carried her own bottle of Naked Pink with her everywhere she went. Naked Pink was the hot color in those days; this was when cremes were first introduced

and this was a bluish-pink, soft shell-color with a shine like ceramic. So Ellen Ross had these tiny hands (she was only about 5′2″, so everything she had was tiny) with these long, elegant fingernails, and she was the envy of Waco, Texas. Obviously, this girl had been born a lady, and the rest of us were left to eat our hearts out.

René filed my nails to a proper, languid length and finished off with a manicure. (Yes, I *had* to have Fire & Ice for my first manicure.) If you could only see me now, Ellen Ross. The nails were a little thicker than real nails, but to the normal eye there was no difference between my nails—and Ellen's. The cost was $40; I tipped $5 and made a weekly standing appointment. "Upkeep," René reminds me, "or all this will have been in vain."

Besides the psychological thrill, there is a physical adjustment. For the first day or two the nails felt funny—I was conscious of them being there. You also have to learn to move differently: because the Pattis are thicker you lose a bit of dexterity, buttons are sometimes harder to maneuver, phones must be dialed with pencils, and fingertips are used where nails were used previously. It's harder to pick your nose with Patti Nails, and impossible to get to a blackhead.

You become accustomed to the nails quickly and soon learn to gracefully accept compliments about your hands rather than blurt out the truth. And you learn the best use of long nails yet invented: drumming them on the counters of stores where the sales help is driving you crazy. The clacking of nails could drive anyone up the wall and is a marvelous weapon.

My own nails grew out underneath the Pattis. A weekly manicure ($3.50) plus regular repair service (at $3 the Patti-Nail) maintained my new bogus beauties until my own nails were grown out, which took about three months. It cost just under $100 just to keep the Pattis going until my nails were at the right length, but it was worth it. By now, all my friends agreed I had exquisite nails. My own nails, when they were finally unveiled, turned out to be very strong at a longer length. (René says this is common; once you get your nails past the bad medium length, they're often stronger in the longer edition.) I was so proud of my newfound glamour that I gladly did everything René told me to keep it going, and if you'll stay with me, I'll be happy to pass along the good advice.

René's Careful Lessons for Beautiful Hands

1. Have a manicure every week, without fail.
2. Wear rubber gloves when doing the dishes, but not all the time: humidity is bad for nails and you can't see what's going on in there and how you may be offending your nails. (I never wear gardening gloves for this reason.)
3. *Never* dial a phone with your fingers.
4. Oil every night with cuticle oil, olive oil or baby oil. Just paint the oil all over the nail and cuticle and rub it in. Do as often as you think about it; you can never do it too much.
5. Use hand lotion as often as possible, whenever possible. Most men aren't too crazy for this one: Use lotion when you go to bed at night, after you do the dishes, when you get out of your bath, and so on.
6. Cover accidents with a Band-Aid and get in for a fix as soon as you can. Save long nails that made clean breaks—they can be grafted (transplanted) back on.
7. Carry a bottle of the color polish you wear with you at all times, so you can apply an instant touch-up to a chipped nail. If you have to miss your manicure, apply a coat of nailpolish to tide you over until your next appointment.
8. Don't pick on your cuticles.

The Dallas Nail Bounty
or
How Your Nails Can Earn You $$$$$

Norm Heinz needed fingernail clippings for the nail transplants that were so popular in his Creative Airs Salon in Dallas, so he took an ad in the local paper offering to pay TOP MONEY for broken nails. He was instantly buried in letters—a thousand the first week, in fact, and about two thousand nail clippings.

So far Mr. Heinz has paid out over $18,000 just for broken female fingernails and has carefully cultivated a collection of some fifty thousand dedicated nail growers across the country.

If you'd like to SELL YOUR NAILS to the Creative Airs Nail Bank, here's how:

Let your nails grow to at least ½ inch or longer. Be sure they're in good condition. If they're not already broken, cut them with a curved pair of nail snippers straight across the nail. Then package them in a small box or envelope and mail them to the address below. When Creative Airs gets the nails, they'll price them and mail you a check the same day. Prices paid for nails vary from 25¢ to $2 per nail, depending on length, quality and which finger the nail is from.

After Creative Airs buys your first set of fingernails, if you want to keep growing nails for them, grow them ½ inch or longer and fairly square on the end, not filed round or pointed.

CREATIVE AIRS (NAIL BOUNTY)
8024 Spring Valley Road (at Coit)
Northwood Hills Center
Dallas, Texas 75240

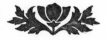

SEVERAL SINFULLY SELF-INDULGENT WAYS TO HAVE FABULOUS FEET

Silky feet feel sooo good that I've moisturized mine with everything from invigorating Weleda Foot Balm (which I get for $2.50 at my local health-food store) to a thick, creamy, chocolate-covered cherry-scented Scholl thing called Cocoa Butter Softening Lotion. I actually slather it on from toes to knees or wherever. Actually, almost any good moisturizer qualifies as treatment material after a relaxing footbath. And speaking of footbaths, a nifty Massage-O-Matic Foot Bath (Model #F600) can be ordered from Hammacher Schlemmer for a mere $39.95.

While you're on the phone with Hammacher Schlemmer, they also have an electric foot massager (the twin-vibrating-disc kind) that felt so good when I tried it I didn't want to leave the store. This mechanical wonder costs $17.95. Best of all, it's compact enough to throw into your suitcase as insurance against travel fatigue.

Rubbing alcohol or any chilled astringent toner is a fine way to remove extra oil while you wake up your foot's nerve endings. Scholl's Anti-Perspirant Foot Spray is the perfect follow-up. One application actually kept my feet AND my socks dry through four strenuous hours of harrowing tennis. Even better, it was a nice change of pace from the normal powder-in-the-socks routine that used to feel like I'd been jogging through a marble quarry. Another neat trick for vanquishing the mid-afternoon doldrums is a cooling blast of Foot Refresher Spray or chilled cologne, an absolute MUST for your travel bag or the office fridge.

Professional pedicures are one way to perk up an otherwise unprepossessing day. For a modest price you can spend anywhere from an hour to a sublime ninety minutes away from ringing telephones or personal pressures, while having your feet lovingly ministered to. It's a joy. You should have a pedicure at least once a month. My favorite New York pedicure parlor is the Thirty East Salon, at 30 East 60th Street, (212)421-7555. Here, for $12, you're assured of being tendered to and polished to your heart's content. The pedicure itself takes an hour, but be sure to schedule another thirty minutes for your toenail polish to dry. Men are also welcome for privately administered pedicures.

West of the Hudson River, you can be pedicured at any one of Elizabeth Arden's plush Red Door Salons. So when you find yourself in Beverly Hills, Palm Beach, Phoenix, San Francisco, Surfside or Washington, D.C., with $10 in your hand and forty-five minutes to an hour and a half to devote to your tootsies, be sure to stop by.

Chicago's Face Place at 102 East Oak Street, (312)642-1333, also comes highly recommended by my devoutly escapist friend Judy. Creative director of a huge public relations firm, Judy regularly manages to carve an hour or so from her busy schedule so she can go get her toes done. For this she gladly pays the $15 and lists it on her expense account as an extremely inexpensive business lunch.

If you can't get your toes to a salon, get Eileen Ford's book, *A More Beautiful You in 21 Days,* Simon & Schuster, $9.95, turn to page 174 and immerse yourself in a cunning cram course on touchable tootsies. Ms. Ford (co-founder and mother superior of the world's largest model agency) has admittedly beautiful feet, and if anybody can turn you on to the secrets of making your own feet lovely, she's the one.

Last but not least—or maybe first and foremost—send to SCHOLL for your 25¢-copy of *The New Foot Book,* which gives you twenty-four compact little pages of straight information on easily accessible treatments for many of the more common, irksome foot troubles. To get your book, send a quarter to:

SCHOLL, INC.
Room 820
150 East Huron Street
Chicago, Illinois 60611

BEAUTY BOOKS TO KEEP IN YOUR KITCHEN

When Beatrice Traven and Robert Goldemberg met several years ago at a cocktail party, she was an author and playwright and the owner of "the world's largest collection of half-used jars and bottles and tubes of cosmetics." He was a chemist who made up just the kind of cosmetics she couldn't resist. While Goldemberg fended off a crowd of women who wanted the real truth about that "miracle" ingredient in their favorite face cream, Ms. Traven was wondering why women couldn't make their own cosmetics in the kitchen.

At first Mr. Goldemberg blanched a bit, mumbling things like, "But that's impossible—there *are* no decent natural emulsifiers to make light creams and lotions ... no *safe* natural preservatives." He worried that cosmeticooks wouldn't have scales and thermometers sensitive enough to handle delicate combinations of temperature and weight. But after a while the idea began to get to him. Thoughts like "What if...?" began playing on his mind. The results were two-fold. First, he married Ms. Traven. Then they put together a wonderful book called *Here's Egg on Your Face.*

She wrote the directions. He figured out the recipes. Spurred on by the success of cosmeticookery and armed with dozens of new kitchen-tested formulas, the Goldemberg-Traven household has now presented us with *The Complete Book of Natural Cosmetics.* Replete with such mouth-watering goodies as Grapefruit Bracer ... Apple Cheeks Toning Lotion ... Lime Tonic and Pineapple Papaya Paw Cream, the book is a must for any dedicated dabbler.

Ms. Traven, by the way, writes so clearly and concisely that the book is fun to read even if you're not planning to rush into the kitchen cosmetics business. The recipes were painstakingly set down in scientific terms, weighed in grams and ounces, aged and tested, then taken right into the kitchen and translated into teaspoons and tablespoons and everyday measuring cups. Then the author remade everything to check the results.

THE COMPLETE BOOK OF NATURAL COSMETICS: An Authoritative Guide To Natural Beauty Aids That Can Be Prepared in the Buyer's Own Kitchen by Beatrice Traven, with Cosmetic Formulations by Robert L. Goldemberg and illustrations by Pam Carroll
Simon & Schuster (Hardcover, $6.95)

It's a Long Long Time From May to September

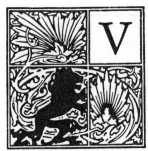

irginia Castleton is beauty editor of the prestigious *Prevention* magazine. She is also a woman who believes in the intrinsic relationship between beauty and nature. So, calling on her years of experience with natural beauty aids like lettuce lotion and sweet almond cleanser, she's given us a helpful, old-world, month-by-month, self-improvement plan called *The Calendar Book of Natural Beauty.*

Recipes for facials, shampoos, conditioners, rinses, hand creams and the like are skillfully blended with lore, legend, exercises, diet suggestions and yummy natural recipes.

THE CALENDAR BOOK OF NATURAL BEAUTY
by Virginia Castleton
Harper & Row (Hardcover, $6.95)

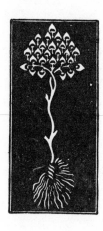
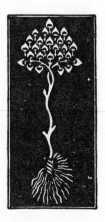

CORNUCOPIA OF COSMETICS FROM THE CORNER STORE

The good things about investing in natural cosmetic wonders like oatmeal and olive oil and mayonnaise is that they're fun to use, convenient and best of all, inexpensive. Besides, if you don't like using them on your face and body, you can put them back into the ice box, or up on the shelf—or—if you're really desperate you can even eat them.

There are, of course, drawbacks to cosmetic groceries. You're not going to find an avocado that's dermatologically tested for strength and safety, for example ... or a strawberry guaranteed not to cause an allergic reaction. It's a very good idea to patch-test your kitchen treatments just to be supersure and supersafe. Put whatever you're planning to use on the inside of your elbow. Cover the spot with a Band-Aid and be patient. Wait twenty-four hours to see that the spot isn't irritated before you rush off and use the stuff all over your body.

Now, most cautions out of the way, the next time you're standing in the A & P feeling adventurous, you might want to consider the following suggestions.

Sitting there next to the Twinkies and the Spaghetti-Os are almost-instant beauty aids ready and waiting to make the transition from your pantry shelf or supermarket shopping cart straight to your vanity table.

Oily/Bumpy Skin Treatments

Garlic Gets 'Em Going

Old wives' tales regale us with the antiseptic qualities of good old garlic. Gypsies used it for treating wounds, pimples and protecting themselves against the invasion of vampires. I don't know how many vampires you've got around *your* house, but if you've got a bump or two you might just want to dab at it with a fresh-cut clove of garlic, then sit back and watch the offending blemish go away.

New scientific research says it's the allincin in garlic that does the trick. Common sense says it's best not to use this remedy before a heavy date.

Buttermilk Basics

If your pores are producing oil like offshore drilling machinery, you should be able to slip into a buttermilk and oatmeal masque and feel much better. Just mix some dry oatmeal and buttermilk into a thick paste. Massage it onto your face and neck. Let it dry, then take it off with a warm, damp washcloth. The extra oil slick should wash away with the remains of the masque, leaving you with lighter, brighter, happier skin.

Brewer's Yeast Beautifier

The trouble with problem skin is that when it's not blotchy from too much circulation, it sometimes gets pale from the lack of it. Brewer's yeast masques are one high-protein answer to pallor. Apply brewer's yeast paste (brewer's yeast and milk), being careful not to get any into your eyes. Relax for half an hour with a good book. Then rinse and kiss that grayness goodbye.

Quick Eggy Facial

This double-duty beautifier calls for one or two beaten whole eggs applied to squeaky-clean skin. Start with your face, and if you have enough egg left over, just keep on going. Two eggs should be enough to cover your neck, shoulders, arms, legs and toes. Unless you're tall, in which case you'll probably need three eggs. Once you're eggy all over, rest somewhere that won't get sticky until your egg-pack dries (about fifteen minutes), then step into a warm, cozy bath. Eggs make your skin very taut when they dry, and make your pores look much smaller when they're washed off.

Treats to Make
Normal Skin Nicer
Cucumber Coolers

There's a mysterious enzyme called erepsin in cucumber juice which works just like the enzyme they use in meat tenderizers. When you use it on your face, what it does is soothe, smooth, cool and soften your skin. So next time you peel a cucumber, save enough long strips of peel to completely cover your face. Lie down for ten minutes, covering the cucumber strips with a hot washcloth. When the washcloth cools down, remove it and the cucumber strips and rinse. If you really like the smell and feel of cucumber enough to want to keep a jar of it on hand, you can whip up several peeled cucumbers in the blender, add a dash of witch hazel (to keep it fresh), store the result in the fridge and *voila!* instant cucumber freshener-upper.

Application of Apples

Students at Michigan State University who ate two apples a day over a three-year period were found to have fewer headaches and skin diseases than students who never ate apples. Women who've used fresh apples to clean off the last traces of soap after washing swear by them as stimulating facial toners. My dentist tells me apples make great natural toothbrushes. With all these good things to say for themselves, it's hard to imagine that apples caused Eve so darned much trouble.

Strawberry Slush

Any strawberries not picture-perfect to serve over ice cream can be mashed into a slush and used to scrub your face with. Use them instead of soap to clean, stimulate and wake up a sluggish complexion.

Surface Salt
(NOTE: Be specially careful with this one; it may be irritating.)

One winter, when I was plagued by flakes and scales, my doctor told me what I needed was a good, thorough thinning. He was not talking about going on a diet; what he meant was a simple salt spray to slough off my huge collection of surface debris. Here's how he told me to do it: "Dissolve a teaspoon of table salt in a small spray bottle full of tap water. Close your eyes and spray your face and neck with the salty spray mist. Let it dry, then gently (GENTLY) rub it off with a wet washcloth." Result: Pink, glowing, dewy skin and no more flakes or scales. Follow with a heavy dose of moisturizer.

Hard-Working Honey

It takes a bee between sixty and eighty thousand trips from flower field to hive to make a single pound of honey nectar. You can reap the benefits of all this hard work by spreading two teaspoons of warm honey on your face before you step into a steamy tub. Honey is a natural humectant, which attracts and holds moisture in your skin. It's also a natural softener. Be sure to rinse well before you leave the tub, or sidle up to some warm toast and have a snack.

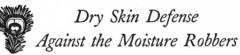

Dry Skin Defense
Against the Moisture Robbers
Polyunsaturated Prettiness

Avocados are sleek, smooth and loaded with polyunsaturated fats. A mashed avocado mixed with a dollop of honey or a tiny bit of fresh lemon juice makes a moisturizing (edible) facial. Leave it on for twenty minutes, then rinse.

Don't Eat That Banana!

Save the calories by mashing up a nice, ripe banana with a touch of heavy cream, spreading it on your face and letting it moisturize and soften you for the next fifteen minutes. After you rinse it off, you can run the inside of the peel over your rough, reddened hands so that they, too, can take advantage of lush, rich banana-oil comfort. If you don't have red, roughened hands you can throw the peel away, or feed it to a needy piglet.

The Handy Moisturizer You Can Cook With

I'd been slathering vegetable oil on my body for years until I read about a dermatologist who so believed in Crisco as a moisturizing protective film, he kept his entire family covered with it. My can of Crisco now travels back and forth between my kitchen and bathroom. At 79¢ the pound, I feel very smug about that.

Help from Hellman's

When you're not using your mayonnaise as a hair conditioner (dab on, comb through, wrap your head in Saran Wrap; rest for fifteen minutes under a hot light; shampoo), you can use it as a rich (somewhat salty) moisturizing mask. Follow the formula for honey masks and enjoy.

A Bagatelle of Baths

Itchy? Try Oatmeal

Oatmeal could have been made to order for cranky, itchy, winter skin. Here's how to make a calming, bleaching oatmeal bath. Grind a cup of dry oatmeal in your blender. Add four cups of warm water (2 cups at a time). Strain the mixture through a cheesecloth square, then add it to your bathwater (the mixture, not the cheesecloth). Now, before getting into the tub, tie up the corners of the cheesecloth into a little sachetlike bag with all the big oatmeal pieces in it, and *voila!* you have a handmade oatmeal washcloth.

Cornstarch Coddling

Dry skin all over your body is uncomfortable. You can soothe that nasty, tight-as-a-kettledrum feeling with cornstarch. Just add two cups to a bathtub full of water, swish around and come out feeling satiny.

Mmmarvelous Milk

Cleopatra, Poppea (Nero's second wife) and Ziegfeld star Anna Held were all addicted to milk baths. They thought milk whitened their skin. We now know it moisturizes. Use one quart to a tubfull. You might also want to have a small bowl of undiluted milk handy as a nourishing, protein-rich facial rinser-offer.

Cider Vinegar Suntan Bath

Jayne Lester of Ironton, Ohio, told me about cider vinegar. We were sitting in the VIP dining room of a swanky resort hotel. Jayne and I had spent the day at the beach. She was healthily tan and glowing. I was lobster-red and in pain. "Use vinegar," she told me. "Pour a pint into your bathtub, add water and you'll feel 200 percent better." She lent me her vinegar bottle. I tried it, and she was right. The pain stopped almost instantly. Within a day or two my tan looked just as good as hers did. I found out later that it's the tannic acid in vinegar that did the trick ... so I might just as well have used lots of teabags. . . .

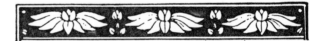

Miscellaneous Groceries For Mouth, Eyes, Fingernails and Wrinkles

Best Beets

Beet juice is the world's least expensive, indelible, natural lip color. The only trouble is it's hard to get off your fingers. Beets come in one shade only and are available (in season) at vegetable counters everywhere.

Bacon and Lemons

Cut off from the mother country, American colonists made do with simple, homemade beauty-treatment formulas like laying bacon strips on their faces to put roses in their cheeks and thwart advancing wrinkles. They also carried small wedges of lemon around to suck on (to make their lips pink) and used undiluted lemon juice to bleach out freckles.

Dunk Your Nails in Olive Oil

Legend says that a ten-minute fingernail bath performed religiously four times each week for a month will strengthen your nails and make them happy. My friend Suzy (with the gorgeous, daggerlike fingernails) says you should do it every time you have a free hand. All it takes is dunking your digits in half a cup of comfortably warmed olive oil.

Develop a Craving for Chamomile Tea

How many other teas can you think of that will settle your nerves, unjangle your upset stomach, lighten your hair and make your tired eyes feel better? Nerve and stomach settling call for a cup of medium-strength tea, taken internally ... like tea, as a matter of fact.

To get your roots lighter, you simply mix up a stronger brew of undiluted chamomile, use it as a rinse after you wash by pouring it repeatedly through your well-rinsed hair, then sit in the sun and dry blonder. Two cotton puffs dipped in CHILLED chamomile, then placed on morning-after or simply awfully tired eyes, will rest them and make them feel nice.

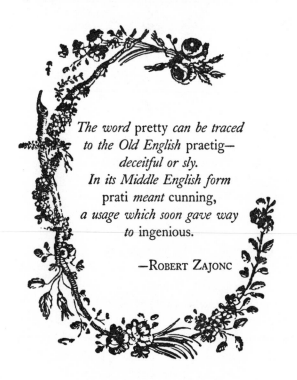

The word pretty *can be traced to the Old English* praetig— *deceitful or sly. In its Middle English form* prati *meant cunning, a usage which soon gave way to* ingenious.

—ROBERT ZAJONC

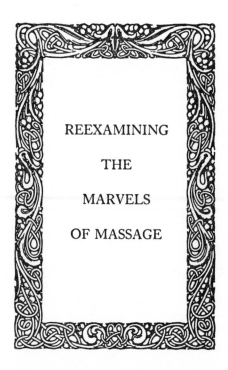

REEXAMINING

THE

MARVELS

OF MASSAGE

Dedicated massage-aholic that I am, I have recently had to face up to the fact that body massage can't really make you beautiful. It can't break down accumulated fat. It can't tone your muscles. It won't even redistribute the weight you've already got.

What massage does is relax you. It breaks up tension and makes you feel good. In some cases it makes you feel very good. Anyway, the better you feel, the better you usually look. So if there is a single beautifying factor under the broad category of massage, it is whatever mysterious thing that makes a relaxed and happy person more attractive than an unrelaxed, tense one.

There IS one area where massage is indispensable, however, where massage really helps get the circulation flowing and where massage can make a real difference. That's on your scalp. Scalp massage can literally make a world of difference in the way your hair looks. That's why I've listed all the best books on massage not under Beauty Treatments, but in the Hair chapter of this book. They are all marvelous, TOTAL treatises, so should you WANT to continue your scalp massage and turn it into a superbly relaxing whole-body experience, please check page 172.

Being Careful About Sun Worship

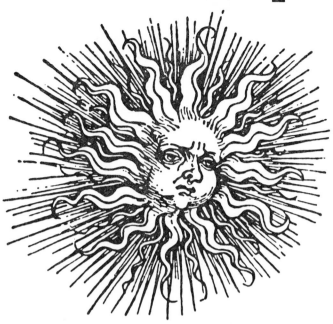

I said to the First Officer, "Gad that sun's hot."
To which he replied, "Well, you shouldn't touch it."

—SPIKE MILLIGAN
A Dustbin of Milligan

Caution: Tanning May Be Hazardous to Your Health

My mother phoned me recently to tell me not to go out in the sun. "What do you mean, don't go out in the sun?" I asked. Because first, my mother is not always right about what she tells me; and second, we'd spent hours, days, probably even months at a time together in the sun, baking at the beach. We were both confirmed beach rats and this was definitely a change of attitude on my mother's part.

"Don't go out in the sun. It gives you cancer," she said. But I know that she gets rabbity about things ... gets a bug in her ear and sometimes gets worried without benefit of facts, so I said, "Aw, come on, Ma ... not sun. Not nice, friendly sun. Sun clears up pimples and it feels good, and besides you look better with a tan."

"Not if you've got cancer, you don't," she told me. And then she told me she had cancer.

Skin cancer. The kind you get from overexposing yourself to sun. So all of a sudden it wasn't nice, friendly old sun anymore. It was something to think about. Seriously.

My mother wasn't the only one who got skin cancer this year. So did my father. And 300,000 other innocent sun worshippers. They won't die from it. Or at least very few of them (about 5,000) will. But every so often their skin will produce small, red, raised sores that look like patches of psoriasis, or hard, red sores that grow inward and spread to vital organs and get deadly. So they'll pack themselves off to the dermatologist, like my parents do. They'll have the red patches burned off, or cut off, or injected with chemicals, and what's left of their skin will look very awful for the next couple of weeks. Then the cycle will start all over again.

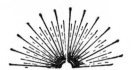

*Mad dogs and Englishmen go out in
the mid-day sun
The Japanese don't care to
The Chinese wouldn't dare to
The Hindus and Argentines sleep firmly
from twelve to one
But Englishmen detest a siesta.*
        —NOEL COWARD
   "Mad Dogs And Englishmen"

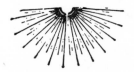

If you cared about your skin, you'd never let it get near the sun. You'd realize that sunlight is never good for grown-ups and that the amount of damage you can do to your skin is directly proportional to the amount of light (sunlight) you expose it to. A few months of intense exposure can do more than centuries of normal wear.

Consider: Sunlight travels 93 million miles from its home and reaches the earth in eight minutes (less time than it takes to broil a steak). And, while we're protected from the shorter ultraviolet wavelengths by the ozone in the atmosphere, the ultraviolet waves that *do* get through affect us every minute we spend outdoors.

If we really cared about our skin, we'd all move to Bergen, Norway. There's a legend that a child born in Bergen can grow up to be seven or eight years old without once seeing sunlight. This, of course, has a wonderful effect on his complexion. And would on ours if we moved there. But I'm not moving to Bergen, and neither are you, right? So let's take a look at what all the ultraviolet light we expose ourselves to can do to us once it gets through to our skin.

The first thing it does to us is irritate us and give us sunburns. It expands our blood vessels and turns us red. It triggers a defense mechanism inside our skin that produces a lot of pigment, makes the cells build up on our skin's outer layer and makes our skin a little tougher. It changes the structure of our skin temporarily. So, okay, you've got a tan, and some temporary structural changes, and if you stay out of direct sunlight for a while, the tan will fade and no harm (no *permanent* harm) will be done.

If you *don't* stay out of direct sunlight and continue to trot out to the beach with your copy of *Vogue* or the latest hot novel, and continue to get sunburned, the pigmentation and cell buildup will accumulate and cause delayed, serious, and often frightening changes later on.

Here's what happens when you burn: Fluid oozes up from an inner layer of your skin and tries to get to the surface. It puts pressure on your nerve endings, swells you up and makes you and your sunburn tender to the touch. It's radiation burn. And if you've got enough fluid struggling around in your system, you're going to get blisters. Then you'll peel, which means that your skin's top layer (the very part of your skin that could have formed a cozy protective cover for you) will peel away and leave you unprotected against further burning. If you expose your body to enough burning rays, it will try to protect itself by making lots of new little cells in a crazy, cancerlike pattern. That's where the real trouble starts.

Actually it isn't the tanning that's the problem. It's the burning part that messes you up. Tanning of the right kind is your body's natural defense against sunburn. But tanning of the wrong kind—the kind that makes you lined and leathery, the kind that makes your skin look like a topographic map of the Andes Mountains—that kind of tanning is really dangerous. That kind of tanning, in fact, is what causes overexposed Australians and Texans and Floridians to look forty years old before they're twenty-five . . . and makes them look sixty-five well before they're past their fiftieth birthdays. The frightening thing is that a fifteen-year-old honey blond in a bikini or a twenty-five-year-old redhead on a ski slope can already have set the stage for sagging flesh at fifty or wrinkles at thirty-five if she hasn't taken care to protect herself.

See, your body has this charge account, this light memory. Your skin cells remember every tiny little bit of light they're exposed to from the day you were born. So every time you get a sunburn or a deep, thick, leathery tan, you are (in effect) saying, "Okay, skin: Charge it." Unfortunately, your skin doesn't send out monthly statements. It doesn't advise you of your balance. So there comes a time (usually all too suddenly) when you have to settle up.

I'm sitting here, in the park, in the sunshine, thinking: "Skin cancer. That's not much to look forward to." And neither are any of the other things that sunlight is going to do to my skin. Like making it look old twenty years before its time, or creating big, brown age spots, or destroying its substructure so that the top layer falls in like a skyscraper built on quicksand. It's not a pretty picture, any of it. And the worst part of all is that none of these awful things *has* to happen. Armed with a little information, a little perseverance and a small dose of fear, you need never worry about doing irreparable damage to your skin.

Danger: Pay Attention

The place to start is knowing who's in big trouble when. You're in greatest danger of wrecking your skin with sunlight if you're a redhead or a blond, or if you have really light skin with a tendency to freckle. Darker-skinned people have natural protection (not 100 percent protection), but Nordic types have to be especially careful. You compound your problems if you're out in the sun a lot, if you ski or play tennis, or sail, or if you live near the equator or high up on a mountain where the atmosphere is too thin to filter out most of the nasty ultraviolet rays. The closer you are to the equator or the higher you are on a mountaintop, the greater risk you run of painful (destructive) burning.

Sun intensity increases about 20% for every 1,000 meters of elevation. For instance, if you were going to ski from the top of Mt. Everest, and remain absolutely protected, you would have to triple the strength of your sea-level sun screen.
—BEDFORD SHELMIRE,
The Art of Being Beautiful

You're also in trouble if the time you spend in the sun is between 10 A.M. and 3 P.M., especially if you're just starting on your tan. The sun is strongest then; hottest; most dangerous.

Where you are, when you're there, what the weather's like and what you're wearing all effect the severity of your burn. So do natural sun reflectors and sun conductors that most of us never even think about. Sun reflectors like snow and sand and even grass bounce the burning rays back at you, increasing your chances of burning badly. Sun conductors let through more burning rays than you think they do; again, no protection.

Percentages of Sun Reflection

Fresh Snow	85%
Dry Sand	17%
Dry Grass	2.5%

Percentages of Sun Conduction

Beach Umbrella	50%
Clouds	30%–50%
Wet T-Shirt	20%–40%

Obviously there's more to this sun-care business than meets the eye. So what do you do? Do you lock yourself up in a closet and never come out? Hardly. Here are all sorts of things you can do to protect yourself:

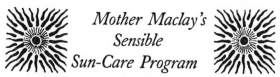

Mother Maclay's Sensible Sun-Care Program

1. You can be aware of the dangers and avoid them. Know when the sun's hottest and stay out of it. Realize that you can still burn on a cloudy day, or while you're swimming, or through the fabric of your beach umbrella. Accept the fact that your physical surroundings can be reflecting light and causing you problems. And never go outside without some sort of protection.

2. You can wear PHYSICAL PROTECTION like hats and gloves and caftans and sunglasses and zinc on your nose and the right kind of protective makeup. All these things physically block the sun's rays from burning your skin. And physical protection from light exposure is one of the major reasons the skin on your bottom looks younger than the skin on your face.

3. You can use a CHEMICAL SUN-BLOCK or a product with a chemical sun-block in it to cut off almost all of the burning rays. There are a host of chemical sun-blocks

around, most of them with long, complicated, unpronounceable names like benzophenone, iso-amyl, glyceryl, homosalate, conoxate, menthyl anthrarilate, digalloyl triolate and triethanolamine salicilate. The concensus of opinion among dermatologists and research chemists is that the most effective sun-block is something called PABA (which is short for para-aminobenzoic acid). Benzophenone runs a close second. Both PABA and benzophenone are gaining popularity and showing up in sun products all over the place. So read the labels . . . that's the first step to controlling your tan.

4. Even if you're not predisposed to burning, you should always use a sunscreen product. SUNSCREENS are for when you're safely past the paleface stage, not before, and you'll find them in lotions, gels, oils, creams and butters.

5. You can and should use an AFTER-TANNING product to stave off flaking and peeling and preserve your body's natural line of defense. After-tans also come in a wide range of formulas, but my friend Helen swears by vinegar. She adds a pint of cider vinegar (high in healing tannic acid) to her bath water and soaks the sting out. One Philadelphia doctor even suggests slathering sour cream all over your suntanned body as an after-tan measure. Personally, I'd rather have sour cream with strawberries.

6. You can cheat and get a SYNTHETIC TAN so you can look bronzed without ever having to set foot in the sun. Synthetic tanners work because they have a sugar called dihydroxyacetone (DHA, for short) in them, which combines with the amino acids in your skin's top layer to stain it temporarily brown. Synthetic tans last for several days, don't wash off, and are much safer than sunburn. Almost anything is safer than sunburn.

TOTAL BEAUTY CATALOG DIRECTORY OF WHO'S DOING WHAT ABOUT SUNCARE

SUN BLOCKS

MANUFACTURER	PRODUCT	SIZE	APPROX. PRICE *
Almay	Sun Block Gel	1 oz.	$1.75
Bonne Bell	Sun Block	2 oz.	$2.00
Clinique	Sun Block	2.5 oz.	$5.00
Coppertone	Super Shade	4 oz.	$3.50
Doak Pharmacal	Solar Cream	1 oz.	$3.37
Dome Laboratories	Uval Lotion	2.64 oz.	$2.85
Estée Lauder	Ultra Violet Screening Creme	2 oz.	$5.00
Germaine Monteil	Super-Moist Sun Block	4 oz.	$4.50
Irma Shorell	Sun Sensitive Creme	1.9 oz.	$6.00
Person & Covey	Sol-Bar	2.5 oz.	$3.25
Key West Fragrance and Cosmetic Factory **	PABA Absolute Sun-Screen	1 oz.	$2.75
Key West Fragrance ** and Cosmetic Factory	PABA Absolute Sun-Screen	1 oz.	$2.75
	Waterproof Fishermens Absolute Sunscreen	2 oz.	$3.50
Sea & Ski	Block Out	2 oz.	$2.25
Texas Pharmacal	A-Fil Cream	1.5 oz.	$1.95

* IMPORTANT NOTE: All prices are approximate and subject to change without notice.

** For mail order information and pamphlet, "How to Get a Good Suntan," write:
Key West Fragrance and Cosmetic Factory
P.O. Box 1643
528 Front Street
Key West, Florida 33040

SOMETHING TO THINK ABOUT

Your skin responds as a total unit. Because it's an organ, injury to one small area will affect the whole system. When you injure an area of your skin and it's unable to perform its vital functions, the UNinjured skin will increase what it's doing until the injured part heals. Healthy skin has a limit to the amount of extra work it can carry on, so if too large an area is out of commission, the healthy skin will collapse along with the injured part.

Special Sunscreens For Lips, Ears, Nose and So On

MANUFACTURER	PRODUCT	SIZE	APPROX. PRICE
ALO Cosmetics	ALO Lip Shield	.15 oz.	$1.25
Caswell-Massey *	Hamol Ultra Lipstick		$3.00
Christian Dior	Lipgloss with Sunscreen		$3.50
Coppertone	Lipkote by Coppertone	.22 oz.	$ .49
	Nosekote by Coppertone	7/16 oz.	$1.09
Elizabeth of Sweden	CARIB-TAN Save-a-Lip	.12 oz.	$2.00
Fabergé	LipSlick Lip Gloss		$2.00
Frances Denney	Lip Moisturizer		$3.50
Miller Morton	ChapStick Lip Balm	.15 oz.	$ .59
Physicians' Formula	Protective Lip Care		$1.50
Sea & Ski	Snootie Extra Protective Cream	1 oz.	$1.25
	Lip Savers (Flavored)		$ .59

* For complete Caswell-Massey catalog and mail order information write:
  Caswell-Massey Ltd.
  320 West 13th Street
  New York, New York 10013
  Send $1.00

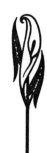

| Shiseido | Dewy Satin Lip Emollient Stick | .15 oz. | $4.00 |
| Texas Pharmacal ** | SunStick | | $1.24 |

Sunscreens (for Medium Protection)

MANUFACTURER	PRODUCT	SIZE	APPROX. PRICE
Alexandra de Markoff	Allevia Sunscreen	6 oz.	$5.00
Almay	Full Filter Sun Lotion	6 oz.	$4.00
ALO Cosmetics	Fashion Tan	4 oz.	$3.75
Bain de Soleil (for extra protection)	Bain de Soleil (WHITE)	3⅛ oz.	$2.50
	Bain de Soleil Super Filter Suntan Lotion	4 oz.	$2.50
Caswell-Massey	Ultra-Sunscreen PABA	8 oz.	$5.00
Clinique	Suntan Encourager	5 oz.	$5.00
Coppertone	Shade Suntan Lotion	2 oz.	$1.49
Doak Pharmacal	Derma Pack Sunscreen	⅞ oz.	$2.25
Elizabeth Arden	Sun Shielding Cream	3.5 oz.	$3.50
Estée Lauder	Moisturizing Sun Lotion (tinted)	5 oz.	$4.50
Fabergé	"Great Skin" Day Care Moisturizer with NMC-12	4 oz.	$4.00

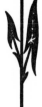

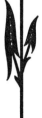

** For booklet SUN & CONSEQUENCES write:
    Texas Pharmacal Company
    P.O. Box 1659
    San Antonio, Texas 78296

Helena Rubinstein	High Protection	4 oz.	$5.00
Irma Shorell	Moisture/Tan Formula	1.9 oz.	$6.00
Leeming/Pacquin	Swedish Tanning Secret for Sun Tan and Protection	4 oz.	$1.75
Princess Marcella Borghese	Super Sensitive Face Cream	2 oz.	$5.00
Sea & Ski	Sea & Ski Suntan Lotion	2 oz.	$1.10
Ultima II	Highly Protective Tanning Lotion	8 oz.	$4.50

After-Sun Specials

MANUFACTURER	PRODUCT	SIZE	APPROX. PRICE
ALO Cosmetics	After Tan	4 oz.	$3.75
AR-EX Products	Chap Cream	4 oz.	$3.00
Bain del Soleil	Apres le Soleil	8 oz.	$2.50
Elizabeth of Sweden	CARIB-TAN After Tan Lotion	4 oz.	$4.50
Charles of the Ritz	Weather Rescue Cream	6 oz.	$6.00
Coppertone	Tan Care by Coppertone	6 oz.	$2.50
Estée Lauder	Apres Sun	5 oz.	$4.50
Germaine Monteil	Super-Moist After Sun Soother	8 oz.	$5.00
Orlane	Astrale Solaire	1.2 oz.	$7.50
Texas Pharmacal	Lubriderm Lotion	4 oz.	$1.55
Ultima II	Moisture Replacement Lotion	8 oz.	$5.00

Synthetic Tanners

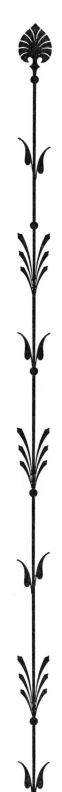

MANUFACTURER	PRODUCT	SIZE	APPROX. PRICE
Coppertone	QT Quick Tanning Lotion (w/sunscreen)	4 oz.	$1.69
	Sudden Tan Bronzing Lotion	4 oz.	$3.25
Sea & Ski	Indoor/Outdoor Tanning Lotion	4 oz.	$2.80

Bronzers To Be Used Instead of Makeup or With It, or To Get That Finished Look While You're Really Tanning

MANUFACTURER	PRODUCT	SIZE	APPROX. PRICE
Almay	Near Nude Bronzing Gel	3 oz.	$4.25
Bain de Soleil	Bain de Soleil Bronzer	2 oz.	$3.00
Bonne Bell	Bronze Glo	3 oz.	$3.50
Clinique	Bronze Gel Makeup	2 oz.	$7.50
Estée Lauder	Go-Bronze	2 oz.	$5.00
Fabergé	Bronze Baby	4 oz.	$2.50
	Tigress Body Bronzer	3.5 oz.	$2.50
Love Cosmetics	Love's Face Gel	1.13 oz.	$2.00
Orlane	Maqui Bronze	1.3 oz.	$5.00

*Sunburn is very becoming—but only
when it is even—one must be very
careful not to look like a mixed grill.*
—NOEL COWARD,
"The Lido Beach"

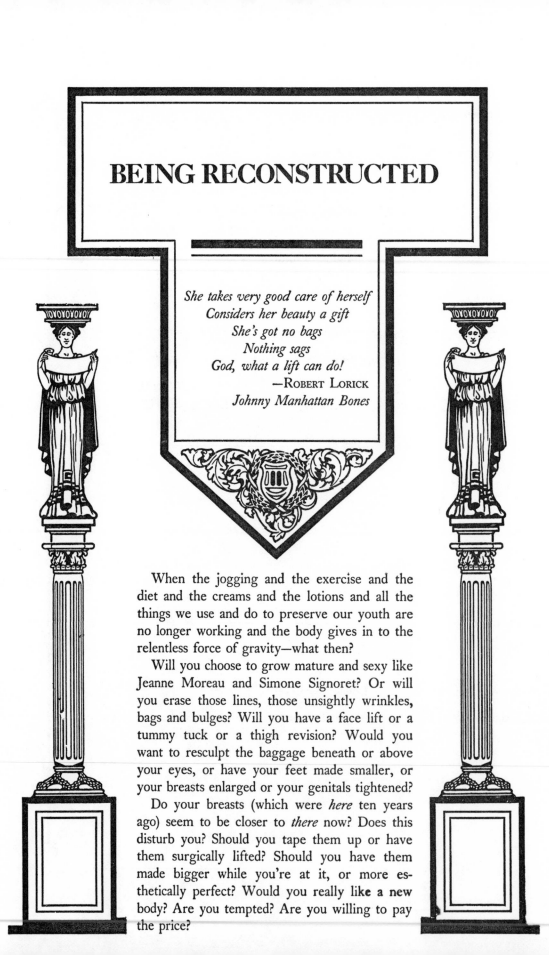

BEING RECONSTRUCTED

She takes very good care of herself
Considers her beauty a gift
She's got no bags
Nothing sags
God, what a lift can do!
—ROBERT LORICK
Johnny Manhattan Bones

When the jogging and the exercise and the diet and the creams and the lotions and all the things we use and do to preserve our youth are no longer working and the body gives in to the relentless force of gravity—what then?

Will you choose to grow mature and sexy like Jeanne Moreau and Simone Signoret? Or will you erase those lines, those unsightly wrinkles, bags and bulges? Will you have a face lift or a tummy tuck or a thigh revision? Would you want to resculpt the baggage beneath or above your eyes, or have your feet made smaller, or your breasts enlarged or your genitals tightened?

Do your breasts (which were *here* ten years ago) seem to be closer to *there* now? Does this disturb you? Should you tape them up or have them surgically lifted? Should you have them made bigger while you're at it, or more esthetically perfect? Would you really like a new body? Are you tempted? Are you willing to pay the price?

Can you *afford* to be replaced, repaired, re-sculpted, remolded, remade? Can you afford *not* to? Will a replacement you that looks better than the original improve your market value? Will it make keeping your job, or finding a new job, easier for you? Will it lift your spirits and buoy your confidence?

Each day at lunch, or over cocktails, or at coffee-break time in the office, there are new and thrilling tales of operations, dishy gossip or proud reports from people who think of plastic surgery not as a last resort ... but as a sensible alternative, or merely necessary maintenance.

My friends have all had plastic surgery. I know at least three women and one man who've had their eyes tucked. It's tough to find an original nose in my peer group. New chins are popping up like crocus in springtime. Josanne had her nose, eyes and chin done last year. Next year she's going back for cheekbones. Elsa had her rear end rearranged in Rio. Barbara has new, smaller, more attractive breasts. Luciana Avedon says there's a midget in Rome who's constructed completely from the fat plastic surgeons removed from one prominent socialite.

Everybody's doing it. The walls ring with incidents. Plastic surgeons' names are traded with an enthusiasm we once reserved for swapping baseball cards ... and the question on everybody's minds, if not already at the tips of their tongues, is: Can any of us afford to grow gracefully old anymore?

Phyllis Diller Says "Do It!"

Phyllis Diller decided, after seeing herself on television, that a new face was definitely in order:

"I did a Sonny & Cher show and I saw a close-up of me that I'd never seen before. I was wearing a dog-collar necklace and my neck hung out over it like a horrible growth. And the bags under my eyes had reached the point of no return. So I called my skin specialist and said I wanted to have a face lift. Actually, I did it to protect the public."

Miss Diller had everything done ... everything except her forehead. "I had nothing wrong with my forehead, but my nose was in very bad shape because of a very bad accident I had when I was younger. So that was the major thing. The doctor did three things to my nose. He straightened a deviated septum, opened the closed side, and shortened it. The rest was a straight lift. He lifted the chin and the face, took out all the extra skin and sewed it all back together. Plastic surgeons call it redraping. They literally take it down and put it back up like window dressers.

"It took about a year for my face to be completely healed and one side was numb for about six months, but I'm fearless. I trust. I have great faith ... and I don't panic about things like that. If I had one thing to say to anybody about having a face lift, I'd say—it's great ... I'd say DO IT!"

❧ Stop! ❧
Take This Important Test

Stand in front of a mirror. Place your index and forefingers on each side of your face, just below the temples—in the hairline. Now, lift up and back toward the crown of your head. If you like what you see, you'll probably be fascinated with the following diary of what happens during an actual face lift.

The Exciting Story of My Operation

by Stephen Lewis *

It began (not the operation, but the reason for it) in Detroit, where I was taping Lou Gordon's syndicated talk show. During a break that would later be filled by a commercial, I glanced at the monitor and saw, in the most literal sense, a side of myself that I'd never seen before—a full

* Over ten million copies of Stephen Lewis's books have been sold, and his works have been translated into eleven languages. His most recent novel is *The Best Sellers*, published in July 1976 by Fawcett/Gold Medal.

profile. The break ended, the cameraman changed his angle (the *real* me, I told myself) and the taping continued.

"What's the matter?" Lou's very attractive wife asked me when it was over.

"I'm the matter," I answered. "I never realized I looked so terrible!" I explained about what I'd glimpsed, mercifully briefly, on the monitor.

"You look fine," Jackie insisted. "You've seen yourself on TV before. You've done lots of shows—"

It was true that I'd made about four hundred stops along the talk-show trail, trying to plug my books, be an interesting person and look good. At that moment I was convinced that while I might have done all right at plugging and being interesting, I'd probably looked awful—at least in profile. I couldn't even tell myself that I knew it wasn't true, since I never watch myself on TV, listen to myself on the radio or read my own books, just on general principle.

A few days later I was seated across the desk from Dr. Louis Parrish, a terrific man who has kept me reasonably sane and surprisingly healthy for several years, describing what had by then become my "traumatic experience."

"You know what you look like," Dr. Parrish said. "And you *know* that you don't think you're a bad-looking man."

I didn't disagree, but I explained that I thought I looked like two different people: *me* from the front, and someone else from the side. I had to admit that from the front I'd done all right, modeling clothes as a teenager when I came to New York, and then writing about how to look good (at one very diversified and understaffed publishing company, I'd been the sports and beauty editor, responsible for both baseball and hairstyle magazines; at the height of the season, I was so overworked that I practically had Mickey Mantle giving tips on washes and sets!).

The office visit ended with my asking Dr. Parrish to recommend a plastic surgeon. He did,

reminding me that (1) I'd just been on a long road trip, was very tired and shouldn't rush into anything; and (2) plastic surgeons like to be called cosmetic surgeons, just in case I was going to rush. I called the "cosmetic" surgeon for an appointment.

As I waited, two weeks later (cosmetic surgeons book very far in advance; the "early" two-week consultation appointment was a favor), I remembered people I'd known in high school. There had been several Donna Donazettis and Marilyn Birnbaums who had gone away on mysterious two-week "vacations" and returned with bobbed noses so identical they might have come from a mail-order catalog. Then, too, there was the girl who went swimming too soon—the nose job and the high diving board had met with disastrous results. I *liked* my looks—from the front, anyway—and I was a man. What, I asked myself, was I doing at the plastic/cosmetic surgeon's?

Common sense provided part of the answer.

I was doing just what I'd done for several long, painful months in the dentist's office when I'd had my teeth capped—namely, facing the reality that looks are important in our society, particularly in terms of a public career. The rest of the answer was provided by the doctor.

"I want my same nose," I explained. "I want to look the same way I do now, only from the side . . ."

He seemed to understand, and told me that it was a matter of "refinement" of the nose (it wasn't shortened, just thinned) and a silicone implant in my chin. He told me that it wouldn't hurt, that people wouldn't know I'd had it done (I guess I've blown that one) and that it would cost about a thousand dollars, give or take a few hundred . . . give, I think.

I was told to make an appointment with a medical photographer, a man whose talent lies in taking merciless pictures in which the head is aligned with something called the Hamburg (or was it Frankfurt? or Buchenwald?) plane. No retouching, no flattering lighting. The medical photographer makes his counterparts at the driver's license and passport offices look like Avedon!

I went back, embarrassing photographs in hand, to the cosmetic surgeon's. I was told that I'd have to be in the hospital for two and a half days, and that the doctor was booked up for several months. If I liked, I could have my name placed on a standby list. I stood by, and someone must have chickened out: I went to the hospital.

One of my weaknesses is the delusion that Dr. Joe Gannon of "Medical Center" cannot perform an operation unless I'm watching the television. Another delusion that comes from watching television is the one that all hospitals look like "Medical Center." Suffice it to say that when I checked into one of Manhattan's most prestigious (and oldest—it goes with the prestige) hospitals, my first thought was whether or not I would get time off for good behavior.

I'd also thought about being very noble and having the operation secretly. One look at the private room I'd asked for (it looked like solitary) convinced me that I'd rather have flowers than be noble. As a result, I spent every moment from the time I checked in till the time I went into surgery (the following day, at noon) on the phone and/or visiting.

Of the operation itself, I remember very little—not surprising in view of a Seconal, another less identifiable pill and an injection. I remember waking up in the operating room, hearing construction- (or destruction-) like noises that seemed to be coming from the general area of my face, and hearing the doctor say that it was almost over.

I woke up bandaged and stoned, and went back to sleep.

Then I woke up bandaged and hurting. There was no pain in my nose. As a matter of fact, there was no feeling at all, since during its "refinement" my nose had been packed with cocaine ... oh, well. But my chin—where an incision about half an inch long had been made and a small silicone implant had been inserted,

sutured to the bone for "anchoring," and then been sewn up—hurt, quite frankly, like a son of a bitch.

The pain would have been better managed had I told the doctor that I had a very high tolerance to medication. He later told me that I had the highest tolerance of any patient he remembered—which explained why I couldn't sleep, couldn't eat the mush (you don't open your mouth too much right after a chin implant) I was fed, and couldn't do anything except ache. The doctor said I should have told him that I took sleeping medication regularly, and he was probably right. On the other hand, I thought he should have asked. Come to think of it, I also thought about Ann-Margret, who'd fallen during her nightclub act around this time, and of how she glowingly told the press how her husband, Roger Smith, had made liquid pizza. Ann-Margret had a broken jaw through no fault of her own; I had a numb nose and an aching chin because I'd asked for it. And I didn't have Roger Smith making me liquid pizzas—just a nurse giving me mush and telling me that even though I hurt and couldn't sleep, she couldn't give me any medication ... any *more* medication, that is.

I must admit that on the night after my operation, I decided at 3:45 in the morning that I'd rather be miserable at home and got dressed, leaving the hospital in a blaze of bandages, mink and Vuitton. I should also admit that I had a black eye—a shiner the likes of which I hadn't seen since Roy Stuckey and I fought it out to the finish in seventh grade, and which I was to see in the mirror for the next three months. Hemotomas (black eyes, hospital-style) frequently accompany nose "refinements."

A day later, the bandages came off. I didn't think I looked any different, except that my hair was filthy and I hadn't shaved (at least I had an excuse). After a few days, the stitches came out of my chin and the pain subsided. But I made a big mistake.

My own attitude, reinforced by the doctor,

had allowed for physical discomfort, but not for the factor of stress, in emotional terms. My body mended, but my nerves were shot to hell. As I recuperated, not feeling lousy, really, but not feeling well, I was depressed. I was a bastard to everyone I knew, and particularly to those I loved. The only defense I have is that I couldn't help it: During surgery, even relatively minor, elective surgery such as mine, the body is the victim of physical trauma. The mind reacts. Nobody told me, but I later saw the same thing happen to friends who had cosmetic surgery.

Be prepared . . . and prepare your friends.

The swelling went down. The black eye lingered, and when, a few weeks later, over dinner, the plastic (the hell with "cosmetic") surgeon told me that it looked awful, I left the restaurant rather than stomp him.

But now I look like the same man from the side (better) and the front (the same as it was). I don't have to be conscious of camera angles when I do TV guest shots, which lets me be myself, such as I am. The change isn't dramatic, but then I didn't want dramatic change . . . I wanted to look like myself, only more so. The black eye is gone.

No, most of my friends and relatives don't even know I had the operation, except for those I told. I had a few follow-up visits with the doctor that included some injections directly into my nose, which sounds worse than it is and helps reduce swelling. I cut the scar under my chin when shaving at first, then nicked it, but now I don't even know that it—or the implant—is there.

Several of my friends, men as well as women, have had work done, ranging from nose refinements to face lifts, and I think all of us feel more comfortable with ourselves, which is what any form of self-improvement is all about. The successful author in my most recent novel, *The Best Sellers* (Fawcett/Gold Medal), had everything from her face to her behind lifted—the author's form of catharsis, I suppose.

Would I do it again?

When the time comes, I will. At twenty-eight, I'm not too worried about the eventuality of the need for a face lift or eye job, but I've found a way to minimize (I think) those worry lines and wrinkles that stem from tension. I've left New York and moved to Houston, Texas, in the hope (realized) of a more relaxed, laid-back life-style.

And Houston, when the time comes, has the world's best cosmetic surgeons.

YOU DON'T HAVE TO WAIT TILL YOU LOOK AWFUL

Top Dermatologist Talks About Plastic Surgery

Dr. Norman Orentreich (associate clinical professor of dermatology at New York University School of Medicine, medical director of the Orentreich Medical Group and director of the Orentreich Foundation for the Advancement of Science, which is involved in dermatologic research and research on aging) is interviewed for the *Total Beauty Catalog* by Dianne Partie (registered nurse, medical writer and frequent contributor to *Vogue* and *Mademoiselle*).

DIANNE PARTIE: *You've told me that when you refer patients to plastic surgeons, you try to match the personality to the need. Can you tell me more about that?*

DR. ORENTREICH: I try to match personality *as well as* need, so the personalities mesh and the patient's need and the doctor's skill mesh. And I find, interestingly enough, that personality is as important as ability, because almost all doctors are equally well trained.

DP: *But you feel that communication is really important . . .*

DR. O: Yes, there are some patients who say, "I just want someone who's technically competent . . . and I want to be able to relate to the physician and have confidence in him."

People vary considerably in what they need. Now, my feeling has always been to match them up. There are some doctors who are very conservative—vest-wearers, inside and outside. There are others who are very easygoing, and they relate to a patient that way. Now if you take a patient who is very formal and has lived a very formal type of life, you'll try to match her with someone who (when she visits his office) will make her feel comfortable.

If you send someone who lives a very casual life-style to someone who's lived a very conservative, rigid form of life, she'll feel uncomfortable in his presence.

What I'll frequently do is send a patient to two doctors. I'll always give her a choice. I think that's a good thing to do in surgery anyway ... I think you SHOULD see two doctors as often as possible.

DP: *While we're on the subject, are there specific things you ought to do or to think about before you even consult the first surgeon? Things beyond just saying, "I want my face lifted," for example.*

DR. O: That's a difficult thing for people to conceive, because they tend to look at their noses and say, "I want my nose fixed," but sometimes they need their chins brought forward and they can leave their noses alone. And sometimes they say, "I want a face lift," when all they really need is the bags under their eyes removed or some silicone to soften their nasolabial folds.

People considering plastic surgery should try to pinpoint what bothers them cosmetically. In their own minds, they should try to analyze why they want this. Is it just to be more attractive (which is perfectly acceptable) or is it for job security, or because they want to get married? They may have to do something very small to get what they want.

You look at a woman's face, and sometimes you just remove the bags from the lower lids and you'll correct her appearance. Do a face lift, a dermabrasion, and silicone—and skip the eyes, and you'll goof the thing up, or vice versa.

I've seen patients go through eyelid surgery, through face-lift surgery, and say, "Gee, I look old." That's because their skin is like a cloth which has been tightened on their faces, but it hasn't been resurfaced. And if they had only one dermabrasion they'd look considerably better.

I think the mature woman (and I've seen a lot of mature women over the past thirty years in medicine) who looks for help should be aware of some basic concepts of the mature face: The skin of the head, unlike many other tissues of the body, continues to grow as you grow older. Your hands don't get very much bigger, your legs don't get very much bigger, your head doesn't get very much bigger, but the skin of your head is one or two sizes bigger than your head needs to be. It's like wearing a dress.

DP: *And that's not just stretching of the skin?*

DR. O: No. It's growth. It's not the effects of gravity (which many people think it is). Gravity manifests it, demonstrates it, but it's not being caused by it. In fact, there are some animals like the rhino mouse, which starts out as a perfectly normal mouse and as it gets older, its head becomes so large with skin that it's called a rhino because the skin is all wrinkled (like a rhino's) over its head. This characteristic of aging happens in many species. And in human beings, if you look at them carefully, you realize that their skin has become larger. What actually happens (without your realizing it) is that it thins slightly and gets a broader surface area. Like taking a lump of dough and flattening it out. The reason you don't notice this thinning is that the fat layer underneath the skin thickens; that's why people look pudgy. But if you have a person who's not pudgy and look at the skin, you realize you can do very little for it except redraping. And face-lifting is redraping the skin.

Another thing that happens with maturity and aging is a loss of tissues in certain areas of the body: below the eye bag, right on top of the cheek. Many people get a depression between the corner of the nose and the corner of the mouth which is caused by both loss of tissue and muscle-skin forces, and causes a folding which produces a bend and more tissue loss. That loss of tissue can't be replaced by anything but augmentation with something like pure, medical-grade silicone.

The third thing you have to realize is that the surface of the face gets more exposure to the elements than anything else. You must realize that all the time you're outside, sun and weather work on your skin, and it begins to show changes we interpret as aging. These are basically upper-third-of-the-skin changes. And to correct the damage you really need to resurface that skin by dermabrasion.

So all three of these procedures—redraping, replacing lost tissue and resurfacing—can be done for the same person, and all make for terrific improvements. Yet when I look at someone's head, I realize that one of these procedures, if it is done first, will do more good than the others, and that in some people one or two of these procedures will do very little good. Now sometimes you'll say, "Do all three," and sometimes you'll say to someone, "Well, you don't really need a face lift, you need a new surface." Or someone will come to you for dermabrasion and you'll say, "You really have a nice skin, what you really have is loose skin; it's redundant; we have to redrape it." Or you'll say to someone, "Your skin isn't bad, it's really firm. But what you have is a hollow under your cheek that

needs to be filled in to give you a nice contour. The deep area between your eyes and the globella area make you look like you're frowning all the time. It makes you look old. A few injections of silicone will correct that."

So many times you have to look at a face and realize that it's a caricature. And caricatures are an excellent way of demonstrating what I mean. With a few lines you can see a whole face; that's true of most people. Certain things stand out. A good surgeon who has cosmetic concepts in mind looks at a head and says, "What is the LEAST I can do to make that individual look best?"

Now, that doesn't mean you can't do one, two, three or four things for them, but most people have economic limitations and, more important, time limitations. I find that many people say, "I'd love to do the surgery, but I can't take two weeks off." So you want to do for that patient first what will give her the biggest lift . . . I'm talking about EMOTIONAL lift. And later on you can do the other things. Something else you have to realize is that you'll get a very disappointed patient if you do the very best face lift and what she needs is dermabrasion, and vice versa.

DP: *People in the New York area have dermatologists like you available to them. But what does the person do who's not living in a major center like this?*

DR. O: I think she herself has to look at herself and say, "How will I look if I wear a lot of makeup? Now I don't like a lot of makeup, but let's say I put a lot of makeup on my face to cover up all the brown, all the fine wrinkles, all the little blood vessels, all the light spots, all the dark spots—so that I wasn't multicolored anymore . . . Just what would that do?"

One of the things that happens with aging is that your skin doesn't have a uniform color. Look at babies; their skin is all one color. But look at an older man or woman and you've got light areas, you've got dark areas, you've got pink areas, gray areas ... And it's the mottling appearance that gives the appearance of aging. So if you put an artificial surface on your face and say, "How do I look?" and say, "Gee, I look great and I'd like to have that look without makeup, and I really think I'd like myself that way ..." Then I'd say, "Do a dermabrasion."

If you look at someone and you put a strong light source over the head, the person might say, "I look AWFUL. I look tired, my nasolabial folds are very marked..." Now those are the lines that you can wash right out with silicone. You bring them out of the shadows. It's the shadow that you see. The caricature. Don't grab your face in front of a mirror and pull from your cheeks. Put your fingers in front of your ears and pull up and back—that's how you're going to look after a face lift. All a face lift can do is work from this area. So if you do that, you can in a sense duplicate the effect. So these are the things, the sorts of things you can do at home to determine whether you need a face lift, silicone or dermabrasion.

DP: *To change the subject just a little, can I ask what kind of procedures most models have done?*

DR. O: Most models come in for contour correction and skin resurfacing. By the time they're with a major model agency, they don't need their noses fixed, they don't need their chins straightened—they wouldn't have gotten to that point if they did. They come to me either for hair care, or because they start to break out. But the biggest thing I think I do for models from the point of view of helping them over the years is erase shadows. Some models, even at a very young age, under lights will throw shadows in certain areas—between the eyes,

under the eyes, the nasolabial folds, that sort of thing. You know, thirty is young, but for a model thirty is a very difficult time, and it's very possible to extend the useful working life span of a model for a decade or more by the appropriate, judicious use of corrective procedures to replace lost tissues, to resurface the skin.

DP: *Is there any such thing as preventive plastic surgery? If I have my eyes done now, does that mean they won't get wrinkled?*

DR. O: No. There is preventive skin care and there are preventive things you can do ... For example, I think you can reduce the wrinkles on your face by having a less expressive face. The enigmatic Asian is a case in point. I think that people who don't raise their eyebrows, who don't squint or otherwise show extreme expressions, will not show as many wrinkles. Generally smokers who hold cigarettes in their lips will get wrinkling above the upper lip more often than people who don't smoke, or who don't hold their cigarettes that way. People who have worried looks end up with *frozen* worried looks.

Men have a very effective method of preventing early signs of aging. They shave. Have you ever noticed how an older man will have very soft skin where he shaves? Well, he's doing a microdermabrasion every day. Women can get the same result with epidermabrasion ... By using something as simple as the Buf-Puf, a woman can literally remove some of the very early damage changes. But that's about the only way I know that's truly preventive.

I would say a woman should have a cosmetic procedure done when she's ready for it. When the morbidity of the operation, when the time spent, the money spent and the risks inherent during the surgery and the degree of her incapacitation warrants her doing it. She needn't put it off until she's worse. That much I will say. You don't have to wait till you look awful.

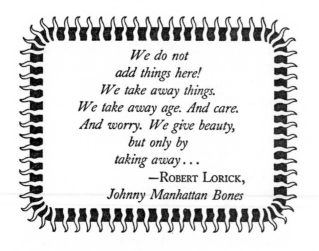

*We do not
add things here!
We take away things.
We take away age. And care.
And worry. We give beauty,
but only by
taking away...*
—ROBERT LORICK,
Johnny Manhattan Bones

THE OPERATIONS

No longer is cosmetic surgery a nifty nose job or a fabulous face lift. It's everything. Dr. Robert Allyn Franklin, for instance, who plys his plastic surgery trade in a futuristic Los Angeles beauty pavilion designed by the architect of Brasilia, recently advertised the following forty-eight hour beauty weekend:

Arrive Friday, have your nose bobbed, bags under your eyes removed, wrinkles erased, size and firmness of breasts taken care of, and be back home before the weekend is over. Price: $2,500.

A competent plastic surgeon can (for a price, and the price varies widely) correct drooping upper eyelids, baggy lower eyelids, double chins, crepey skin or dewlapped necks, pendulous breasts, sagging bellies, jodhpur thighs and drooping buttocks. And that is just the beginning. The thing to remember is that the discomfort, expense and difficulties tend to increase as you work your way down the body. Eyelid operations are the simplest, and the ones involving breasts, bellies, thighs and buttocks are the most difficult.

Dr. Ivo Pitanguay said of his patients, "The youngest group comes in for nose or acne, the oldest for face-lifting, and in between are the breasts and the bellies." Whatever category you fall into, here's what the cosmetic surgeons can do for you:

Feature	Problem	Cost	Operation Time	Hospital Stay	Scars
eyes	drooping upper lid	$500–$2,500	4 hours	outpatient, 24 hours, or 2 days	hidden in natural fold under brow bone or underneath bottom lashes
	baggage beneath	$2,000			
eyebrows	drooping eyebrow	$800–$1,750			
ears	Mickey Mouse or protruding	$500–$1,500	1 hour	24 hours or 2 days	behind ear or inside it
nose	bumpy, large, small, short, long, thin, fat, crooked, wide, etc.	$500–$2,500	2 hours	3–5 days	inside nostrils

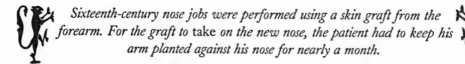

Sixteenth-century nose jobs were performed using a skin graft from the forearm. For the graft to take on the new nose, the patient had to keep his arm planted against his nose for nearly a month.

chin	weak or small (augmentation)	$250–$1,000	1 hour	office visit	underneath or inside
	reduction of protruding chin	$1,000–$2,500	1–3 hours	1–2 days	inside mouth
	double chin	$500–$1,000	1 hour	1–2 days	underneath
face	Total	$2,500–$5,500	4 hours	3–7 days	hairline and ears
	Partial	$1,000–$1,250	various	3–5 days or outpatient	
neck	crepey/wattled	$1,000	2 hours	3–5 days	in hairline at nape of neck

BUYER BEWARE: TIJUANA SILICONE ROT

According to Rae Lindsay (The Pursuit of Youth), *some unscrupulous Mexican doctors use industrial silicone injections to enlarge breasts. This silicone (which costs about 20¢ a gallon and is otherwise used for floor waxes, adhesives and water-repellant coatings) is highly dangerous and causes ugly complications, not the least of which include amputation, strokes, blindness, gangrene and death.*

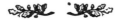

breasts	drooping (lift)	$500–$1,500	3 hours	3–5 days	underneath
	small (enlarge)	$500–$2,500	2 hours	outpatient, overnight	underneath
	too big (decrease)	$750–$2,000	2 hours	2 days	around nipple and beneath breast
stomach	slack	$1,000–$4,500	2 hours, general anesthesia	7–10 days	bikini line
waistline	love handles	$1,000–$2,000	2–3 hours, general anesthesia	7–10 days	like belt at waist
thighs (outer)	breeches	$1,500–$2,500	2–3 hours	7–10 days	below bikini line
thighs (inner)	heavy	$1,000–$3,000	2–4 hours	7–10 days	zigzag from knee to groin
bottoms	lackluster	$2,000	2 hours	7–10 days	in fold of buttocks
hands	wrinkled	$400–$800	1 hour	1–2 days	pinky side or in bracelet line
arms	batwings	$500–$2,000	1 hour	outpatient, 24 hours	armpit to elbow
genitals	tightening	$750–$3,000	2 hours	7–10 days	not where you'd notice

INTRIGUED? INTERESTED? WHAT TO READ BEFORE YOU SEE THE DOCTOR

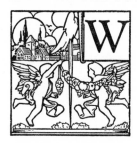

Want to find out more about plastic surgery? Get right over to the library, then, cause there are bunches of really excellent books on the subject. And the more you know about what goes on, and how the operations are done, and how much they cost, and how long they last, the better prepared you'll be to find your own plastic surgeon and ask the right questions. Reviews of the best books I've seen on the subject are listed for a variety of reasons. Some are here because they are good general reference works, or because, while the *whole* book doesn't necessarily deal with plastic surgery, it does include a section or information that directly relates to the subject.

Body Sculpture—Beauty Surgery

by Simona Morini
Delacorte Press (Hardcover, $10)

Simona Morini holds a doctorate in classical philology from the University of Rome. She's been a translator, a journalist and a language teacher, and she's written what has come to be a classic work on cosmetic surgery. She describes advances in and the current status of cosmetic surgery with compassion and warmth, and she's managed to unearth solid, detailed, interesting information as well as interviewing fifteen plastic surgeons, giving us case histories of nose, hand, ear, oral, face, breast, thigh and abdomen patients, and much much more.

Consultation With a Plastic Surgeon

by Ralph Leslie Dicker, M.D., and
Victor Royce Syracuse, M.D.
Nelson-Hall
(Chicago; Hardcover, $9.95)

This is the best $10 investment you can make if you're interested in getting all your questions answered *before* you visit a plastic surgeon. *Consultation with a Plastic Surgeon* is presented in a question-and-answer format just the way a meeting with a plastic surgeon would be carried on. There seem to be thousands of questions (questions that were actually asked by hundreds of thousands of plastic-surgery patients) and Drs. Dicker and Syracuse answer all of them frankly and clearly, and go so far as to include prices as well.

How to Win in the Youth Game: The Magic of Plastic Surgery

by Kurt Wagner, M.D., and Helen Gould
Prentice-Hall (Hardcover, $7.95)

A beautifully written book, *How to Win in the Youth Game* manages to blend the poetic, the philosophical and the utterly practical into a book that's both fun and reassuring to read. An excellent source book for the literarily inclined, Dr. Wagner and Ms. Gould discuss principles, techniques, costs, benefits and risks involved in ALL types of plastic surgery. Naturally, they cover such familiar surgical procedures as work on the eyes, nose, chin, face and hairline—but they also talk about treatment for more interesting problems, like how stomachs sagging from weight loss or any other reason can be tightened up, how protruding ears can be pinned back and how flabby arms can be slimmed down. Eighty-five before and after photographs, plus numerous line drawings showing surgical procedures, put *How to Win in the Youth Game* in the profusely illustrated category.

The Youth Doctors

by Patrick McGrady
Coward, McCann & Geoghegan
(Out of Print)

This book is out of print now, but my friend Parker, who writes lots of medical-type articles for a magazine called *Moneysworth*, says he thinks *The Youth Doctors* is one of his best sources for technical plastic surgery information . . . so rush to your library and look it up.

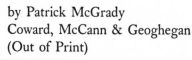

The Miracle of Cosmetic Plastic Surgery

by Richard B. Aronsohn, M.D., and
Richard A. Epstein, Ph.D.
Sherbourne Press
(Los Angeles; Hardcover, $12.50)

This book doesn't fool around—no namby-pamby line drawings here. *The Miracle of Cosmetic Plastic Surgery* is full of the scariest postoperative, prerecuperation photographs I've ever seen.

Plastic Surgery: Beauty You Can Buy

by Harriet La Barre
Holt, Rhinehart and Winston
(Hardcover, $5.95)

Award-winning writer Harriet La Barre explains each operation step by step: the techniques involved, extent of scarring, length of treatment, amount of pain and possible complications. Like, she tells you how much weight to lose before a face-lift operation and why; how to care for your skin afterward to make the results last longer (the bad news is that face lifts aren't permanent) and how to cope with such worrisome problems as what will my family and friends say?

Ms. La Barre also gives special attention to teenagers and their plastic surgery problems, including the right age for each operation, parents' attitudes and qualms and the perplexing When should you, when shouldn't you? questions. Acne, the numero-uno teenage beauty problem, also gets discussed in depth, with particular emphasis on dermabrasion (which is literally planing the top layer of skin to reveal a new, smoother layer underneath). According to Ms. La Barre, it's the most successful and least known method for curing or inhibiting acne.

Did you know . . .

- The operation for a relatively receding chin takes fifteen minutes and some nose corrections take only forty-five minutes to do?

- Wrinkles on an upper lip can be erased in a five-minute operation?

- Hospital insurance very often covers reducing an oversized bosom?

If not, it's all covered in *Plastic Surgery: Beauty You Can Buy.*

Doctor Make Me Beautiful!

by Dr. James W. Smith and
Samm Sinclair Baker
David McKay Company (Hardcover, $7.95)

Doctor Make Me Beautiful! tells you everything any reader of any age or sex might want to know about corrective and cosmetic surgery. Written by an eminent plastic surgeon and a writer who has himself had plastic surgery, the book includes such chapters as:

"How Necessary Is Cosmetic Surgery?" "Self Analysis Test: Are YOU a Good Candidate for Cosmetic Surgery?" "Finding a Cosmetic Surgeon," "What is the Right Age for Cosmetic Surgery?" "Can You Have Cosmetic Surgery for the Asking?" and "Your Consultation with the Cosmetic Surgeon."

It also covers the important facts about what "total" face lifts entail and what they can do for you; eyelid-lift surgery; chin reshaping; reshaping, enlarging and lifting your breasts; reorganizing your nose; trimming your bottom, abdomen and thighs; and how to hold back the signs of aging.

 ## The Pursuit of Youth

by Rae Lindsay
Pinnacle (Paperback, $1.75)

"Look Younger: Cosmetic surgery . . . reconstructive surgery . . . nose bobbing . . . face lifts . . . body lifts . . . breast augmentation . . . silicone . . . cellulite . . . wrinkles . . . bags . . . fat . . . and other problems." That's what it says on the back cover of this seriously helpful book.

What it doesn't say is that Rae Lindsay has managed to perfect the art of making technical operations perfectly understandable. She not only gives you a wealth of fascinating background information about plastic surgery, but describes the actual surgical procedures for nose jobs, eye lifts, total face lifts, chin-skin surgery, breast augmentation, breast reduction, built-in girdles, waistline operations, thigh and buttock lifts, bat-wing corrections and genital alterations.

Ms. Lindsay has also devised a practical directory that answers the questions WHO, WHAT, WHERE and HOW MUCH? The purpose of the book is to give a detailed analysis of current and future antiaging techniques, and at that it is investigative, well written and superbly valuable. If you're at all interested in plastic surgery, run right out to your local bookstore and ask them to order *The Pursuit of Youth* for you.

Winning the Age Game

by Gloria Heidi
Doubleday (Hardcover, $8.95)

Winning the Age Game is a 345-page guide to escaping the middle-aged-matron syndrome and enjoying a truly ageless body and soul. It's a virtual well-spring of moral support and great information. The chapter on plastic surgery ("Lowdown on the Big Lift") deals with face-lifting primarily, but even so, if you've been wavering about taking the plunge, the information here can be invaluable.

The Medically Based No-Nonsense Beauty Book

by Deborah Chase
Alfred A. Knopf (Hardcover, $10)
Pocket Books (Paperback, $1.95)

Trained in biology and basic medical science, Deborah Chase has produced a beauty book crammed full of authoritative and useful facts on everything from clearing up your skin to the pros and cons of plastic surgery. In her chapter "Cosmetic Surgery: Features to Fit Your Face," she discusses, explains and illustrates facial problems that can be helped by the artful wielding of a scalpel.

The Easy Way to Good Looks

by Shirley Lord
Thomas J. Crowell (Hardcover, $10)

Ex-*Vogue* beauty editor and currently vice president of Helena Rubinstein, author Shirley Lord insists, "Age is totally unimportant. The years are ... irrelevant. It's how you cope with them." She goes on to say that coping with them is easy and sets out to prove it in a straightforward, no-holds-barred style full of scientific dirt, simple how-tos and a smattering of gossip. She spends quite a bit of time and space on plastic surgery, noting, among other things, that different countries are noted for different kinds of lifts: "South America is famous for body lifts. Eyes are the Tokyo specialty. Russia has made great strides in hair transplants and New York is now tops for face lifts."

BIG-NAME PLASTIC SURGEONS AROUND THE WORLD

Ivo Pitanguy	Rio de Janeiro, Brazil
Hector Marino	Buenos Aires, Argentina
John Mustardi	Ayr, Scotland
Percy Jayes	London, England
Hugo Obwegeser	Zurich, Switzerland
Jan D. Strombeck	Stockholm, Sweden
Karl Schichardt	Hamburg, West Germany
Hiroyama Takeshi	Tokyo, Japan
Claude de Fourmentel	Paris, France
Paul Tessier	Paris, France
Hunter Fry	E. Melbourne, Australia

REAL,
TRUE STORIES
OF PEOPLE WHO
ENJOYED
THEIR
OPERATIONS

"Elizabeth's" Eye Lift (A Pseudonymous Report on One Woman's Surgery)

When I asked my friend "Elizabeth" if I could interview her about her operation, she said, "Sure. But if you use my real name, I'll break your fingers." Here then, is "Elizabeth's" story:

Q: Why did you want to have eye surgery?

A: I hated the way I looked.

Q: How *did* you look?

A: I was just verging on looking bad—what I mean is that the bags under my eyes were making me look *old.* I also didn't want to wait until they got really bad, because I didn't want to go through the stage of having my friends say: "You've had something done—you look ten years *younger."* Neither did I want to hear, "You look rested!" I didn't want to hear any of that. I didn't want to look *rested,* I wanted to look *pretty.*

Q: When you went in for your consultation, did the doctor agree you needed work done?

A: He said I could wait and do it later on. That was the only negative thing he said.

Q: Can you describe the procedure?

A: I checked into the hospital in the afternoon, and had surgery done the next morning.

The doctor took out a little blob of fat in the top lid at the corner of my eye. Actually, I always liked it, and thought it gave me an oriental cast. But if that oval lump loosens, it pulls the upper lid down, and that looks awful, so he pinched it out with one stitch in the corner of each eye. Then he trimmed the bags off, and stitched everything up along the lower lash line. I stayed overnight after the surgery, but that was about it.

Q: Is there anything special you had to do after the operation?

A: Yes, you're supposed to lie down and not go out for a few days. You shouldn't bend over so the blood rushes to your head. You shouldn't move or shake your head a lot. You shouldn't wear contact lenses, and you can't wash your hair yourself.

Q: How soon after surgery do the stitches come out?

A: They came out fairly quickly. I went twice—first to remove the stitches along the lash line. The second time was to take out the corner stitches, which stay in longer.

Q: Was there any bruising?

A: Well, you have a thin red line under your lashes for a while, but a little mascara covers that pretty much. Ten days after, I looked perfectly normal.

Q: Are there any dangers involved in this sort of procedure that we should know about?

A: Yes. Too much skin can be removed from under the eye so it's pulled open at the bottom. You can repair it with a skin graft from behind the ear, but it's complicated. Second, if the work is done too tightly, your face compensates for the tightness of the skin under the eyes by forming deep crow's feet that bend into the cheeks. Which is again something you don't really want.

Q: How much did it cost to fix your eyes?

A: The whole business, not including medical photos (befores and afters) and the initial consultation, came to around $1200.

INTERESTING NOTES

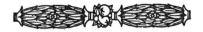

In 1950 there were a handful of surgeons in New York City who performed face lifts in total secrecy for the astronomical sum of $15,000 to $20,000. Today there are about seventy-five certified plastic surgeons in New York; their prices for a face lift range from $1,000 to $3,000.

In Russia . . . you can have a new nose for $75 and a face lift for $150, all skillfully done at egalitarian clinics.
—RAE LINDSAY, *The Pursuit of Youth*

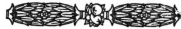

Famous People Who Have Not *Had Plastic Surgery (Nor Do They Plan To)*

Coco Chanel *(who admitted in her eighties that if she ever needed it, she would certainly have it done)*

 Jeanne Moreau
Anna Magnani
Elizabeth Taylor
Mae West
and

The Countess of Castiglione (Napoleon III's mistress), *who at the age of 39 triple-locked herself into her Paris apartment, broke all her mirrors and never came out again rather than reveal her declining beauty.*

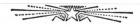

You are only as good as your last plastic surgery.
—PRINCESS LUCIANA PIGNATELLI,
The Beautiful People's Beauty Book

FREE BROCHURES

Both the AMA and the American Society of Plastic and Reconstructive Surgeons will be happy to send you brochures on cosmetic surgery if you send them a self-addressed, stamped #10 (letter size) envelope. Here's where to write:

"Aesthetic Surgery Booklet"
American Medical Association
535 North Dearborn Street
Chicago, Illinois 60610

Question & Answer Booklet
The American Society of Plastic and Reconstructive Surgeons, Inc.
1110 West Main Street
Durham, North Carolina 27701

Free Pamphlet on Plastic Surgery

Dr. E. B. Frankel, medical director of the Cosmetic Surgery Center Medical Group in southern California, will be happy to send you a FREE booklet telling you all about the group's Cosmetic Center, including vital information on breast enlargement and reduction; face, eyelid and eyebrow lifts; nose, chin and ear reconstruction; tummy, buttock and thigh lifts; chemosurgery; dermabrasion and tattoo removal. For your FREE booklet, WRITE:

FREE BOOK
Cosmetic Surgery Center Medical Group
5203 Lakewood Boulevard
Lakewood, California 90712

DOCTOR'S-EYE VIEW
Have You Ever Thought About Having Everything Done at Once?

There once was a lady in her early forties who decided that she'd rather have a new body than continue along with her old one. So she went to Dr. James O. Stallings for a total body lift. Here's Dr. Stallings's description of her operation:

She had a face lift, an eye lift. I trimmed the fat from her upper arms. I lifted her breasts and made them larger. I took off the excess fatty tissue and stretch marks from her abdomen, tightened her abdomen, repaired a hernia around her navel. Then I did a thigh lift and buttock lift all at the same time.

The operation took six hours, and the patient was up walking the next day. She left the hospital a week later and did marvelously well . . .

Dr. Stallings says that people are often unaware that plastic surgery can help correct so many different types of physical problems. He suggests that anyone considering plastic surgery ask the following questions to see if there is any additional way plastic surgery might help.

1. Do you feel a need to improve your appearance?
2. Is there some aspect of your appearance that makes you uncomfortable or self-conscious?
3. Is this proving to be a real problem in your dealings with other people?
4. Are you unhappy with your facial appearance—especially your nose or your chin?
5. Do you have difficulty breathing through your nose?
6. Do you feel the signs of aging make you appear older than you feel?
7. Do baggy eyelids make you look dissipated or old?
8. Do you have excessive frown lines, smile lines or wrinkles?
9. Do you have a receding chin?
10. Do you have acne scars?
11. Do you have jowls?
12. Do your jaws fit together properly?
13. Do your ears protrude?
14. Do stretch marks and a flabby abdomen make you feel "old before your time"?
15. Do heavy thighs and buttocks make you feel ungainly or out of proportion?
16. Do you have flabby arms?
17. Do you feel your breasts are too small . . . too large?
18. Do you realize that age alone is no barrier to having plastic surgery?
19. Do you have scars or deformities that make you appear less attractive?
20. Do your hands look and work normally?
21. Do you have burn scars?
22. Are you troubled by impotence?
23. Are you becoming prematurely bald?
24. Are you in a good state of general health?
25. Do you find that your present appearance is a deterrent to your business, social or personal success?
26. Are you aware that plastic surgery can help you if you are overweight?
27. When was the last time you were complimented about your looks?

Dr. Stallings and his staff have assured me that they will answer your questions about plastic surgery. So if you'd like to know what Dr. Stallings can do for you, or if you are seriously interested in the extensiveness and variety of operations and procedures now available to you, WRITE:

JAMES O. STALLINGS, M.D.
207 Crocker
402 IBM Building
Des Moines, Iowa 50309

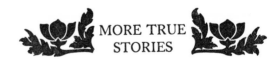 MORE TRUE STORIES

See Elizabeth Taylor's "Plastic Surgery" in Glorious Technicolor

The Films Incorporated brochure lists it this way: "Trying to regain her lost youth, a fat, baggy, middle-aged housewife enters a clinic in Italy where complete plastic surgery (body sculpture) is performed. She emerges looking like a gorgeous, 35-year-old Elizabeth Taylor."

The film they're talking about is Paramount's 1973 feature, *Ash Wednesday,* which is probably the most realistic portrayal of head-to-toe plastic surgery ever put on film. All the surgical procedures filmed at Dr. Ralph Troques's clinic in Paris are brutally graphic, and were very well received by women who saw the film in theaters. Unfortunately they made the men in the audience very nervous, and sometimes even actually sick.

Be that as it may, if you or your women's group would like to *RENT* a 16-mm color print of this R-rated film starring Elizabeth Taylor, Henry Fonda, Helmut Berger and Keith Baxter, you can do so for $150. All you have to do is make arrangements with one of the three major FILMS INCORPORATED offices around the country.

FILMS INCORPORATED (WEST)
5625 Hollywood Boulevard
Hollywood, California 90028
(213)466-5481
FILMS INCORPORATED
(SOUTHEAST)
5589 New Peachtree Road
Atlanta, Georgia 30341
(404)451-7445
FILMS INCORPORATED (NORTH-EAST)
440 Park Avenue South
New York, New York 10016
(212)889-7910

I've always thought God was the best sculptor.
—MARIO RIVOLI, Fine Artist

The Painful Truth About My New Chin
by Karen West

By the time I was ten years old, I'd already forgotten when it was that I first decided I wanted to be an actress. When I told my family about my plans, my father (not quite certain how to put his misgivings) blurted: "But you're not beautiful enough to be a movie star."

Indignant, I told him I didn't want to be a "movie star," I wanted to be "an actress." Six years later I announced my plans to have my nose restyled. Lacking my parents' permission, it was several more years before I actually did the deed.

At the final examination after my nose surgery, the surgeon suggested it might be a good idea to complete the job by putting an implant in my somewhat tiny chin. Still glowing in the aftermath of my nose job, I put it out of my mind . . . almost. Actually, it haunted me. So five years later I went back to the doctor to find out what getting a new chin entailed. Surprised to learn that it was relatively simple and didn't even mean a hospital stay, I made the appointment.

On July 23 of that year, I went back to the doctor's office for the operation. Having already been told that the implants come in three sizes (small, medium and large), I asked what size I needed. The doctor said I should trust his artistic judgment, as well as his surgical skill. Then he gave me a local anesthetic (about six injections of novocaine), which was the only painful part of the procedure (so far). The nurse then placed a covering over my face that had a hole in it to expose my chin. The covering had a hole in it, that is; my face was (till this moment) intact. The nurse then told me not to move my head and the surgery began.

A small incision just below the chin-line, a medium-sized implant inserted, the incision neatly closed, and forty-five minutes after I'd entered the treatment room, I was ready to go home. Two pieces of surgical tape held my face immobile, protecting my new chin, and I had a prescription in my pocket for codeine (should there be any pain after the anesthetic wore off).

Two hours later I phoned the corner drugstore in desperation to get the prescription filled. By midnight, the pain was so intense I was imagining it had always felt that way. At nine

A.M. I took a taxi to the doctor's office. He gave me another prescription for demerol. I went back home, took the demerol and the codeine and three aspirin and the pain still cut through it all.

I finally threw out all the medication, killed a pint of Scotch and no longer cared about the pain. By the third day after surgery, only a slight ache remained. By the sixth day, I was looking forward to having the tape removed and the stitches taken out. Once that was done, it took several more weeks for the swelling to go down completely. Four months later it no longer surprised me when I saw my new reflection in a mirror or a darkened store window. It still pleases me. I think it pleases my father, too. At least, he says it does.

 GETTING IT DONE FOR LESS

For those of us who really need or want plastic surgery, but can't beg, borrow or steal the money to do it, there are university hospital teaching clinics across the country where we can be operated on by qualified residents (under the direction of a big-name plastic surgeon) for next to nothing. Here's how it works:

You call your local teaching hospital and ask for the plastic surgery clinic. The clerk gives you an appointment. You'll then be interviewed by one of the residents. There's a nominal charge for clinic visits—something like $8.75. The resident then examines you. He determines if you're a good candidate for surgery, and if you are he explains the procedure and just what he's going to do. Then he gives you a projected time for your operation, arranges for your admission to the hospital and calls you to make the final arrangements. You go into the hospital on the day he's told you to, you're operated on by him, he handles your follow-up visits and that's that.

There's a fee for the use of facilities (approximately $250), but you have to remember that two days in the hospital (even as a clinic patient) costs somewhere around $600. Still, if you're only paying, say, $200 for an abdominoplasty (tummy surgery) instead of $2,000, you'll probably have cash left over to cover your hospital bill.

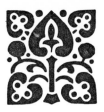

The Less-Than-$15 Face Lift

How would you like to have a sneak preview of how you'll look once you've had your face lifted? How'd you like to see, without trouble or considerable expense, those laugh lines gone—those eyes wide—those cheeks high and smooth again?

Then step right this way, folks, and let an expert tell you about a temporary face lift.

Dick Smith hardly gets involved with beauty makeup anymore. He's the man responsible for the extraordinary character makeups you've seen in films like *The Exorcist* and *The Godfather* (both I and II). But, like many film makeup men, Dick Smith has known about and worked with temporary face lifts for years. Here's what he told me about getting your face lifted temporarily:

"A temporary face lift is actually a very delicate little harness arrangement made up of two small, oval tabs of thin silk or plastic tape, which get attached to the skin between the top and front part of the ears and the hairline. The tabs are glued on, and a thin thread (attached to the corners of the tabs) is tied to an elastic band,

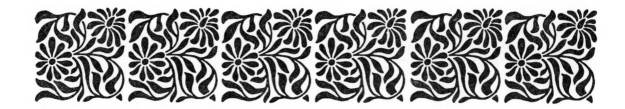

which is then secured and tightened across the top of the head and hidden in the hairdo.

"Lifts can also be used further down on the jawline, below the ear, back near the corners of the jaw. The elastic is then run, not over the top of the head, but around behind the neck. This helps the lower jawline and neck area.

"Another thing to do with a temporary lift is to put it up in the temple area, which is like giving someone a simulated oriental eye, the purpose being to lift a droopy eyelid and bring it back to normal.

"Lifts are great, but if you do them badly, it looks like a terrible face lift. Like an aging actress who, when she talks, gets these diagonal lines running from her mouth up toward her ears ... which is literally where her skin has been pulled back too tight, and you get these strange lines that don't look quite natural."

You can buy temporary face lifts at beauty salons, in department stores, in theatrical makeup stores, by mail order or through ads in those movie magazines you find at the beauty parlor.

One of the people now marketing two different types of face lift is Mark Traynor, a leading television makeup authority and president of Mark Traynor Cosmetics.

The TRAYNOR TEMPORARY FACE LIFT ($6.95) is a harness-type device (like the one Dick Smith described). It's easy to use,

comfortable to wear and is quickly concealed with a little help from your hairdo. Each Traynor Kit comes with a set of elastics, ten tapes (enough for five face lifts) and a tube of special adhesive.

The second Traynor goodie is called an ISO-METRIC BEAUTY BAND ($12.50). This is an adjustable black silk velour headband that puts even tension all around the perimeter of your hairline, pulling up your temple area, around your eyes, and even lifting your lower jaw in a very gentle, very even, very subtle way. It lifts, smoothes out lines, widens your eyes and gives a younger, more rested look to your entire face.

To get your Traynor Temporary Face Lift or Isometric Headband, write:

MARK TRAYNOR COSMETICS
12 East 33rd Street
New York, New York 10016
Face Lift: Enclose $7.45 ($6.95 for lift, 50¢ postage and handling)
Headband: Enclose $13.25 ($12.50 for band, 75¢ postage and handling)
NO CODs PLEASE

HANDLING YOUR HAIR

Hair is the first and only thing you can change about yourself immediately. *The easiest way to make yourself look ten years younger is to get yourself a haircut. In three minutes in the bathroom with a pair of hair shears, you can cut bangs—hide wrinkles, and face the world showing a well-lipsticked mouth and a great pair of eyes.*
—SUZANNE FLYNN, Beauty Editor, *Seventeen* Magazine

A few weeks before the storming of the Bastille, Marie Antoinette showed up at Versailles with a miniature replica of the French man-of-war *La Belle Poule* riding in her enormous, intricately curled and constructed, powdered hairdo. The hair itself (following the fashion of the day) was carefully groomed to look like an ocean of crested waves. It stood just about four feet high (which, when you think about it, is just about as tall as a small child).

Centuries later, *avant garde* poet Tara Osrik shaved her hair off completely and lacquered her skull a bright orange.

Somewhere between these two extremes, we find ourselves—searching the counters and combing the salons for the ways and means to keep our crowning glories acceptably glorious. The problem, more than anything else, is TIME. And perhaps, in a more minor way, HELP. No longer do we have devoted and capable handmaidens trained to duplicate the fury of an angry Atlantic Ocean in our hair. Nor do we have the time to spend countless hours in the salon being permed, straightened, colored, waved, combed, tufted, arranged and blown dry. Still, very few of us want to take Tara Osrik's way out and shave it all off.

The answers to having nice, healthy, shining, touchable "rich-girl" hair lie somewhere between the salon and the shower with side trips into the beauty supply store and the five and dime. The products and services are there in abundance. The basic knowledge about hair itself and how to avoid disaster with it can be had for the price of a book or two, or a trip to the library. My own favorite hairy secrets are all in the following pages.

My whole life is governed by washing and setting my hair ... and makeup.
—BARBARA WALTERS, *People* magazine

Up From Confusion

Seems that every time you turn around, someone is telling you something different about your hair. The magazines tell you one thing. The latest book tells you something else. Your hairdresser has yet another slant on the subject. So where do you start? In my case, I started with a book called *Natural Hair Care Comix,* which was written by two women who were on very friendly terms with their hair. They did the book because they wanted to explain that getting your hair back to its natural, healthy, childlike condition was neither a mystery nor a complex operation. The book is deceptive in that it looks like it is written for little kids. In other words, it's a comic book. But don't let this put you off for a minute; the information in it is wonderful. In fact, I kept thinking what a great primer it would have been for a high school hygiene class. My copy of *Natural Hair Care Comix* is so dog-eared the pages have started to crumble because I keep going back to look things up about brushing, shampooing, conditioning, dandruff, split ends, graying, baldness, massage and haircutting tricks I can perform right in my own living room.

NATURAL HAIR CARE COMIX & STORIES
by Mary Lee and Suzanne Perelman
Straight Arrow Books (Softcover, $3)

To Crystal, hair was the most important thing on earth. She would never get married because you couldn't wear curlers in bed.
—EDNA O'BRIEN, *Winter's Tales*

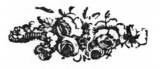

Katherine Everett Doesn't Need to Wear Curlers to Bed

Katherine Everett straightens her hair more than anyone else does. Or at least that's what *she* says. Katherine has what I would consider perfect hair. In other words, she looks like she stuck her tongue in a light socket and frizzed. I think this is perfect hair because my own baby-fine crop refuses to hold a set for more than thirty-five seconds under any circumstances. Naturally, Katherine thinks that *I* have perfect hair. Anyway, Katherine has made an in-depth study of getting her hair straight, and getting rid of those hundreds of lovely ringlets.

Ten years before she discovered hair straightener, she used TONI HOME PERMANENTS to get her hair flat. The trick was to use the perm as directed, but to comb her hair *straight* rather than use the curlers. She had moderate success with this, but discovering that she could apply straightener safely at home changed her life and made her a straightener convert. Her current favorite is put out by MAX FACTOR, but she's used EVERYTHING.

"The first application is almost always safe to do, if you're scrupulous about following the directions..." she says, blithely flying in the face of hundreds of hairdressers who will all tell you never to straighten your hair at home. "The one thing you have to remember is to put megatons of conditioner on when you wash it (every time you wash it) or you'll think your hair was magically turned to cardboard."

Katherine's other trick for keeping her hair plumb-line straight is to comb it straight after she washes it, wrap it tightly in a hairnet and dry it under a hood dryer. She uses a MAX HATTER ($22.95) because it has a 15-foot cord, and she can go to the cupboard and get a cup of Vienna Coffee without having to take the thing off or interrupt the drying process.

Pam, whose hair isn't quite as curly as Katherine's, found that smearing "pounds" of DIPPITY-DO SETTING GEL on her wet hair, putting clips into it so it was completely plastered down, then sleeping on it was effective, if somewhat sticky. Her other answer to the "What am I going to do with my awful hair?" question was: scarves.

 SHAMPOOING

Wash and Wear Hair

Scalp experts say most shampoos are too harsh to use constantly. "We've gotten used to bubbles," one of them told me, "but bubbles themselves don't have much to do with getting your hair clean. They're just an esthetic addition to the shampoo compound. So if you want to clean your hair without killing it—especially if you're washing it every day—add an equal amount of water to the shampoo before you start. You won't get the sort of lather you see on television commercials, but your hair'll be around longer."

My friend Ellen's favorite shampoo product is AMINO-PON (by Redken). She says it makes her hair thick and shiny and leaves it smelling good. Besides, she gets a tremendous bottle of Amino-Pon for about $5.95, which gets her through four months of everyday washing and makes her tremendously happy. Now Ellen isn't an expert, but in informal talks I had with over a hundred hairdressers, six out of ten of them recommended Amino-Pon, so Ellen must be doing something right.

The oddest· item that came across my desk about shampoos was the clipping from a Western poultry show where one of the participants (a man who owned a prize-winning chicken) said that he used Prell Shampoo to keep his chickens white.

I had no idea anyone would go so far as to shampoo a chicken, but—since my own hair very often looks like a collection of feathers—why not? The American public spent $497 million on shampoos in 1975; I wonder how much the chickens spent?

 Set Your Hair With Jello

If you ever run out of setting gel, try unflavored gelatin. (Jell-O will do the same job, if you like scented hairsets and don't mind reeking of Black Cherry.) Just follow package directions, let it set, apply it to your towel-dried hair and set as usual. The only trouble with using gelatin is that it has a shelf-life of about three days before it grows an interesting red fungus. Nevertheless, KNOX UNFLAVORED GELATIN (at approximately 33¢ for four ¼-ounce packages) should get you through at least five years of emergencies.

 Gonna Wash Them Rocks Right Out of My Hair

Washing your hair with rocks may seem strange at first, but Lynn Beck says it's an experience that grows on you. And she should know, because she's single-handedly responsible for making rock hairwashing popular again after a five thousand-year lull.

Her secret (the secret of the ages, actually) is RASSOUL. RASSOUL is a natural phenomenon in the mysterious East ... a rocky blend of herbs, spices, rose water and orange water that makes a lovely low-suds conditioning shampoo. And, if you want to use it elsewhere, it also makes a nifty cleansing facial masque.

Here's what Princess Luciana Pignatelli has to say about RASSOUL (she spells it funny, but you know those Italians):

> Jhassoul is made from Moroccan earth and should be diluted with water into a greasy liquid paste before use. You rinse your hair, apply the paste, wait until it dries like mud, then rinse the hair again. As it dries, you begin to suspect that jhassoul is made from camel dung. It is not, though even if it were, I would use it. The hair comes out so baby-soft and shiny.

RASSOUL (by TRUE EARTH COSMETICS) comes packed in an ecologically sound 12-ounce terra-cotta-colored paper bag (or in a handmade pottery cannister that looks like it was taken directly from a pharaoh's vanity table). You can buy RASSOUL in health food stores, or in selected department stores everywhere.

> *In the 1700s women's hair was styled once every three to nine weeks in the summertime . . . less often in winter. When a woman went for three months at a time without being able to comb her hair out, she had to cope with some special problems. Not the least of which was the hairdresser's ritual of "opening a lady's head." This happened every month or so and consisted of the hairdresser getting into the hairdo to kill the wildlife that had nested there in spite of Milady's daily applications of poisonous pesticide compounds.*

Pampering Poor-Pearl Hair

There's a secret shampoo for long, fine, wispy, baby-type hair that's been an underground favorite with folks who want more shine and less splits. It's called Windsor and it's made by Helene Curtis. The secret ingredient is a lustering agent that's held in colloidal suspension until the shampoo hits water . . . then it goes right into the hair shaft. Helene Curtis claims to have been the first company to market shampoo (a soap that's specifically made for the hair). They did it in the 1930s. Windsor is sold in beauty supply stores for about $3.98 a pint, but the best part is that it's concentrated, so that the pint mixes up into a whole gallon, which should last you about a year of constant washing.

> *Ten teams of oxen draw much less*
> *Than doth one hair of Helen's tress.*
> —John Florio

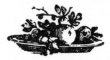

BEAUTIFYING TREATMENTS
Several Sensuous Ways to Get Your Scalp to Tingle

Trichologists (people who specialize in scalp and hair treatments) always start their good works with a brisk, thorough, scalp massage which sometimes goes as far as including the neck and shoulders. The point is to untense you and get your circulation going, because healthy scalps mean healthy hair.

You may not have a trichologist around the corner, so you might want to know how to massage your own scalp. Unfortunately, once you raise your arms above your head, your scalp locks. This makes it very hard to do a good job unless you're bent over at the waist watching the blood rush into your eyeballs.

My answer is to seriously think about talking a good friend into learning the art of massage.

Not only will sharing a massage with a friend make your scalp feel better, it will do wonders for your entire disposition. You needn't run out to the nearest massage parlor for lessons (what do THEY know?) because the following books are all terrific.

MASSAGE: THE LOVING TOUCH
by Stephen Lewis
Pinnacle (Paperback, $1.95)

Touching—for therapy, for sensual communication, for relaxation. Stephen Lewis tells you how to massage, teaches you how to touch and tells you why. If you liked Stephen Lewis's plastic surgery story (page 000), you'll love his massage book.

HOW THE BODY FEELS
by Byron Scott
Ballantine Books (Paperback, $2.95)

An interesting blend of the medical and the sensual/physical methods of massaging the tension and aches out of each part of the body from head to toe.

THE MASSAGE BOOK
by George Downing, illustrated by Anne Kent Rush
Random House—The Bookworks (Oversized Paperback, $4.95)

This is a book about energy, with a lot of practical information covering everything from using your hands to building a massage table. It was written by George Downing, whose own techniques were developed for the Esalen Institute in Big Sur and who searched in vain for the ultimate massage book to recommend to his students ... so he ended up writing his own.

SWEDISH MASSAGE WORKBOOK
by Dr. Sidney Zerinsky, $5.95
Order FROM:
THE SWEDISH INSTITUTE
160 West 71st Street
New York, New York 10023

Dr. Zerinsky (director of the Swedish Institute) gives you all the fundamentals of a proper Swedish massage (which can be so relax-ing it will actually put you right into a deep, restful, dreamless sleep). He also diagrams easy-to-follow, traditional manipulations and sets out a host of complementary exercises you can do in conjunction with massaging.

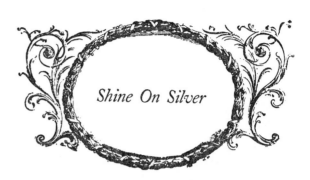

Shine On Silver

Curly hair is more porous than straight hair, and it reflects light differently than straight hair does. When I got my first East African Afro permanent, I was mortified that my hair didn't shine anymore. The only thing that made it look shiny was standing under a 10,000-watt light bulb. You can rent a 125-pound, 10,000-watt, 100-amp Mole Richardson light from movie equipment rental houses for about $12.50 a day, but I wouldn't advise trying to plug it into your wall socket.

Alberto VO 5 also makes hair look shinier. It's less expensive than renting movie lights and won't wreck your wiring.

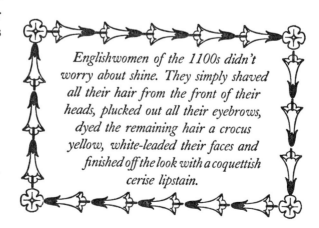

Englishwomen of the 1100s didn't worry about shine. They simply shaved all their hair from the front of their heads, plucked out all their eyebrows, dyed the remaining hair a crocus yellow, white-leaded their faces and finished off the look with a coquettish cerise lipstain.

Mint Condition

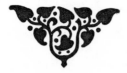

Ten years ago no hairdresser worth his scissors had anything nice to say about conditioners. They all told me they wouldn't give a conditioner to their enemies. They all said that conditioners attracted dust from the air and made it stick to your hair. Yet, with all the damage we've done to ourselves by blowing our hair dry every morning, conditioners are now essential, necessary parts of the hair ritual. Without them we'd all look like haystacks.

Dr. Myra Barker (who travels constantly in her work for Pantene) says that more women ask her questions about the effects of blow dryers and other heat appliances than ever before.

"All a woman really needs is a shampoo and a conditioner," she says, and Pantene puts two special conditioning ingredients in every one of their hair products to take care of almost any problem that might crop up. One special Pantene addition is pantyl (a derivative of vitamin B_5). It's a conditioner that penetrates the hair shaft, smoothes the hair cuticle and makes your hair more shiny and manageable. The other special extra ingredient is called thytantriol, which helps regulate your hair's moisture balance and goes a long way in fighting the rainy-day "my hair's all frizzly—I can't go outside" syndrome.

If you're worried about the damage your hot comb or blow dryer may be doing to your hair, or if you have any other questions about taking care of, conditioning, treating or anything else, all you have to do is explain your specific problem to the PANTENE people. Don't just say, "My hair looks dreadful, can you help me?" but rather, "I've got more split ends than the Green Bay Packers. They seemed to start only this summer, and they're getting worse every second. What can I do about them? P.S.: I body-surf a lot." PANTENE will happily answer all questions addressed to:

Doris Bach
Consumer Relations Manager
PANTENE
340 Kingsland Street
Nutley, New Jersey 07110

While We're Talking About Conditioning

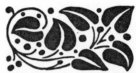

Your hair gets more abuse in the winter than it does in the summer. Think of the changes it has to go through: It's 80 degrees in Saks Fifth Avenue and 20 degrees outside on Fifth Avenue—so your hair expands and shrinks violently.

In practical terms, this means that you need two different conditioners: one for summer, and one for when it's dreadfully cold out. The large-molecule conditioner that fits nicely into stretched summer hair is FLEX, by Revlon. Put it on, leave it in for twelve minutes, then rinse it out.

For winter, WELLA BALSAM CONDITIONER by WELLA works wonders. It's made of smaller molecules that sneak into your hair shaft in just sixty seconds. (Step out from under the shower. Count to sixty by elephants.)

By the way, if you swim a lot and hate to use a cap, but also hate what the water does to your hair, you should use a conditioner before setting foot in the surf. Undiluted FLEX is fine for salt water, so is VASELINE. And if you swim in chlorinated pools, undiluted BRECK PINK CREME RINSE will both protect your hair and soften the water.

Two Vegetarian Answers To the Conditioning Dilemma

Bambé Levine (beauteous ex-beauty editor and ski instructress in the Italian Alps) conditions her hair with mayonnaise. She slathers it through her damp, lovely blond locks, wraps it up in a hot towel and swears it's the ultimate replacement for shine and body. She discovered mayonnaise not because she was a confirmed vegetarian (that part came later), but because she happened to be standing in her kitchen one day, making a BLT on toast, and musing on the benefits of egg protein, when she caught a glimpse of her hair (reflected in her kitchen mirror) and decided to get right into her economy jar of Hellman's Mayo. She's been at it ever since.

Unlike Bambé, Paul McGregor is a *devout, committed,* 200 percent vegetarian. He's also the man who created the shag and whose nimble shears have clipped the tresses of such famous names as Faye Dunaway, Goldie Hawn, Lee Grant, Julie Christie and Jane Fonda. So, when Mr. McG set out to develop a system of hair care, he avoided animal derivatives like the plague. Result: PURE BODY—a shampoo, conditioner. and hair builder all based on soya protein and polyvinyl pyrollidone. You can order the whole organic batch for just about $10 (in check or money order), but best write Mr. McGregor first to make certain the price hasn't changed.

PAUL McGREGOR/HAIRCUTTERS
15 St. Marks Place
New York, New York 10003

Why Not Use Rosemary Instead of a Conditioner?

My friend Rosemary thought this last suggestion was exploitive until I explained it was rosemary oil I was talking about ... Honestly!

Pure oil of rosemary (the herb) shines up your hair, doesn't get it sticky and smells like—well, some people *like* the way it smells. Others think it's kind of medicinal. That's a personal choice, of course, but putting a drop of pure rosemary oil on your natural-bristle hairbrush before stroking it through your hair can be a lovely organic experience. Rosemary, being a stimulant, can also wake you up in the morning while it permeates your bedroom with its strong, herby fragrance.

You can order rosemary oil from the following friendly suppliers, but please note that prices on all natural herbs and oils vary greatly because the plants and flowers they come from get scarcer and labor costs (to gather and distill them) get greater by the minute. So it's wise to write first and ask for current price information.

APHRODISIA
28 Carmine Street
New York, New York 10014

HARVEST HEALTH, INC.
1944 Eastern Avenue S.E.
Grand Rapids, Michigan 49507

HAUSMAN'S PHARMACY
6th at Grand Avenue
Philadelphia, Pennsylvania 19127

HERB PRODUCTS CO.
1012 Magnolia Boulevard
North Hollywood, California 91601

INDIANA BOTANIC GARDENS, INC.
Hammond, Indiana 46325

KIEHL'S PHARMACY
109 Third Avenue
New York, New York 10003

NATURE'S HERB COMPANY
281 Ellis Street
San Francisco, California 94102

NICHOL'S GARDEN NURSERY
1190 N. Pacific Highway
Albany, Oregon 97321

ORGANIC HAIR CARE CENTER
138 Blithedale Avenue
Mill Valley, California 94941

WESTBRAE NATURAL FOODS
1336 Gilman
Berkeley, California 94706

Down With the Oilies

Living in the city, your hair seems to get oily after every meal. Cutting down on the oilies is a persistent problem that can drive you nuts, especially if you don't have time to dash into a shower every fifteen minutes.

My mother, who never ate fried foods and hadn't seen a roasted cashew or any other kind of nut in years (save, of course, members of the immediate family), always used oatmeal in her hair to get rid of the oil slick. Not the cooked kind (ick!) but the dry stuff, right out of the Quaker Oats package. She figured, and rightly so, that the little oat flakes were absorbent enough to blot up all the oil ... and also that the ton of brushing it took to get all the flakes out of her hair did wonders for it, too.

My blond friend Lyle (without whose research this book would have been about two and a half pages long) says he uses two shakes of talcum powder instead of oatmeal to do the same job. Says its marvelous.

My all-time favorite, fast, dry shampoo is *Psssst,* which sprays in and brushes right out. But if you have a serious misgiving about using aerosol spray products, you might try putting a square of cheesecloth over your hairbrush, wrapping it tight, then brushing your hair with it. The cheesecloth works on the oatmeal principle: absorption. It's not quite as thorough as oatmeal or *Psssst,* but it can pinch-hit for either in emergencies.

... In my area, however, they [barbershops] have gone the way of the butcher shop, replaced by something called the unisex hair stylist—a cross between a barbershop and a discotheque. They are invariably staffed by Frenchmen who seem to have had their hips removed.
—RICHARD M. COHEN,
Washington Post News Service

HAIRCUTTING AND HAIRDRESSING

The Engineered Haircut

Here's a unisex barbering joint that looks more like a Victorian parlor than a discotheque, and has invented—or rather, perfected—something they call the Engineered Haircut.

The rationale is that, more often than not, hairstyles are haphazardly created and usually don't last very long. According to Volumetric principles, the construction of haircuts is based on the desired hair length and the position of the wide stationary bones of the skull: (a) the temporal, (b) the parietal, (c) the occipital, and (d) the frontal. The weight of the hair is then displaced so that the end result is an engineered hair shape that has volume, density and movement.

The place to get this very special shearing is:

VOLUMETRICS
56 Irving Place
New York, New York 10003

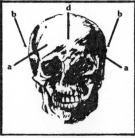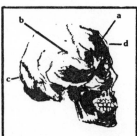
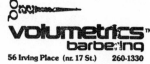

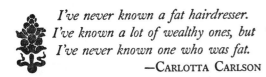

I've never known a fat hairdresser.
I've known a lot of wealthy ones, but
I've never known one who was fat.
—CARLOTTA CARLSON

What Are Those Superstar Hairdressers Really *Like?*

There are three different hairdressing superstars whose names I see once a month, when the magazines come in. In fact, I've seen their names so often over the last ten years or so, I mistakenly think of them as friends. "Oh, there's Kenneth again this month," I'll say as I whip through the fashion pages. Or, "I wonder what Cinandre's doing for spring?" Or, "Whatever *happened* to Vidal Sassoon?"

What do I REALLY know of these men, personally? Frankly, not much. I have my hair cut at a neighborhood salon once every six weeks. True, Kevin, who cuts my hair and cuts it beautifully (for $23, tips included) *did* work at Sassoon once. Still, I can count on the fingers of my left hand the times I've actually taken a week's salary and braved a personal trip through the gleaming doors of the top-name salons.

On the other hand, one week last year I got very interested in finding out just what went on in there, so I arranged a cozy little lunch. Just me and three top beauty editors who are in and out of the big-name salons about as often as I am in and out of the Chinese laundry.

"Who goes to the superstars?" I asked them. "And what is it like?" It took a while for everybody to warm to the task, but somewhere between the soup and the dessert course, they started with Kenneth (the high-priced hair person who became famous for creating Jackie Kennedy Onassis's hairstyle when she was First Lady).

Editor Number One (names have been changed here to protect the vitriolic) said that it was the social woman who went to Kenneth, the woman over thirty-five, or even the young girl whose mother was a steady client.

"She's safe. She's Waspy. She's got that clean, pampered, thoroughly monied, conservative look. The sort of look that Babe Paley and Jackie O have. There are names like Newhouse and Cushing on the register book. The women who go to Kenneth appreciate the low-keyness of the place. The operation is low-key, which their lives are. They all entertain and exist on a very low-key, wealthy level. Sure, they have money; in fact, they probably have *most* of it, but it's not the kind of money that wants to spread it around. Not the sort of wealth that stands up and lets everybody know. They're also secure in that they know that Kenneth consistently has the best clientele. That everyone who waits on them at Kenneth is going to be very nice, but not make a big deal over them when they walk in for a comb-out.

"The salon itself is set up in nice, feminine, intimate, little private rooms. Everything seems small and very intimate here, which is just another extension of the way the clients lead their lives. And I think Kenneth himself fits very well into the picture. He's like that. He's in his mid-forties; he's thin; he's got blondish hair; a tall, thin body; and a very soft-spoken approach. He's just a very nice, well-heeled kind of person. His suits probably come from Dunhill, so he's really not a flashy fashion figure.

"In terms of his stylings, he's keeping up with things that are contemporary, but he tones them down so that they're not freaky. He might be doing the same sort of permanents that Cinandre's doing, but he's toned it down so that it's going to look nice and smooth and soft and flattering. He's still the specialist in soft, smooth, flattering hair. Nothing that makes a blatant statement. Quality rather than flash. Something that's going to last longer and wear better than this year's China Chop or last year's Dutch Bob. Kenneth's work is traditional and classic—and handled with the smoothest velvet approach."

At this point Editor Number Two (who had been only momentarily distracted from her seafood crepe while Editor Number One described what was going on at Kenneth's) put down her fork to tell me the story on Cinandre.

"Cinandre is the direct opposite in feeling to Kenneth. For one thing, André (who started the whole Cinandre style) is an elitist. Not that Kenneth isn't, but André is an elitist on a different level. He's volatile. He's speedy. He wears jeans and maybe a terrific sweater. You'd never catch him dead in a Dunhill suit. But then again, his jeans aren't Levis—they're from Fiorucci, or whatever Italian boutique is making the papers that month. And the cowboy boots are probably from Charles Jourdan. André's from Paris, so he has that sort of attitude that a lot of Americans interpret as Parisian snobbery. You can really compare it to when you go to a French restaurant and somehow you feel like the staff is absolutely doing you a favor by dealing with you. You know, that feeling you get when, even though you're paying an exorbitant amount of money for the meal, they don't really give a damn whether you're there or not.

"Going to Cinandre for the first time can be frightening, because even though you know it's going to cost you in the neighborhood of $50 for André to cut your hair, nobody seems to be helping you into the experience. You go to the girl behind the reception desk and she's cool. The tone is, you can come or you can go, and they don't really care much either way. The place itself is like a factory. I mean, it's light and it's clean and everything, but people are bustling around in their jeans and their sweaters and their chic-ness and there's this tangible electricity in the air. Something about the temperament of the client playing off the temperament of the hairdresser. I've had women call me and say, 'I used to go to Cinandre when they were just starting. When they would set a woman's hair with electric rollers. Now they tell me not to come back because they don't DO that kind of thing anymore.' It's like sweet revenge."

On that note, the waiter came with the coffee, and Editor Number Three shook her perfectly cut mane of chestnut hair and explained about Vidal Sassoon.

"Sassoon is in between," she said. "He's a very precise, careful Englishman. He started the whole splash for geometric cuts and effortless, stylized hairstyles in the mid-sixties, and has just carried it on and loosened it up from there. Kenneth is more formal than Sassoon. Cinandre's more freaky. Sassoon can cut your hair and you'd never have to worry about it again because the cut itself was so wonderful. You could step out of the shower, make several quick passes over your head with a blow dryer—and you'd be set to go.

"The best thing about Sassoon is that he's tried to give you a certain security when you go there. Each hairdresser has an assistant. Most of them are very nice. They go out of their way to make you comfortable. They're not hostile. They're not snobbish. He's tried to create a different kind of classiness. It's hard to pinpoint exactly what's going on at Sassoon, because in one chair there's a young secretary from Queens and in the next chair may be the Duke of Marlborough's daughter, or a little kid, or a young-looking grandmother, or a fabulous-looking model. There's a "now" feeling in the salon. There's someone there who's capable of doing just about anything. There's someone to do something freaky (if that's what you want) and someone to do something pretty. They have all kinds of ways to go now that pretty much defy categorizing. I think the big thing to remember with all the superstar hairstylists is that their mainstay is not the cut you see on the fashion pages every month with their little credit beside it. That's all publicity . . . trendy new cuts that make news. But the bulk of everybody's business is still the styles they do on the women who come back every week. That's where all of them make their money."

The check came just about then and we all collected our coats, thanked each other profusely and walked out into the spring air, our perfectly done hair gleaming behind us.

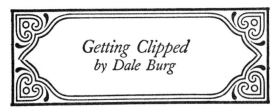

Getting Clipped
by Dale Burg

I, who have appeared without stammering on national television, had a tooth filed *sans* novocaine, and successfully demanded a new air conditioner from my landlord, cry at the hairdresser's. Fairly regularly. Once I came as close as I have ever come to an anxiety attack. I bolted from the chair, but returned to leave a tip.

Why hairdressers intimidate me is a puzzlement. We're talking, after all, about persons who are generally smaller than myself and who are supposedly in a service profession. I have found most hairdressers to be blissfully unaware of the latter. I suspect there's a required course in Disdain at beauty-culture schools.

Perhaps I would feel more in control of the situation were I standing and they sitting, though royalty seems to cope well with the opposite circumstance. Since such an arrangement seems impractical, I have tried to remember some basic rules that will minimize my difficulties.

I try to look my best. Fortunately, this no longer requires wearing one's most trendy outfit. Second only to the French Revolution as an egalitarian gesture was the introduction of the smock at beauty salons. Now you need only make certain your shoes are shined and your panty hose aren't snagged. In addition, you will feel more secure if you're in full makeup and wearing status earrings, even though you will probably be asked to remove them.

It is not necessary to do your hair the night before. Actually, this is a rather futile gesture, since nine times out of ten some assistant will wet you down before you face Monsieur's critical eye. Accept the fact that the wetting down procedure takes place primarily to insure that you are feeling at least somewhat unattractive and less sure of yourself. Another virtue of wetting down, from the hairdresser's point of view, is that he doesn't have to concern himself with what sort of hair you have but can cut whatever style he pleases.

Recognize that you are courting disaster in a unisex salon. My friend Connie was having her hair dyed black. Roots exposed, dye dripping down her face, looking as if she were at midpoint of tar and feathering, she glanced up to see A Movie Star making his way to the gentlemen's part of the salon. She asked to be placed in the back room. "What do you care if (they mentioned his name) sees you in this condition?" she was loudly reprimanded.

Curb the impulse to let the hairdresser know Just Who You Are. He can always top you. If you are the beauty editor of the local paper, he has just treated the beauty editor of *Vogue*. If you are the beauty editor of *Vogue,* he has just worked on Babe Paley. You can't win.

Accept the fact that if you are in a shop where English is the second language, if they are speaking in the first language, they are talking about you. It is always possible that they are saying something flattering. It isn't likely.

Above all, resist the urge to make transparent attempts to ingratiate yourself with your stylist. Once, in an attempt to get in his good graces, I brought two passes to a Barbra Streisand movie to my hairdresser of the moment. As everyone knows, there is no hairdresser in the world who would not wait on line several hours to see a Barbra Streisand movie. The crafty hairdresser I was dealing with pretended the passes were of no consequence. He thanked me in a perfunctory manner, stuck the passes in his pocket casually and, without warning, gave me bangs, just to let me know he still had the upper hand.

It is best always to recognize the caste system in the beauty salon. Never consult with the shampoo lady about anything but the texture of your hair. Never make an appointment with the head of the salon for anything less than a full styling. Even if this means he is only to take the scissors in hand to snip off a single errant hair, it shows the proper subservience.

Recognize that you will always be the loser in any struggle for power. The ultimate gaucherie, of course, is to bring in a picture of some hairstyle you might have in mind. Hairdressers delight in crumpling the photo, tossing it to the floor among the cuttings, and telling you why your hair is too limp or frizzy or otherwise unsuitable for anything like that, letting you know that it is sufficiently difficult to make you look reasonable, much less like anything from the pages of a fashion magazine.

I once merely asked for something simple. Miffed at my interference, my hairdresser trimmed an infinitesimal amount, then stuck me under a dryer without further ado. When I looked in the mirror, I saw a person who appeared to be wearing a stuffed mushroom on her head. I asked him if he liked it. He did. Actually, I think what he felt was supreme indifference; he'd washed his hands of me when I dared to give him instructions. I told him I didn't feel capable of appearing in public disguised as an hors d'oeuvre. Sensing I was properly chastened, he took mercy and started all over again.

If you don't want a henna rinse, say you want a henna rinse. That way, he'll tell you it's impossible and will scrap his original plan to coerce you into having a henna rinse. There is nothing a hairdresser likes better than to exercise his prerogatives in the matter of your hair.

The most important rule of all is never to admit you've cut your hair yourself. This is a sure route into the doghouse. If you come in with your left side in a flip and your right side in a pageboy, they get a big kick out of telling you what a terrible job their predecessor did. But if they find out you have actually dared to take shears to your own head, there's no telling what may happen. You may find yourself in the middle of a double process before you know it.

Finally, always leave them with warm feelings toward you. This can be best done by leaving a suitable tip. If you are in doubt about how much to leave, hand over the entire contents of your pocketbook. That's probably enough.

How Much Do You Love Your Haircutter

Three hairdressers out of five today will modestly admit to being the real-life model for Warren Beatty's love-'em-and-leave-'em hair-bender role in the movie *Shampoo*.

My own personal choice for the real. role model is the late Allan Lance, to whom haircutting was a most intimate operation. He believed that all women were in love with their hairdressers. "When you come right down to it," he used to say, "other than their husbands or their lovers, who else runs his fingers through their hair and tells them they look beautiful? Who else listens patiently to their traumas? Who else is going to give them a big hug when they're feeling awful? A hairdresser makes it possible for every woman to have a lover on the side."

Want to have a more meaningful relationship with your hairdresser? Want to flaunt it (quietly)? Get yourself a tiny, 14-karat-gold blow dryer on an 18-inch gold chain for $120
Write:

Bill Thompson Associates
P.O. Box 6746
Providence, R.I. 02940

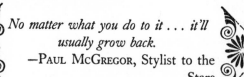

No matter what you do to it . . . it'll usually grow back.
—PAUL MCGREGOR, Stylist to the Stars

Growing . . . Growing . . . Grown

Hair grows at the same speed in the summer as it does in the winter. It grows six inches a year on everybody. It never grows any more than six inches a year on anybody (anybody in good health), *ever.* Hair can grow up to eight feet in length, and if you'd like yours to get that long you should definitely see THE LONG

HAIR EXPERT.

GEORGE MICHAEL OF MADISON AVENUE has thirty-six thousand clients with lush, lovely, long (or getting there), flowing, healthy hair. The first appointment with Mr. Michael costs $25; he sits you down in his sumptuous office with five or so other women and tells you everything there is to know about what hair is, how it grows, how to take care of it and what happened to the poor, misguided pussycats who didn't follow his good advice. He then personally inspects your hair and trims it. Royalty swears by his services. So do the top hair models all over the world.

THE LONG HAIR EXPERT
GEORGE MICHAEL
OF MADISON AVENUE
420 Madison Avenue
New York, New York 10017
(212)PL 2-1177

> *Sudanese called himself a dervish, swallowed a fishhook, cut himself open, took it out again. If an uneducated savage can do that, you can cut your own hair.*
> —GILES COOPER, "Mathry Beacon,"
> Radio Drama

STYLING IT YOURSELF

This very well may be the book that has everything. Susan Sommers Winer got together every single solitary hairdo in the entire world (or so it seems), wrote the simplest, easiest to follow how-to-do-it directions I've ever read, and put them together with wonderfully attractive photographs; then wrapped the whole package into a neat little book called *101 Quick 'N Easy Hairdos*. The book really does include everything: Afros, topknots and tiebacks, upsweeps, shags, rice-bowl cuts, flips, bangs—the works.

Once you get this book, you'll never again have to wonder how to do it, or search around for the right picture in the right magazine to show to your hairdresser.

101 QUICK'N EASY HAIRDOS
by Susan Sommers Winer
Pyramid (Paperback, 95¢)

 Yes . . . But Can You Blow Your Hair Dry?

My survey of the bouquets of blow dryers proliferating in my friends' bathrooms divided them into three distinct categories: the light-weight, long-handled styling combs (meant for styling dry hair); the slightly heavier, slightly more powerful two-or-more-speed styler/dryer (to be used to dry and tame damp hair); and the hand-held gunlike dryer (more powerful, but light enough to be handled without herniating yourself) for use after shampooing.

The minimodels all come equipped with enough attachments to delight any toy freak. The most common combinations were fine- and wide-tooth combs, natural- and plastic-bristle brushes, and (in extreme cases) even a mist-making gizmo.

The larger dryers have speed-drying attachments (to concentrate air flow on a specific area), curl curvers and detachable soft-bonnet hoods.

Literally everybody and his brother seem to be making dryers these days . . . so I went to the professionals and found them unanimous in recommending three things: the heavy-duty, hand-held dryer; the natural-bristle hairbrush; and the human hand. The hairdryer name that came up most often was Continental Pro-Style (Model 060) which, according to Anthony Farish (marketing v.p. at Continental), has everything going for it—1200 watts, a four-temperature control, a year's guarantee and an unbreakable case made of the same plastics and polymers that go into football helmets, so when you drop it on the bathroom floor you're not out a bunch of money. The Pro-Style can be had for in the neighborhood of $29.99 at most major drug and department stores.

The next problem is: Once you have the dryer—do you know what to do with it?

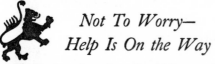

Not To Worry—
Help Is On the Way

Does the thought of wielding a blow dryer give you hives? Don't give it another thought. Bob Bent can solve all that, and HAS solved it in his profusely illustrated book called *How to Cut Your Own Hair or Anybody Else's.* Not only does he tell you about blowing your hair dry, but he also gives you the lowdown on what hair is, what it does, what you can do to it, with it and for it—then he moves right along to give simple, step-by-step instructions for cutting short, medium or long hair—yours or anybody else's (just like it says in the title).

HOW TO CUT YOUR OWN HAIR OR
ANYBODY ELSE'S
by Bob Bent
Simon & Schuster
(Quality Paperback, $4.95)

 ## Gum In the Pigtails?

Glue behind the cowlick? Bob Bent's new book *How to Cut Your Children's Hair,* tells how to solve these maddening minor problems. For glue, for example, you put oil on the trouble spot, then use an ice cube, which you work down with the oil until the offending substance gives up and comes out.

How to Cut Your Children's Hair is written for adults to read (with easy-to-follow directions so they can DO, too) but—and this is an important BUT—it's also designed for children to LOOK AT. All the kids in the book have names, so you can relate to them, and they're big enough to color in (or for your children to color in if they can get the Crayolas away from you). Mr. Bent did the book the way he did because he felt everybody he knew was terrified of getting a haircut as a child; so he thought a book kids

could get involved with would give them a chance to get over their fear.

HOW TO CUT YOUR CHILDREN'S
HAIR
by Bob Bent
Simon & Schuster
(Quality Paperback, $4.95)

Keeping That Afro Attractive—Free

Styling tips on mini, short, curly, rounded and natural Afro hairstyles abound in a FREE BOOKLET by Willie L. Morrow and The Electro Tool Corp. (Sounds like a rock group, doesn't it?) Anyhow, the booklet is full of inside news on how to thin, shape, cut and style—and you can get one free by writing:

FREE BOOKLET
Electro Tool Corp.
1718 Layard Avenue
Racine, Wisconsin 53401

Hair Begins at Forty

One of Gloria Heidi's pet peeves is the "Menopause Bob." She describes it as "that short, teased, shellacked and grouted helmet that's ground out every Saturday afternoon at the beauty salons like so many sausages."

"Hair is sexy," says Ms. Heidi, "and age has nothing to do with it." She preaches the gospel of artistic disorder, quotes George Masters (one of Hollywood's master stylists) on the art of hair *un*dressing, explodes the myth of blunt cutting and reminds us of deathless late-late-show hair dialogue:

> Is that really you, Miss Grundage? Without your glasses and with your hair all soft and loose like that . . . why . . . you're LOVELY.

Ms. Heidi gives us the guidelines and the courage to face up to Mr. Beverly (or any other stylist) and get what we want from him. She also makes the very good point that many of the most glamorous women in the world (all over forty)—women like Merle Oberon, Elizabeth Taylor, Zsa Zsa Gabor, Barbara Walters and the incomparable Marlene Dietrich—have sexy, touchable, ageless, LONG hair. She says ANYBODY can, and she tells you HOW. It's all right there in her beautiful book, *Winning the Age Game,* and so is a raft of wittily written vital information on everything every woman needs to know about looking, feeling and being younger.

WINNING THE AGE GAME
by Gloria Heidi
Doubleday (Hardcover, $8.95)

Want That Gray to Go Away? Take Vitamins!

Premature grayness can be due to a vitamin deficiency. When the Russians fed hundreds of thousands of gray-haired refugees para-aminobenzoic acid (one of the independent B-vitamin complex), they found that the grayness disappeared, and even better yet, the natural color came back.

The following advice is taken from an address called "Treatment of Clinical Achromotrichia with Para-Aminobenzoic Acid," which was given to the members of the Society for Experimental Biology and Medicine at Cornell Medical College by Dr. Benjamin F. Seive.

Dr. Seive claimed that he and his colleagues actually changed the color of the hair of almost three hundred patients from gray to its natural shade solely by giving them PABA tablets. In the talk, Dr. Seive suggested the following procedure for the treatment of premature graying with para-aminobenzoic acid:

"Fifty milligrams daily for a period of ten to twenty days until early changes (yellowing or darkening) are observed. Then 100 milligrams daily." Dr. Seive emphasized that it is most important that the vitamin not be given in a single dose, but in divided doses throughout the day.

You can get PABA anywhere you get your other vitamins.

BE MINDFUL OF THE MOON

Get your hair cut when the moon is in Taurus or Capricorn but not when it's in Virgo (which is barren). For faster growth, get your hair cut when the moon is in a water sign like Cancer, or Pisces. To find out WHERE the moon is, get yourself a copy of THE CIRCLE CALENDAR, $2. You can order one (between January and March) from:

SAMUEL WEISER, INC.
·734 Broadway
New York, New York 10003

Include 45¢ postage and handling for first item ordered, 10¢ for each additional item. New York residents add local sales tax.

Or send $2.35 to:

CIRCLE BOOKS
Heart Center
1041 North Main
Ann Arbor, Michigan 48104

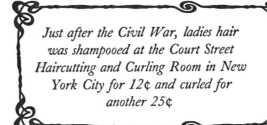

Just after the Civil War, ladies hair was shampooed at the Court Street Haircutting and Curling Room in New York City for 12¢ and curled for another 25¢

I Can't Do a Thing With My Hair!

If you can't do a thing with YOUR hair, you should pick up a copy of a hair-styling magazine. There are two on the market. Both are quarterlies, both are published by pretty much the same staff, and both cover trendy, fashionable and practical hair advice with good pictures and illustrations and easy-to-follow directions. You've probably seen both of them at the beauty salon—they're the tattered copies hidden under *Vogue* and *Harper's Bazaar,* right next to the dryer . . . Anyway, if you haven't seen them, here's where to write for your very own copies:

HAIRDO ORIGINALS
Modern Day Periodicals, Inc.
257 Park Avenue South
New York, New York 10010
Single copy, $1; subscription, $4 per year

HAIR STYLE
Beauty Secrets, Inc.
257 Park Avenue South
New York, New York 10010
Single copy, $1

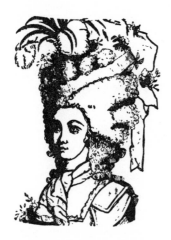

Where Were You *During the Belle Epoch?*

My friend Veronica was right in the middle of writing a novel the year the Belle Epoch hairstyle came into fashion. By the time she'd finished writing her book, the hairstyle was gone. She still gnashes her teeth about not learning how to construct that glorious topknot. Since I couldn't explain how to do it with full professional expertise, I called Vincent Nardi, the fabulous Italian who runs the Doing Your Own Hair course at the New School in New York City. I reasoned that if anyone could tell us how to deal with a hairdo, Vincent could. Here's what he said:

"The Belle Epoch is easy. Stand somewhere where you have a bit of room. Take your hairbrush in your hand. Bend over at the waist so your nose is just about parallel with your knees. Brush your hair from nape of neck toward the floor. When your hair is thoroughly brushed, catch it up into a high ponytail right at the crown. Use a cloth-covered rubber band so you won't break your hair all off.

"Once you've got the rubber band tight, pull it away from your head a little so that it rests about an inch from your scalp. This makes the bulk of your hair look full and graceful. (If you leave the band tight to your head, you look like someone out of a 1950 high-school yearbook.)

"Next, wind the ponytail around itself into a cruller shape, or a doughnut, twisting as you go. Secure the newly twisted ponytail with bobby pins. If you're like most of us, your hair won't be all one length, so you'll now have small sections of loose hair that have freed themselves at the nape of your neck and possibly around your cheeks or on your forehead. Don't let these disturb you. Set them in pincurls (with setting gel) and when they're dry, just remove the pins and let them fall naturally."

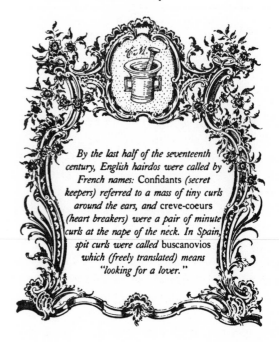

By the last half of the seventeenth century, English hairdos were called by French names: Confidants *(secret keepers) referred to a mass of tiny curls around the ears, and* creve-coeurs *(heart breakers) were a pair of minute curls at the nape of the neck. In Spain, spit curls were called* buscanovios *which (freely translated) means "looking for a lover."*

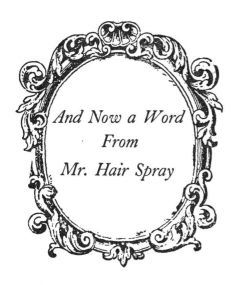

*And Now a Word
From
Mr. Hair Spray*

Seven years ago there were something like a hundred different brands of hair spray on the market. Then came the "natural" look, and most stores carried no more than twenty or thirty of the best-known brands.

Hair sprays are made up of three basic ingredients: holding resins, alcohol and a propellant (to get the other two ingredients out of the can). Or at least hair sprays *used* to be made of those three things. Now, in response to growing ecological pressure, there are "natural" pump sprays around which don't use freon or any other propellant and which *look* terribly expensive. For example, the 8-ounce NONaerosol AQUANET costs 79¢. Well, so does the 16-ounce spray can. So I called Richard Barrie, president of the Rayette division of Fabergé, who makes AQUANET, and asked why the smaller size costs the same as the big one. "No propellant," was the answer. "You get 40 percent more sprays from a nonaerosol. And it weighs less because there's no propellant in the package."

Mr. Barrie also told me that AQUANET is the strongest, longest-holding and least-expensive hair spray around ... and that you can get a 1-ounce purse spray AQUANET for as little as 39¢.

Beauty-Supply Houses Are Heaven's Gift to the Hair Nut

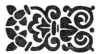

Huge bottles of shampoo. Enormous cartons of rollers. Clips by the gross. Hairbrushes. Dyes. Bleaches. Tints. Wigs. Falls. Dryers. Stylers.... You name it, and it's probably available at your beauty supply store.

There are sixteen hundred of these wonderful places across the country. They're there to service hairdressers and salons, but enterprising civilian consumers (like you and me) can very often wander in off the street, pay cash and take advantage of the 25 to 30 percent discount if we're cagey and gutsy enough.

The trick is to look like a hairdresser. Try to go when you need something more than a card of bobby pins. And, MOST IMPORTANT, make friends with the owner. In extreme cases, the management will ask to see your beautician's license. But most often you can get away without it.

My friend Sabina (who recently discovered the beauty-supply racket) got a tremendous bargain on a professional hair dryer and a pint of Green Out Shampoo (made by Colorful Products), with which she removed the nasty green tinge she'd picked up in her chlorinated pool. She also got a huge box of professional rollers and a natural-bristle hairbrush—and the whole shopping bag of stuff she walked away with cost her considerably less than what she would have paid in a discount drugstore. Beauty-supply stores are also fabulous places to pick up on things like 150-watt infrared light bulbs (THE NEWEST WAY TO DRY CURLY HAIR). They can be screwed into any lamp, so you can dry your hair while you're having breakfast and reading the latest issue of *Forbes*.

So indulge yourself. Look up your nearest beauty-supply shop under "Beauty Supplies" in the Yellow Pages ... then wear your trench coat and your slouch hat, and the rest of your spy costume ... and enjoy.

Getting The Brush

KENT OF LONDON makes the best natural-bristle brush I've ever seen ... and I'm not the only one. Countless spontaneous tributes to the excellence of every type of KENT brush are delivered to KENT's offices every year.

Take the retired chemist, for example, who wrote that he was ninety-two years old, and that on the completion of his apprenticeship seventy-two years ago, he had had a KENT hairbrush presented to him—and that he had used it every day since.

Or take the case of the retailer from Edinburgh who wrote in that one of his customers had a KENT baby's hairbrush which had been in use for sixty-five years by three generations of her family, and that she was hoping to use it on the fourth generation.

My favorite KENT brush is their Model LHS 5, which has a satinwood, dome-shaped back, and a full head of light-colored natural bristles. It retails for approximately $49.50 and will last forever if you don't abuse it. Even if it only lasts ten years or so, you've had the use of a magnificent instrument for less than $5 a year.

KENT makes thirty-seven different styles of natural-bristle brushes for women. They range in price from $13.50 all the way up to $80.00.

There are two other types of status brushes on the market I'd like to mention: DENMAN and MASON PEARSON. The DENMAN brushes ($4–$10) feature nylon pins on rubber-cushioned backs and are especially good for blowing your hair dry because they're built to withstand the heat your blow dryer puts out.

MASON PEARSON's mainstay brushes ($6.50–$37.50) are sleek, black ovals with natural and plastic bristles imbedded in soft, red, rubber bases.

If you can't find any of these lovely brushes in your nearest quality drugstore or in a department store nearby, write to the companies directly. They assure me they'll be happy to give you the name of a brush dealer in your area.

KENT OF LONDON
British Empire Building
620 Fifth Avenue
New York, New York 10020

DENMAN BRUSHES
Sekine Company
200 Park Avenue South
New York, New York 10003
ATT: Hal McGahey

MASON PEARSON HAIR BRUSHES
7 Main Street
East Rockaway, New York 11518
ATT: Bea Grossman

My Kingdom for a Fine-Tooth Comb

Luckily, fine-tooth combs don't cost kingdoms ... and anyway, fine-tooth combs aren't recommended for combing your hair. Especially if it's wet. Combing wet hair is a delicate operation for which you need a WIDE-tooth tortoiseshell comb. SPEERT #15, a 7½-inch comb that is handmade in Switzerland, is a perfect honey for combing wet hair and sells for about $2. A smaller version on the same theme to carry around in your purse is the SPEERT #14, which measures 4½ inches, has the same wide teeth as the #15 and costs approximately $1.50.

SPEERT also makes marvelous tortoiseshell bobby pins which don't break or bend your hair as much as regular metal-type bobbies. They come twelve to a package and sell for about 50¢ each.

By the way, if you're still using rubber bands ... Stop It! Rubber bands are a disaster.

They make friction points in your hair, which in turn heat it up, which makes the hair cells big and easily breakable. Before you know it you've got a severe case of the splits and the frizzies.

SPEERT makes hundreds of beautiful tortoiseshell barrettes, clips, hair ornaments and interlocking combs that do the same job as rubber bands, but without the damage.

Ask at your drugstore. If they don't have a big SPEERT display, write to SPEERT, and they'll tell you where to find their products.

SPEERT INC.
315 West 35th Street
New York, New York 10001

Some Combs Are Just for Show

The most beautiful combs I've seen anywhere in the last five years look as though they should cost fortunes. Some are ebony-black laced with gold or mother-of-pearllike designs. Some are coral and green feather designs.

They're wonderful for putting in evening bags or leaving out on top of the bureau. Last year I gave one to everybody I know as a Christmas present. And the best part of all is that these luscious, handmade-in-India combs are extremely affordable. They're made of inlaid plastics, come in various colors, patterns and sizes, and even have their own accompanying hand mirrors and toothbrushes.

pocket-size tiny comb	$5.00
small half-round comb	$6.00
long, skinny purse comb	$5.50
fancy bureau comb	$8.00
curly hair or Afro comb	$7.00
large-handle comb	$48.00

colors and patterns: white striated with brown, coral/green, black/gold, green/white, and brown/white check pattern.

All combs can be ordered from:

JENNY B. GOODE, INC.
1194 Lexington Avenue
New York, New York 10028

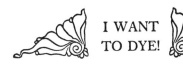

I WANT TO DYE!

Auburn tresses went out of fashion in England with the death of the Red-Haired Queen. A pity it was, too, because the English had just perfected a hedge-privet and radish hair dye. When the fashion changed, women took to coloring their hair gold-blond with rhubarb and white wine, or honey and gum arabic. White complexions were in fashion, too, and were effected by covering the face with poppyseed oil and dusting it with pulverized ash of pig jawbone. In 1660, Samuel Butler wrote this of English womanhood:

Not ten among a thousand weare
Their own complexions nor their
    haire . . .

Left-Handed Implements

Left-handed people have terrible problems with right-handed scissors because the blades are angled only for right-handed use and won't cut worth a darn when used by a south-paw. To solve this annoying problem, June Gittleson (president of THE LEFT HAND) offers several interesting versions of left-handed barber shears and some nifty little nail scissors all with sturdy reversed blades, powerful leverage and fine-ground edges. THE LEFT HAND's catalog (which includes things like left-handed catchers' mitts, left-handed water carafes, left-handed address books and left-handed boomerangs) can be yours if you'll send $1 to:

THE LEFT HAND
140 West 22nd Street
New York, New York 10011

The Egyptians didn't have any choice. They HAD to use all that natural stuff. WE, on the other hand, believe in the benefits of pure, unadulterated chemistry.

—Spokesperson for Clairol

If you really want to, there are all sorts of ways to dye your hair. You can spray yourself with a temporary Nestlé (metallic based) color, for example. Or use a Grecian formula to get rid of gray. You can get yourself a temporary rinse from Roux or a Finger Painting Kit from Clairol. You can even dye your hair with food coloring. You can use a single process, a double process or a semipermanent rinse. You can be frosted, streaked, highlighted, naturalized, marbelized, framed, haloed, tortoise-shelled or dimensional-shaded. What's more, you can do all these things at home and save yourself enough money to invest in something that matches your new hair color.

Think of it this way: The same frosting can cost you $100 (at Leslie Blanchard's) or $30 (in your neighborhood salon) or $6.50 (in your bathroom). Add to this price schedule the fact that most hair-coloring products are discounted like crazy, and doing your hair at home becomes almost too tempting to miss.

Discounting also makes shopping around a must. Basically, the price depends on the store. I've seen a hair-coloring kit in my local drugstore for $4.50, and right across the street somebody's got the same one for $2.95 and down the block someone else has it for $3.40. The thing to remember is that the major companies have no control over what price your store sells their product for. They can only suggest a retail price. This means the field is wide open, and that diligent legwork very often pays.

Now, it occurs to me that (since only one out of every three women in the country over the age of sixteen dyes her hair) there are two out of three of us who may be confused about what all these terms mean. Just what IS single-process color? And what kind of a commitment am I making if I do it to my hair? It was this sort of question that drove me to Harriet. Harriet has (by her own admission) been changing her hair color regularly since she was fifteen. She insists that blonds really DO have more fun, and she works for one of the major manufacturers of hair-coloring products in the United States. Some little while ago, Harriet sat by my side, squinted evilly at my graying roots, and helped me draw up the following vital information.

Harriet's Home Hair-Coloring Handbook
Single-Process Color

Single-process color is just what it sounds like—a single process that allows you to change the color of your hair in one operation. You can lighten it as much as five or six shades, or darken it as much as you want, or simply cover gray.

Single-process color is permanent, peroxide-based, and you can pick it up in two forms. The first is a *shampoo-in formula* that comes with color, developer and bottles all in one tidy package. The second is a *cream formula,* which is fine for just covering gray or simply retouching roots, but is a little more complicated to buy. With cream formula, you have to buy your developer and your bottles separately. The price is about the same: Shampoo-in runs about $2.75, cream formula plus developer comes to about $2.50.

It should take you about an hour to change your hair color. That's an hour from start to shampoo out. The disadvantages depend on what it is you want to do. Which means that if you want to change your entire hair color noticeably, you'll have to touch it up every four to six weeks. The severity of the change you make determines how often you'll have to touch up. For instance, if you're using a shade that's very close to your natural color, then you won't have to bother so often because your regrowth won't be as noticeable as if you went five or six shades lighter.

Double-Process Color

Double processing allows you to go the full range from very dark hair to very, very light. It's a major, drastic change. Double process involves a phase which everybody in the industry calls prelightening. This is merely a fancy way to say bleaching—in other words, removing the natural pigment from your hair. When your natural pigment is gone, you use a product called a toner to deposit whatever nice, soft, shade you want. You have to use a double-process method whenever you want to go from dark brown to light blond (for instance) or whenever you want to lighten your hair five or six shades. Figure that there's about a twenty-shade difference between dark brown and light blond, and proceed from there. Double process is also the answer if you want to have very close control over the shade of blond you wind up with.

The only disadvantages to double process are that it takes about twice as long to do (something like two hours), it's lots harsher on the hair (because of the bleaching) and it requires more frequent touch-ups. Remember that when that dark brown grows in at the scalp, it's going to contrast with your light blond, and you're going to have to cover it again every three weeks or so. How often you'll really need touch-ups depends a lot on how you wear your hair. If you have a part and you wear your hair simply, your roots are going to show more quickly than if you've got a soft, tousled kind of fluffy hairstyle where regrowth won't be obvious quite so quickly. The price range for double-process products (for both lightening kit and toner) is in the area of $5 or under.

Semipermanent Colors

Semipermanents have no peroxide in them, so they can't lighten hair. Their primary use is for covering gray, but they can also be used to enrich and give very subtle highlights to your own natural color. Semipermanents are marvelous for a woman who really doesn't want to color her hair, or for someone who really likes her own shade a lot but is getting some gray that she'd like to get rid of. Semipermanents come in two formulas: shampoo-in, which is best for covering gray; and foam, which is not as runny and is generally acknowledged as being more fun to use. Either formula will run you between $2.20 and $2.50. The only drawbacks to using this method are that semipermanents wash out in four to six shampoos, and you can't make much of a color change with them . . . but for some people, these disadvantages are plus points.

Temporary Rinses

The sad part is that temporary rinses don't do much of anything. In fact, they're primarily used by blonds who find that their hair is getting a little brassy between color treatments, so they'll use a temporary rinse to cut down on the brass.

I'm forever reading in newspapers and magazines things like: "Before you go into a drastic and permanent change, try a temporary rinse and see if you like it." Well, that's meaningless, because you simply can't do enough with a temporary rinse to find out if you like something. They are useful in toning down brassiness in lightened hair, but that's about it.

Metal-Based Combs and Lotions

Most of these metal-based hair colorings are used to coat the hair shaft and cover up the gray. Some of them are "instant" and some of them work over a period of weeks and seem to miraculously bring back your natural color. The trouble with them is that they cause an unreliable metal buildup on your hair, and if you're not careful or if you've been using the product for an extended period of time, you can end up with an interesting, off-beat green tint.

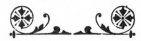

Haircoloring Sprays, Vegetable Dyes and Food Colorings

The sprays are really temporary rinses that coat your hair and give you dramatic effects that you can't normally get with temporary products. You can, for example, put ribbons of platinum blond into your flame-red hair on Wednesday night, then wash them away on Thursday morning. This is not natural-looking color, but it sure is fun, cheap ($1.50 for a 4-ounce can) and easy to get rid of. This sort of temporary color works sort of like water-based paint, coating your hair, then washing off as soon as you get into the shower. Beware of rainstorms.

Vegetable dyes and food colorings merely stain the hair. Most vegetable-coloring products, as a matter of fact, are derivatives of henna. Their major benefits are that they give you body and sheen. Their major defect is that it's hard to control the color. Vegetable dyes and food colorings (like the kind you put into Christmas cookies) can cost anywhere from 39¢ to $5.

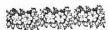

Multicolored Treatments or Special Effects

This broad new category covers a multitude of things, a lot of which are merely terminology. What one person calls frosting another will call tortoiseshelling or sun lightening or gosh knows what all. There are a million terms for the multicolored treatments, but certain rules apply to all of them.

The most important of these rules is that with multicolored special effects you work only on certain strands. You don't color the entire head. This means that within the perimeters of not making one major drastic change, the sky is pretty much the limit. For example, you can frost a very dark head with very blond streaks (for $6.50), if that's what you want. Or you can lighten up a light brown and bring up natural-looking blond highlights with a ($4.50) hair-painting kit, or you can encourage reddish or golden brown highlights in your dark auburn hair with a ($4.50) fingerpaint set. It's all up to you.

The wonderful advantage to multicolored treatments is that your roots don't show as obviously when they're growing in, so you don't get that awful, obvious line of demarcation. Also, you can create special effects as often or as infrequently as you want to. If you want to do them once every six months, that's fine ... you're not committed to a regular touch-up schedule.

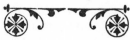

I regard one's hair as I regard husbands; as long as one is seen together in public, one's private divergences don't matter....
—SAKI (H. H. MUNRO), "The Secret Sin of Septimus Brope"

The Ever-Popular "Does She or Doesn't She?" Question

Joan Crawford did (in the early fifties) and so did floral designer Irene Hayes and interior decorator Melanie Kahane. Grace Pelham did it in the 60s, and by 1972, when Cybil Shepard did it, hundreds of models and celebrities and millions of American women just like you and me already HAD.

If anybody is still in doubt about what all

these women were doing—they were coloring their hair. Now almost everyone colors her or his hair, including Richard Burton and Dave De-Busschere. So if you do NOW, or you haven't YET but you're seriously thinking about it, CLAIROL wants you to know that they're ready, willing and able to help you. Thrilled, in fact. They actually *are* ... I've been up there and they are kind and patient and darling. They'll answer your questions personally and graciously if you call them at (212)644-2990, Monday through Friday between 9 A.M. and 5 P.M. (New York time). And, if you're in New York, you can drop in for a personal consultation. No muss. No fuss. No charge.

Having a problem with coloring? Clairol will help with that, too. They'll even send you the right product in the right color. All you have to do is fill out their hair-coloring questionnaire, send them a swatch of your hair, and enclose 50¢ for haircoloring and $1 for a hair-painting or frosting kit. To get your questionnaire, write:

HAIRCOLORING INSTITUTE
Consumer Relations Department
CLAIROL
345 Park Avenue
New York, New York 10022

Before you seal the envelope to Clairol, you might want to ask them for a copy of their book *Healthy, Happy Hair.* This will cost you $1.75, in return for which it will deliver lots of basic information on the hair you have (fine, coarse, thick, thin, straight or curly), the different cuts you might want to have and the coloring facts you'll need to know to lighten, darken, change your color or get rid of gray; it'll also give you a valuable section called "Special Considerations for Black People," which goes into Afros, braids, naturals and straighter styles.

What do you say to a teen-age
daughter who has saved up from a
really skimpy allowance and wants to
become a blonde?
—Press, Elmhurst, Illinois

Create a New Light In Your Life

Get yourself a hair-painting kit. Why shell out $65.00 at the salon when you can easily paint your hair at home for $4.50? Wait a minute. What *is* hair painting anyway?

The French call it *balayage,* but no matter what you call it, hair painting is simply the delicate process of making ribbons of highlights on the top layer of your hair. It's as simple as finger paints (even though you do it with a special brush), and it takes about fifteen minutes to spark up mousey brown hair or take the dirt out of a dirty blond. Besides, it never needs to be retouched (no roots, you know) and you can do it every few weeks or whenever the mood strikes. Hair painting is yet another goody from Clairol. The Clairol QUIET TOUCH Hair-painting Kit (for brush-on hairlights) is at drugstores everywhere for just about $4.50.

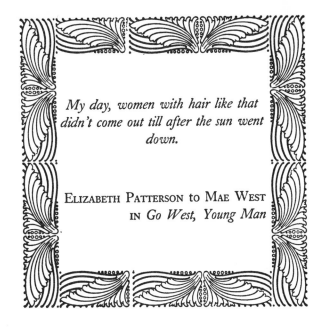

My day, women with hair like that didn't come out till after the sun went down.

ELIZABETH PATTERSON to MAE WEST
IN *Go West, Young Man*

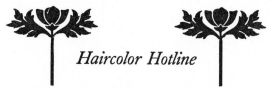

Haircolor Hotline

L'OREAL's consumer relations people get thousands of calls and letters from women all over the country with hair-coloring problems or questions that need personal, and sometimes *immediate,* attention. They're also happy to help students who are doing term papers on hair coloring or research people who need technical advice. Just about the only things they won't divulge are trade secrets. If you'd like to speak to someone at L'OREAL, call (212)697-5115 and ask for the consumer relations department. If you'd rather have your question answered in writing, send it to:

> L'OREAL
> Consumer Relations
> 530 Fifth Avenue
> New York, New York

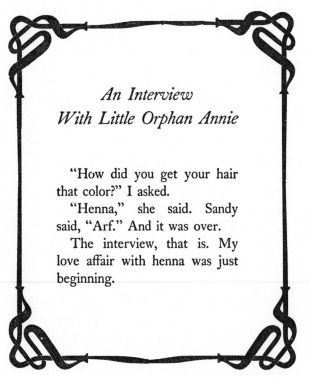

An Interview With Little Orphan Annie

"How did you get your hair that color?" I asked.

"Henna," she said. Sandy said, "Arf." And it was over.

The interview, that is. My love affair with henna was just beginning.

Henna is a totally natural hair color that's made from dried leaves and flowers of the eastern henna bush. When you get it from the herb store, it's powdered and looks like a fine green sand. But wet it, and from spinach green it turns a lovely amber color and takes on the consistency of mud-pie materials.

Once you get over any initial objection to the way henna looks, you'll be able to think of all the marvelous things it'll do for your hair ... like turning it a deep mahogany red or a bright frizzeldy orange. The first time I used henna I was completely caught up in the way it smelled—just like new-mown hay—so I didn't even think about the fact that it was a superb conditioner, or that Mohammed dyed his beard with the stuff. I just sat there in the sun on my terrace (oh, all right, on my fire escape) and let the mud dry till it caked. The result (after about three hours of letting my dark brown hair bake) was a deep purple copper color, plus masses of body and shine. A jam jar full of henna will cover a wild, curly mass of medium-length hair, and you can alter the coloring process by the length of time you leave it on or by adding things like lemon juice (to make the final effect orange-bright) or grape juice (to get a funky purple) or coffee (to deepen the red).

For medium brown hair, two hours under a henna pack will turn you a deep red. For light brown hair, an hour will give you a sort of Irish setter color. For blonds, an hour will make you look like your hair is on fire. If you'd rather just condition with henna than color with it, it does come in a colorless version made specifically for blonds, but all other procedures are the same: Mix to a muddy consistency with water (or lemon juice or whatever), apply till it covers your hair completely, let dry for an hour (or longer), wash out and revel in being a redhead.

You can, by the way, dye your *skin* with henna (which makes an interesting semipermanent eyeshadow and a natural finger-and toenail polish that turns your nails amber-pink and lasts for weeks.

You can order henna from natural herb suppliers (like those on page 000) or you can buy Egyptian henna in a profusely illustrated cannister at your drugstore, or you can search out a health food store that carries TRUE EARTH COSMETICS. TRUE EARTH henna comes in 3-ounce paper bags or in handmade (ancient-looking) pottery cannisters.

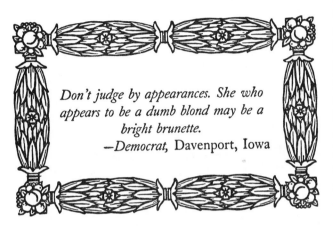

Don't judge by appearances. She who appears to be a dumb blond may be a bright brunette.
—*Democrat*, Davenport, Iowa

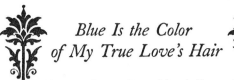

Blue Is the Color of My True Love's Hair

According to Irene Frangides (editor of *American Hairdresser* magazine), blatantly phony hair color is on its way back. Brassy blonds, flamboyant reds, maybe even greens and blues. To make things even more interesting, the new whiz-bang colors will go with carefully constructed hairstyles—constructed like buildings ... intricate erections, really—like Marie Antoinette's boat hairdo. Seemed to me a far cry from the free-swinging, geometric, "let-the-wind-blow-in-my-hair" look I'd just gotten to know and love, so I asked why we were going back to *paper-mâché* hair. "Because," said Ms. Frangides, "with the economy the way it is, no woman wants to look like she just woke up and blew her hair dry anymore. She wants to go to the beauty parlor and have the $15 she spent there really SHOW."

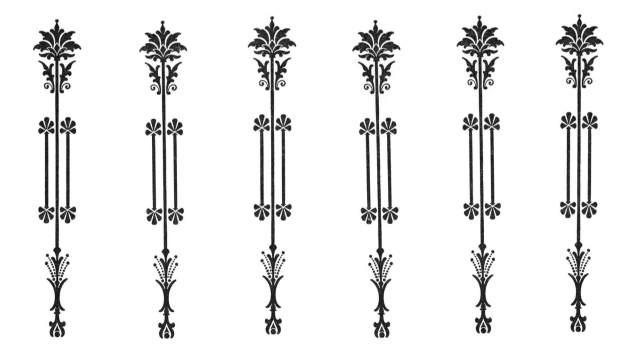

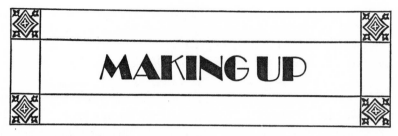

MAKING UP

Every woman has the potential to be beautiful. There ARE no ugly women. There are only women who don't do the right things for themselves. With the right help, every woman can get heads to turn when she walks down the street. If women took the time to find out what's best for them, you'd have a world full of very pretty ladies.
—Statement attributed to a not atypical executive vice president at Revlon, Inc.

Watch closely now, because the American cosmetics business is changing faster than a hot cat hightailing it over a back fence in the dead of night. In fact, beauty is a business firmly rooted in change and surrounded by an atmosphere where everybody's looking for a breakthrough.

Breakthrough. It's an interesting word. If it were used in medical circles, *breakthrough* might mean finding the cure for colds, cancer, or the bubonic plague. In the beauty industry a breakthrough is a product or a concept or a method of application that changes everything.

Like great, inspired poems, breakthroughs don't just happen. They're the result of the right people being in the right places when the channel to the cosmic consciousness opens up, and for one split second they can put together all the elements in history and come up with something new.

Needless to say, breakthroughs are just about as exciting as having 200,000 volts of direct electrical current zapped through your brain. People have been known to work twenty-six-hour days for months perfecting a breakthrough concept that came to them in an instant.

Now, you get one breakthrough (like the kind of blusher that's applied with a brush instead of a powder puff or your index finger) and, if it's really hot, the way blusher was when it was first invented, it tends to expand itself into other areas. Blush-On changed the way we applied our eyeshadow, changed the way we put on our lipstick, and so on.

So breakthroughs are one way cosmetics change. Another (and stick with me now, because this is a bit more subtle) way we change is that the *words* we use to describe what we want out of a product stay the same—but the product changes. Suzanne Grayson, the woman who was directly responsible for developing Blush-On, told me this story about lipsticks, and I'm going to repeat it here because it made me stop and think about all the changes I've lived through in direct relation to what I put on my mouth to make it prettier.

"If you were to look at consumer surveys back in the 1950s, where they asked women 'What is most important to you in a lipstick?' the answer was always *color*. And after that, that the lipstick should be creamy and moist and should stay on and not dry the lips and not be greasy.

"They said that in 1950 and they're saying it today. Only the evaluation of what is 'creamy' and 'moist' and 'nondrying' and 'stays on' is totally different. A 'creamy lipstick' in 1950 would be a terribly dry lipstick today. So the words have stayed the same, but the frame of reference has changed and lipsticks have gotten creamier and creamier and creamier ... and softer and softer and softer."

To add about a cup and a half of confusion to the fact that there are constant changes and no firm definitions to lean on, the beauty business is based on specific, peculiar and extremely personal nuances. What looks fabulous on ME may not work for you at all. OK, that's a BIG nuance, as is my predilection for red eyeshadow, and your avowal not to be caught dead in it. But consider this: Consider the change the ingre-dients can make in a product you use. Consider that not only can the difference of 1/10 of a percent of a certain ingredient completely and drastically change the way a product performs, but that the process of putting that product together can change it just as radically. This brings up questions we consumers never have to think about, like: "Do you add the bismuth oxychloride to the eyeshadow *before* you add the talc ... or after? And if after, how LONG after?" These are crucial questions, and the answers are critically important to the way your eyeshadow performs.

Testing is also one of those crucial questions we just never think about when we're standing there in the drugstore looking for a new liquid foundation. Would you feel better about the stuff you're buying if you knew it wouldn't even *get* to the drugstore unless it had survived test conditions that would make your teeth curl?

A lipstick is kept in a room at a constantly uncomfortable temperature of 120 degrees, and if it can survive this kind of treatment, you can be sure it'll live happily on your dressing table for anywhere up to three years without breaking down, getting moldy, or being contaminated by use.

OK. So beauty is a business of nuance and a business of change and a technical business that's not based just on puffery and sham and illusion. And if all that is true, there is a lot to know about this beauty business of ours, and a lot you can do to get the most out of it.

For one thing, you can know about things to be careful of. You can follow label directions carefully because they're there for a purpose. You can be wise about ingredients, which may take a little work, because ingredient-labeling regulations are a little strange and the words are confusing, but there are books around to help, and you can get your hands on them. You can find out how professionals test products—what they look for—and then you can apply what you need from that information to make your own tests at the counter or at home.

You can experiment like crazy and be aware of the companies that make experimenting easy as well as fun and won't send you to the poorhouse in a hand basket if you make a mistake. THAT's what you can do . . . and while you're at it, you can read the rest of this chapter and pick up some solid, practical information on special carrying cases, drugstores, application equipment and Lord knows what all.

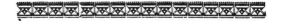

Beauty is a form of genius—is higher, indeed, than genius, as it needs no explanation.

—Oscar Wilde

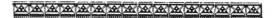

GIANTS OF THE BEAUTY BUSINESS

Three Gossipy Books on the Beauty Business

Dear K.T.,

These are my three absolute favorite books on the beauty business, which, as you know, is inhabited by some special breed of insanely dedicated and driven eccentrics. They all worked very hard. All of them demanded ultimate loyalty from their people.

They were all completely competitive. They all hated each other (at least publicly). They were all a completely fascinating collection of drives and compulsions and quirks that will hold you spellbound when you read about them.

Helena Rubinstein (the ultimate Polish-Jewish mother figure) had an empire built on skin cream and a priceless collection of paintings. She accessorized her bowler hats and maharanee jewels with the brown paper bags she carried her lunch in.

Elizabeth Arden rubbed her creams and lotions into the flanks of her thoroughbred horses . . . Charles Revson put sex into the makeup business . . .

These are the people who serve as raw material for my favorite bedtime reading, and they're all covered so bloody well that you must RUN, do not walk, to your bookstore and get all of them. Here's a rundown on each:

Madame: *a book which faithfully recreates the whirlwind of chutzpah who was Helena Rubinstein. Written with love and not a little bitchiness by Patrick O'Higgins (Madame's secretary, bodyguard, social director, guinea pig and most unabashedly benevolent critic).*

MADAME
by Patrick O'Higgins
Dell (Paperback, $1.50)

Miss Elizabeth Arden: *The fabulous, rags-to-riches portrait of the bizarre life of beauty's bitch-goddess that takes you into her laboratories, her office, her salon and her bedroom to reveal a world that was hers and hers alone (almost).*

MISS ELIZABETH ARDEN
by Alfred Alan Lewis and Constance Woodworth
Pinnacle (Paperback, $1.50)

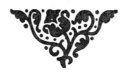

The Man Who Built the Revlon Empire: Charles Revson was the kind of powerful, controversial, ruthless, self-made American businessmen I just can't get enough to read about. He didn't give a damn about winning friends and influencing people with his charm. He had the guts and the brains and the merciless energy to take a bottle of nail polish and a psychic understanding of female fantasy and carve a multimillion-dollar business out of American womanhood with them.

He was a power broker, a philanderer, and a hypochondriac who wended his way through a world of top models, big spenders and cut-throat businessmen, earning himself the reputation of the world's biggest son of a bitch. He couldn't remember his first wife's name, he walked out on his second, and gave Lynn (the third Mrs. R) $30,000 in a tin can for their tenth anniversary.

His sex life was strange. His business life was stranger. Still, there are literally hundreds of men and women who remember him as the most vital, positive influence on their careers and their lives.

When he died, he owned one of the world's biggest yachts and was king of one of the world's most glamorous empires. Andrew Tobias has written a gossipy, revealing story about the man and his genius. It's called Fire and Ice, *and I would thoroughly recommend reading it the next time you need a little injection of excitement.*

FIRE AND ICE
The Story of Charles Revson—
the Man Who Built the Revlon Empire

AN UNAUTHORIZED BIOGRAPHY
by Andrew Tobias
William Morrow & Company (Hardcover, $10)

Yours Covered in Moisturizer,

Terry Vaughn...

Malibu, California

SEND FOR THESE FREE CATALOG HITS NOW

**THE HERBARY AND
POTPOURRI SHOP**
Box 543
Orleans, Massachusetts 02653
Soaps and cosmetics using herbs and other
organic properties

JENNY'S GARDEN
235 East 53rd Street
New York, New York 10022
Natural organic cosmetics

MEADOWBROOK HERB GARDEN
R 138
Wyoming, Rhode Island 02898
American distributor of Dr. R. Hauschka's
cosmetics

THE SOAP BOX
Box 167
Woodstock Hill, Connecticut 06218
Unique soaps, shampoos and cosmetics—
profusely illustrated.

HOW I FOUND MY MILLION DOLLAR FACE IN A FIVE-AND-TEN-CENT STORE
by Bambé Levine

Take back your mink cream. Take back your
poil oil. What made you think that I was one of
those goils?

I grew up in Great Neck and what did *I*
know? Royal bee balm at $100 a shot. Placenta
emollients from some unknown donor. Neck
creams. Elbow lotions. Deep-pore potions. I was
innocent to it all. I swear.

Mother told me: "To look beautiful you gotta
spend." And now it's hard to go on a Maybelline
diet after a history of: "Here. Take, dahling. Go
to Erno Laszlo and BUY! Ya should look beautiful and get MARRIED ... such a gorgeous kid
like you."

But today I'm poor. Like an agnostic mouse.
I'm poor. Off on my own. Out of a job. So now
it's Woolworth's. Lamston's. The five-and-dime
circuit. *I'm* not proud.

I reasoned: I've always known how to communicate with women. And I think they know how
to communicate with me. After all, where would
I be today without Estée (Lauder), Helena
(Rubinstein), Elizabeth (Arden) or the adorable
Marcella (Borghese)? But I'll let you in on a
secret. They've nothing to compare with the
delights of (Lady) Esther, Hazel (Bishop), Helen
(Neushaffer) or even Monica Simone ... bless
her cheap heart.

Everyone knows you buy color and consistency. That's all that really matters. "It's all in
the application, my dear." Think for a moment.
Instead of spending $4 for a rod of Biba mascara
or the like, you can eat a large lunch, go to the
movies, get a manicure, take a taxi instead of
waiting for the bus, or put the money toward
something you *really* want. How absolutely
logical!

You don't ever have to spend big bucks to
look great. I'll prove it to you with a step-by-
step you wouldn't believe.

First, you invest $1.25 for a jar of *Elizabeth
Post* moisture cream (moisture is a MUST under
makeup). Besides, a rumor went around several
years ago that Post was really Arden in drag. I
don't know if this gossip was ever resolved, but
who cares. When you dip your finger into the
richest concoction this side of the East River;
what does a label mean, I ask you?

"Neck," I always heard. "Don't forget about
your neck. That's where the tell-tale signs of age
begin. You must nip them in the bud." *Germaine
Monteil* was fine for high school (when my
mother could afford it), but when you're a career
girl (even if it is by default), you can't afford to
take too many chances. I've learned to love
Johnson and Johnson's Baby Cream and smear up
each night before I bed down. Look, Ma. No
wrinkles!

For my next testimonial, may I sincerely

recommend one of Woolworth's most popular brands of liquid foundation, *Fresh'n Lovely* by *Maybelline*. For $1.49 you can afford to buy an extra bottle for your summer tan. The color range you wouldn't believe.

Contour your face with a dab of *Tangee* rouge at 49¢ and a dash of *Cecila's Brush 'n Blush* at $1.00. If you really want to go to town on your cheeks, dust on *Angel Face* powder by Ponds—a real steal at 69¢, and I couldn't live without it.

Eye shadows? Ummm. It's hard to decide, since the selection of inexpensive shadows is so vast. For both quantity and quality, I heartily recommend *House of Westmore's 4-Shade Palette* affair; the $1.59 is well spent for a two-year supply of mixing and fixing. *Cutex Frosty Powder Shadows* (at $1.25) also come in myriad colors to suit any mood or fancy. And then of course there are . . .

Lashbrite pencils. House of Westmore Crayons. On and on and on. Who could go wrong?

Eyelashes are out (even though you can still get them at the 5 & 10). My advice is that if you're still addicted, pull them off immediately and throw them away. They're tacky. Get rid of them. The same for eyeliner, which went (or should have gone) the way of the ocean liner and is now as *passé* as glitter sweaters and bell-bottom pants.

The kiss. How will you taste when kissed? Bubble gum? Jasmine? Teardrops? Rain? The people at *Italian Labs* (who else would be so tuned in to love) have developed lip potions which will make lips quiver well into the night. In flavors, yet. At 89¢, a cheap price to pay for such pure pleasure. Even Hazel Bishop has come a long way since her first indelible lipstick, and every cosmetic manufacturer from here to there has an answer to lip magnetism.

Take BACK your expensive mink cream. Turn the other cheek at *Beauty Checkers*. Sue me. Sue me. What can you do me, if I learned to love the finer but CHEAPER things of life.

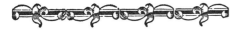

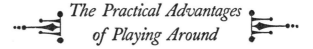

The ideal makeup is one that makes you look completely perfect. You can't make a mistake with it. It looks terrific. It's a joy to use (a really sensual *experience). You don't have to be an expert to put it on, and, even if you use it wrong—you can't mess it up.*

—SUZANNE GRAYSON,
President, THE FACE FACTORY

TRUTH IN MAKEUP

The Practical Advantages of Playing Around

A product manager in the cosmetics industry earns her keep searching for the perfect product. A product manager is a cross between someone who likes getting drill presses for Christmas gifts and a five-year-old girl playing dress-up. She's a little bit of scientist, a little bit of chemist and very much a woman. Technically, product managers involve themselves in almost every phase of making the over 200,000 products on the market today. They dream them up, get them made by chemists, test them, refine them, have a say in what kind of box, bottle, jar or tube they come in, find names for them and bet their jobs on YOUR ACCEPTANCE of the finished product.

Like scientists and mathematicians and astro-physicists and astrologers, product managers talk to each other in their own special language. They sit in front of a mirror with a lipstick and judge its slip, drag, mass, coverage and transfer. Each kind of product has its own particular qualities, the qualities product managers define with funny words like *playtime*. And, oddly enough, once you have a working vocabulary of these technical words and the concepts behind them, it's easier to define what a product is doing (or not doing) for you . . . so that the next time you're standing at the makeup counter playing in the testers, you can tell the saleswoman you want a foundation with more coverage, or a lipstick that stays on longer, and thereby cut down on expensive mistakes caused by lack of communication.

The problem is that even though cosmetics have been around since ancient Egypt and product managers have been speaking to each other in technical terms for well over thirty years, there was never a "Webster's Dictionary of Cosmetic Conversation" or anything that would give the civilian population a clue to what was going on. So product managers might just as well be speaking in tongues, for all the good it did us. Well, that's silly; why shouldn't any one of us be able to judge cosmetics with the tools and words the pros use? And because I'm annoyed by such gaps in the information banks, I went and talked to some of the best product people in the business, and we sat down and developed "The Product Manager's Phrase Book."

The Product Manager's Phrase Book

Bleeding. Color flow, especially applied to the lipstick that runs into those little lines above and below your mouth.

Caking. This word is usually used to describe the small particles that form on top of your lipstick that you end up biting off. Also used to refer to makeup.

Coverage. The hiding quality in a makeup or a lipstick. Products with good coverage tend to mask imperfections and even out skin tone.

Drag. Drag is a feeling of resistance as you apply the product. It's *not* a negative term. The more drag a lipstick has, for example, the easier it is to outline.

Feathering. See *bleeding*.

Flaking. When a mascara is too dry, small chunks of it will flake off onto your cheeks.

Grabbing. Color that bunches up where it's first applied, then spreads unevenly, is said to be grabbing. This sort of thing happens mostly when you use a powder rouge over a cream or liquid foundation.

Lengthening. Product managers test lengthening qualities by putting one mascara on their left eyelashes and another on their right. They then compare the end result to see which is longest.

Mass. Mass means the amount of material deposited on your skin. It's different from coverage (hiding) in that you can have lots of mass with very little hiding. A lip gloss (even a dark one), for example, can have lots of mass and very little coverage.

Overall Effect. Overall effect is a very personal feeling. Three different sorts of effects *can* be described by the words *dewy*, which means glowy, not dry; *matte*, which is a nonshiny, pancake effect; and *lustrous*, which is a frosted, pearly effect.

Playtime. Playtime refers to blendability. It was best defined by Dr. J. J. Mausner, director of research and development for Helena Rubinstein, as "The time available to you to apply your makeup and get the effect you want from it before it sets into its final situation." For example, an eyeshadow is very mobile when it comes out of its container. It slides comfortably around on the surface of your lid and moves with the pressure of your finger on the applicator you're using. But after a while the wet stuff dries out and you can no longer move the shadow around or blend it. It's no longer "playable with." After twenty or thirty seconds the average eye makeup has set . . . which is why it stays in place and doesn't fall onto your cheeks. That's the intention with all makeup—to stay in place—but you don't want that to happen before you've blended it and spread it around, so playtime is the period between first putting the product on and final setting time.

Running. See *bleeding*.

Separation. Specifically applied to mascara. It means the space created between your eyelashes. A mascara with good separation doesn't clump your lashes all together.

Slip. Slip is the opposite of *drag*. The easier the slide is, the better the slip ... whether you're talking about foundation or eyeshadow or lipstick. Imagine a kid going down a children's slide. If he's wearing jeans he'll slide down easily. If his legs aren't covered he'll stick all the way down. The more difficult the slide, the less the slip.

Smear. If you touch your lipstick and then find it above or below your lip line (or anywhere else on your face), that's smearing. The same thing is used to describe what happens when you touch your mascara before it's completely dry and then find it on your cheek or above your eye.

Smudge. See *smear*.

Stain. The color left on your mouth after you wipe your lipstick off. Or, similarly, the color left on your cheek after you tissue off your blusher.

Tack. Tack is an interesting word used in lipstick testing. Basically, it means the sticky feeling you sometimes get when you press your lips together, then separate them slowly.

Transfer. Makeups that don't dry down completely transfer onto towels when you pat your face dry. Lipstick that comes off on your wine glass. Mascara that doesn't dry completely leaves tracks above your eye or on your cheek. All these things are *transfer* and they're different from *smear* because they don't involve the direct application of the human hand.

Transparent. Light goes through the product, like sun through a window.

Translucent. Light passes through but there's more coverage, like sunlight through frosted glass or shoji screens.

Wear. The length of time the product stays on. Lipstick wear depends both on the type and formula of a product (gloss or stick) and on what you do with your mouth. If you smoke a lot your lipstick will not wear as long as it would if you didn't smoke. Foundations generally wear all day long, unless you're particularly oily skinned and you're not using an undermakeup oil blotter or a specially prepared oily skin-type makeup.

Cream eyeshadows don't wear for very long, but the new powder creams wear virtually forever (or at least all day) without creasing or smudging.

Factory Fact-Lets

Big vats filled with pink, blue and brown liquids bubble industriously on the stove. Mason jars filled with powders in every conceivable color line the shelves. The technician lets me peek over his shoulder, and as I watch the birth of an eyeshadow, I feel a strange urge to be coated from guggle to zatch in maddening mauve, wild grass green or passionate plum. The colors look good enough to roll around in.

At the main Estée Lauder plant in Long Island, some twelve hundred people work with an equally staggering number of complex machines to put their secret formulas into bottles, compacts, tubes and boxes. Walking through the factory, you can see:

• Color-compounding and quality-control rooms which all face north, because north light is not distorted by sunlight. (So if you want your makeup to look its best and most natural when you're in natural light, put it on in front of a north-facing window.)

• Lipsticks that come to the packaging department in Baskin-Robbins-sized drums as a solid mass of color. The people in the packaging department liquify them, pour them into lipstick molds, let them solidify, then feed them down an assembly line where women in hairnets wave the finished sticks at a mixture of gas and air. This adds sheen to your lipstick and takes out any minor imperfections.

• Your favorite 5-ounce lotions mixed in three hundred- to one thousand-gallon kettles big enough to swim in.

The more time I spend in cosmetics labs, the more I think they'd make spectacular sets for science fiction movies. I wonder why nobody's done THAT yet?

 A fair exterior is a tacit recommendation.
—P. W. LONERGAN

*Experimenting is the only way to
learn about cosmetics.*
—PHYLLIS POSNICK,
Beauty Editor, *Vogue* magazine

Phyllis Posnick's
How-Not-to-Make-Mistakes Manual

1. Don't assume a makeup will look the same on your skin as it does in the pot. It won't—it'll probably look lighter.
2. Don't buy anything just because you liked the way it looked on the model in the magazine centerfold. Try it out first to make sure you'll be happy with the way the color and formula work for *you*.
3. Read the labels. Don't think they're kidding when they say Avoid Eye Area. The cosmetic companies go through great trouble and expense to test, research and retest their products. They do it for your protection, and they print cautionary tales on their labels. Reading and paying attention to them is not only good common sense but could save you untold problems.

Five Popular Misconceptions
About Eye Makeup

Your favorite color says a lot about you, but when it comes to eye makeup, you may be working under some popular misconceptions. Here's a tiny TRUE/FALSE Test that may give you a whole new way to look at your eyes.

1. *Eye shadow that matches my eye color makes my eyes look larger.* [True/False]
(False. This is an outdated idea that should have gone the way of the buggy whip and the hoop skirt. Eye shadow color is meant to be worn as a fashion accessory. It should pick up and extend the color of whatever it is that you're wearing. The idea is that if your shadow blends with the rest of your outfit, it's automatically more flattering not only to your face but to your total visual image.)

2. *When it comes to eye shadow, I'm always safe with blue, green, turquoise or aqua.* [True/False]
(False. The trouble with these popular eyeshadow colors is that they're not found in the natural color of your skin. Also, because they're vibrant, they can be very difficult to wear flatteringly. If you've been wearing nothing but these colors for the last two years or longer, it's probably time to experiment with ginger, or mocha, or even a light gray.)

3. *I'm scared of shadows like yellow and pink. They're too way out for me. Besides, you have to be very young to wear anything that vivid.* [True/False]
(False. Colors like lilac, violet, pink, peach and yellow are the same colors that show up in natural skin tones, so they automatically create a soft, natural look. They're also good for softening the vibrancy of blues and greens and for creating warm, natural highlights.)

4. *Frosted shadows look brassy. Besides, they always turn cakey before the evening is over.* [True/False]
(False. First, because frosted shadow is not just a *nighttime* experience anymore. The new ones are sheer enough to wear all the time. Second, because new technology has made frosty shadows almost totally foolproof. Aziza [the eye-makeup people] even came up with a new way to put color and frost together permanently, so that the shadows wear longer, look truer and can be counted on never to go chalky.)

5. *It's the eye-shadow color (not the mascara) that brings out the color of your eyes.* [True/False]
(False. Mascara acts like a light filter on a camera. With blue or green eyes, dark blue or dark green mascara intensifies the color of the iris as ambient light filters down

through your lashes. With dark eyes, blue or burgundy mascara gives depth to the iris, while sparking up the white of your eye.)

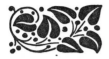

Million-Dollar Woolgathering

Usually it happens on a rainy Wednesday morning—or any other morning when, staring into a cosmetic drawer so messy only starlings would nest there, I lean back in my chair, close my eyes and fantasize the perfect product.

"It would be *small*," I say to myself. "Small enough to fit in my handbag without displacing the credit cards, cigarettes, sunglasses or car keys." Then I think about that for a while. Maybe I open my eyes and look back at all the nonsmall items that clutter my cosmetic life; the pots and the tubes and the jars and the packets.

"Yes." I say to myself, "it would be small—and—it would do *everything.*"

This, of course, is code. When I say, "It would do everything," what I am really saying is that I'd give almost anything to have a foundation, a lipstick, an eye shadow, a blemish cover, a mascara, and a blush-on all rolled into a 1½″ × 2″ aesthetically pleasing package. Oh, yes . . . and the colors should all be perfect. That goes without saying. In fact, if I could magically and in an instant be transformed from just getting up in the morning plain to stupendous—that, too, would be fine.

It hasn't happened yet. That's not to say it's impossible. Or that it isn't going to happen. But right now there are still minor problems with the production of the kind of product that I want. Like (for example) there's no supplier in the world who can make a container to hold so many different chemical compounds without disintegrating. (The case, that is, not the supplier!) And even if there were such a container, if I *really* wanted to have so many different products

in such a tiny package, I'd constantly have to refill the thing. Naturally, the minute the refilling stopped being fun, I'd stop thinking I'd got my hands on the perfect product and I'd go right back to staring into my cosmetic drawer.

In my fantasy (there with my eyes glued to the bottom of that dumb cosmetic drawer) I am not alone. Millions of women across the country are sitting in similar positions staring into THEIR cosmetic drawers, or their medicine chests or wherever it is that they keep their makeup. But the interesting thing is that in the nonfantasy, REAL world the pros are staring, too—and they're even more interested in turning up with the perfect product than we are.

There are some major differences between us and the professionals. The professionals, for openers, are not alone (they have a whole corporate structure to keep them company). They also have a lot more products to stare at, and their careers are riding on the kind of answers they come up with. So instead of peering into their medicine chests or vanities, the pros make long, thoughtful inspections of their product lines and their competitors' product lines, and when they've finished (and worked up a good stinging headache from the profusion of products on the market), they call in help.

In other words, they call in product managers and creative talents and marketing people and say, "OK, if you could have any cosmetic thing you wanted in the world . . . if you could make the perfect whatever . . . what, exactly, would it be? What would it do for you? What would it look like? How would you put it on and take it off? What kind of package would it come in? What would it cost?" (And on and on like that until EVERYBODY has a stinging headache.)

This search for perfection is merely another version of what you do or what I do on those rainy Wednesday mornings when we stare into our cosmetics drawers, with two notable important exceptions: one, the pros take this creative woolgathering deadly seriously. And two, the pros have a formal name for it— 'blueskying."

Blueskying is kind of like brainstorming, and one of the best people I know at the art is Cathy Cash Spellman (executive vice president of a relentlessly creative marketing firm called Spellman and Company).

"Blueskyers are expected to be wild," says Mrs. Spellman. "We're expected to be unusual. We're expected to come up with literally anything. Could be tomorrow's greatest convenience, or tomorrow's biggest bargain, or tomorrow's most sinful luxury. What our clients ask us to do for them is to shake out our thinking caps and polish up our long-distance vision ... and suggest all the things we can see in our mind's eye."

Since Spellman and Company's client list includes some of the weightiest names in the beauty business, Mrs. Spellman couldn't talk to me about the near future at all, because that's SECRET. But she did tear out a page from the *very far future* section of her blueskyer's notebook and allow me to reprint it here.

Before you delve in, however, I feel I have to warn you that all these suggestions are for the very far future. They are geared for people growing up maybe two or more generations from now. Consequently, some of them (or even ALL of them) are going to sound pretty strange to you. Therefore I urge you to pause for a moment and consider just how ridiculous cleavage makeup and false eyelashes and hair spray (or even matching lips and fingertips) might have sounded to an American woman in 1776, who just barely relied on beetroot for lip coloring and thought that rouging one's cheeks was an outrage.

They laughed at Christopher Columbus. They asked Alexander Graham Bell whom he was going to call. When *your* great-grandchildren ask you what it was like in the old days, are you going to have to tell them that you laughed at:

Mrs. S's Bluesky Makeup Notebook
or,
What's In Store for the Day After Tomorrow?

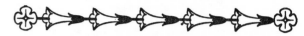

Spray Paint for Faces. Colorless stuff that goes on colorless and changes according to your own body chemistry. Spray face colors that look like clear gels but turn out to be just the right skin tone once you've put them on.

Antipollution Makeup. Because, as the pollution gets worse, we're going to need antibiotics or anything else we can get to smear on our bodies to keep them from absorbing all the horribleness.

Antibacterial Disease-Fighting Makeup. Much like antipollution makeup, but specifically geared to combat germs and bacteria.

Scalp Makeup. With increased social and business pressures incumbent upon them these days, women are beginning to lose their hair. So instead of getting false hair or wearing wigs, why not decorate the scalp? If you are completely bald and have lots of space to work with, you could decorate your head to match your body (like they do in Africa).

Internal Skin Tints. You take this pill, see, and it colors your skin from the inside so you look healthy. You could be darker or lighter all over with no muss, no fuss and no streaking. You could have a winter tan, or turn green or become just about any color that pleased you.

Healthful Makeup. If the womb-to-tomb dwelling really happens and we're all going to be inside all the time, we're going to have to give our bodies the nutrients that they'd normally get from being out in the fresh air and sunshine. That means vitamin D makeup and other makeups that replace healthy outdoor elements for an indoor culture.

Ear Makeup. We're already puncturing multiple holes in our ears and sticking things into them ... so why not an all-out effort at ear *decoration?* Ear makeup could either match eye makeup (like scalp makeup) or be designed to coordinate with the shade of your shoes, gloves, bag and hat.

Elastic Makeup. Antiaging makeup that freezes your face into a perpetual expression of youth, or allows you to pull back the wrinkles and glue them down. This could be every woman's answer to plastic surgery. One major drawback would be what to do when you peeled it off at night.

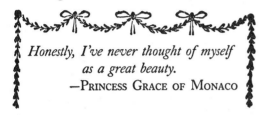

Honestly, I've never thought of myself as a great beauty.
—PRINCESS GRACE OF MONACO

YOUR CHANCE TO BECOME THE HIGH SCHOOL COVER GIRL OF THE YEAR AND WIN $1,000, TOO!

Ever been told you're pretty enough to be on a magazine cover? Ever dreamed about an all-expense-paid trip to New York, where you could try modeling, meet celebrities and be a contender for a $1,000 educational scholarship? Dreams are only a contest away, because once a year the search goes on for the lucky teenager who'll be chosen High School Cover Girl and have her picture on the cover of *Co-ed* magazine.

The national contest, sponsored by *Co-ed,* the classroom magazine, and the Noxell Corporation, makers of Cover Girl makeup, is open to all girls in grades seven through twelve. The winner is the girl whom the judges think typifies the American ideal of charm, personality and good grooming.

Ten semifinalists selected from four regions of the country (Northeast, Southeast, Midwest, Far West/Canada) are brought to New York, put up in an elegant hotel and swept into a whirlwind of glamorous activities. They have their hair styled by top New York stylists, get makeup tips from the experts and are photographed by a famous photographer. Each girl will also get a special fashion outfit, a model's kit of Cover Girl makeup and a $50 savings bond, and the national winner becomes High School Cover Girl of the Year and gets the grand prize: a $1,000 scholarship from Noxell and her picture on the cover of *Co-ed* magazine.

If you're in grades seven through twelve and want to enter, submit one full-length and one close-up photo and a statement in seventy-five words or less describing your daily grooming routine and the beauty aids you consider most important. Write your name, address, school grade, weight, height and measurements on the back of both photos and statement. *Co-ed*'s editors will judge your statement for originality and clarity and will count it equally with good grooming, charm and poise shown in the photos in the selection of the semifinalists. Entries, which become the property of Noxell Corporation, should be mailed to High School Cover Girl Contest, *Co-ed* magazine, 50 West 44th Street, New York, New York 10036 before the contest closing date, April 30.

MEN WHO WORK IN THE BUSINESS

Men who work in the cosmetics business have to develop uncaring attitudes about what the public thinks of them, because if they don't have a very secure image of themselves, they can get a little nervous. Here's a story a marketing director of one of the large companies told me:

"When I started in this business, I never had tissues around for testing lipsticks, so I would wipe my hands on my handkerchief. Once, when my wife had brought a suit of mine to the cleaners, she was checking the pockets and pulled out this handkerchief with eighteen different shades of lipstick on it. The cleaner was embarrassed for my wife, but my wife said, 'As long as it's here, clean it too.' Then she said, 'My husband has orgies.' So now we can't go back to that cleaner anymore."

MORE BOOKS
Definitions

If you flunked your high-school chemistry course the way I did and are hard pressed to tell the difference between aluminum hydrate and aluminum hydroxide, but you still want to know just what it is that went into your liquid foundation, go get yourself a copy of *A Consumer's Dictionary of Cosmetic Ingredients*. It's like a cram course in how cosmetics are made, and while it's not particularly riveting reading, it's certainly a handy book to have around if you ever need to know what flavor, color, fragrance or chemical made up the major part of your favorite product. It can also be a big help in figuring out what you may be allergic to and avoiding stuff with that ingredient in the future.

A CONSUMER'S DICTIONARY OF COSMETIC INGREDIENTS
by Ruth Winter
Crown (Paperback, $3.95)

Is There a Doctor in the House?

No doctor around? The next best thing is Deborah Chase's *Medically Based No-Nonsense Beauty Book*, which pays off with all the scientific knowledge you'll need to deal with your everyday beauty problems, plus special problems for skin, hair, eyes and great advice on choosing the cosmetics that work for you and on avoiding those that don't. The Westinghouse Talent Search chose Deborah Chase as one of the country's top young scientists ... the Bronx High School of Science gave her twenty-five assorted prizes for original scientific research and New York University trained her in biology and basic medical science—so her qualifications are sterling and her attitude is careful, concerned, thorough and might very well revolutionize your whole approach to beauty care.

THE MEDICALLY BASED NO-NONSENSE BEAUTY BOOK
by Deborah Chase
Alfred A. Knopf (Hardcover, $10)

 I think you could use a little mascara dear. I can still see your eyes.
—ROBERT LORICK,
Johnny Manhattan Bones

Postgrad Course in Total Beauty

When the time comes for a total make-over—a complete new you—and you want to settle in with some reading that combines diets, exercises and a complete (almost) instant make-over beauty program, the book to get your hands on is Eileen Ford's *A More Beautiful You in 21 Days*. Mrs. Ford is the cofounder and head of the world's largest model agency and agent to such famous beautiful women as Ali McGraw, Jane Fonda and Candice Bergen. In the book she tells of how she fell into the trap of middle-age drabness and in desperation figured out a plan to undo the damage in a record-breaking twenty-one days. The book includes menus, exercises and beautifully basic beauty advice.

A MORE BEAUTIFUL YOU IN 21 DAYS
by Eileen Ford
Simon & Schuster (Hardcover, $9.95)

I'm not going to try to make a model or a movie star out of you. I just want to help you make yourself the healthiest and most beautiful black woman you can be.
—NAOMI SIMS

The Beauty of Blackness

Naomi Sims, supermodel turned super-businesswoman turned author, knows how to make herself beautiful. In a word, the lady is striking ... and she's worked at it long enough and conscientiously enough and well enough so she can tell you—straight and clear—how to work it out for yourself. Which is exactly what she does in her book, *All About Health and Beauty for the Black Woman.* She shares not only her own knowledge of beauty but also what she's learned in hours of consultation with doctors, beauticians, cosmetologists, dentists and other pros. In fact, after four solid years of research Ms. Sims has come up with an easy-to-read encyclopedia you won't want to miss.

ALL ABOUT HEALTH AND BEAUTY
FOR THE BLACK WOMAN
by Naomi Sims
Doubleday & Company (Hardcover, $8.95)

> *A sensible girl is more sensible than she looks because a sensible girl is too sensible to look sensible.*
> —*Tribune,* Chanute, Kansas

Model Advice

The *I Hate to Make Up Book* has nothing to do with hating to make up. It's a professional model's guide to getting pretty with less strain and pain than you could possibly imagine. Oleda Baker, who is an international fashion model as well as an author, has pared every phase of making up down to its most basic parts, so that what you get is an expert's guide to city, country, daytime, evening, formal and informal makeup that takes virtually seconds to do. The line drawings are super, the directions easy to follow, plus you get inside beauty information on how to use highlights and shading, how to use corrective makeup, how to make up if you wear glasses and how to cope with pesky false eyelashes.

THE I HATE TO MAKE UP BOOK
by Oleda Baker
Prentice Hall (Hardcover, $7.95)

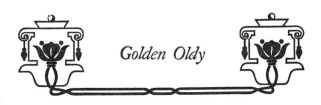

Golden Oldy

First published in 1899, *Harriet Hubbard Ayer's Book: A Complete and Authentic Treatise on the Laws of Health and Beauty* is a sincere, amusing and sometimes dictatorial trip down memory lane. By the time she published *Health and Beauty,* Ms. Ayer had divorced her husband, fought her daughter's father-in-law for her business, and battled to have herself released from a mental institution (to which she'd been committed by her daughter and ex-husband)—a brave and forthright woman. *Health and Beauty* is based on her years of research, travel abroad and in high society and her own rather acute observations. Scanning persons (her word) from head to foot, Ms. Ayer indulged in the first total make-overs (which she illustrated with some of the funniest pictures I've ever seen in the area short of the *Harvard Lampoon*'s spoof of *Cosmopolitan*). She also covered dyes, creams, cures for corns, exercises, massages (quite up to date), how to sleep without nightmares (illustrated), how to read character from the features and, in Appendix A, an amazing article on how "Catherine Lane, a human wreck, was restored to health and beauty without drugs or stimulants of any kind." This wonderful 543-page manifesto, available in a sensitively done reprint, would make a delicious addition to your own library or gift to a memorabilia-nut friend.

HARRIET HUBBARD AYER'S BOOK
(A Complete and Authentic Treatise on the Laws of Health & Beauty)
by Harriet Hubbard Ayer
An Arno Press Book published in cooperation with
Quadrangle/The New York Times Book Company (Hardcover, $8.95)

> *There were no distinctive lipstick flavors when Granpa was a young man. He says that when you kissed a girl all you could taste was girl.*
> —*Democrat*, California, Missouri

MARVELS OF MODERN MAGAZINES

Up-to-the-minute beauty advice—all the poop on what's new and what's wonderful. Step-by-step instructions on how to do it—whether the *it* is diet, skin care, exercise, haircuts or the newest way to put on eyeshadow—comes from women's magazines like *Glamour, Seventeen, Cosmopolitan, Vogue* and *Town & Country*. Some of these magazines gather up bunches of fine information and publish them in the spring and fall as sort of distillations of their best beauty material. Watch for them on your newsstands. In the meantime, here are two very special bits of information from two of my favorite magazines:

The Cosmopolitan *Beauty Philosophy*

You can do a hell of a lot with rather mediocre raw material.
—MALLEN DE SANTIS,
Beauty Editor, *Cosmopolitan*

Cosmopolitan is always interested in interesting first-person experiences. Sometimes they're interested enough to buy articles about them. So if you're THAT COSMOPOLITAN GIRL and you've just had your sweat glands removed or suffered through a difficult but thrilling orthodontia or signed into a fabulous fat farm and you would like to write about it, here's how: Sit down at a typewriter and write off a brief letter describing what your problem was, what you did to correct it, what the experience was like, how it turned out in the end and why you think it

would be a neat piece for *Cosmo*. Include samples of other things you've written if you have them, and send the whole lot to:

COSMOPOLITAN
BEAUTY DEPARTMENT
224 West 57th Street
New York, New York 10019

There's no guarantee that *Cosmo* will actually buy your article, but it may make you feel better just telling the pros about what happened.

One of the most interesting beauty articles I've EVER seen was done in the August 1973 issue of *Cosmopolitan*. It was the distillation of *Cosmo*'s silk purse out of a sow's ear philosophy and demonstrated so graphically what could be done with mediocre raw material that it took my breath away. It started with a picture of Samantha Jones (one of New York's really tippy-top models). The picture looked like it had been taken first thing in the morning after a very late night. Sam Jones looked—how shall I say it—AWFUL. We then watched in words and pictures how she transformed herself from really a very plain mouse of a girl (not just a girl you might not notice on the street but really actively plain—someone you might even feel a little sorry for) into a raving beauty, with a very skillful use of makeup. Reprints can be had by sending $1.50 to

HEARST PUBLICATIONS
Back Issue Department (COSMO, August 1973)
250 West 55th Street
New York, New York 10019

Jet-Set Beauty Booklets

Twice a year *Town & Country* magazine puts together an enormously elegant guide to beautifying. They've done wonderful in-depth sections on spas, beauty treatments, health and beauty for resort living, travel, night-life beauty, skin care and fragrance. The nicest thing about these special guides is that they represent the best, most current, most sybaritic goods and services available throughout the world. Names and phone numbers and complete information are usually included where applicable, and reprints are available. Should you want a back issue, write:

Back Issue Department
HEARST BOOK DIVISION
250 West 55th Street
New York, New York 10019

Send check or money order for $1.50 and remember to include the date of the back issue you want. Reprints and tear sheets are available in large quantities. Write Mr. Prumato for information.

MAIL ORDER MAKEUP

You wouldn't believe how many wonderful things you can have sent you through the mail. Fabulous collections of makeup, marvelous carrying cases, nifty brushes, and you can have them all without any more effort than it takes to put a stamp on an envelope and get to your nearest mailbox. Here are the most interesting mail order possibilities I've found:

Cinandre's Selection With a Sensible Price Tag

When the Cinandre people decided that they wanted to make makeup, they sought out the clearest, most vibrant colors they could find, gave them names like Sienna, Henna, Cinnabar, Garnet, Lapis, Belfast and Lynchburg, invented a way to make a small selection of items mixable and matchable so that the combinations were enormous (and the esthetic range was, too)—and then they made the whole collection available through the mail. They carry everything from nail lacquer to brushes at prices that are wonderfully inexpensive—$4 to $6. So here are the areas of absolute excitement:

Cinandre Cheek Gel. $3.50. A sheer, transparent color screen that actually stains anywhere

you put it with a delicate wash of color. Perfect makeup for wearing on Saturday night because it can't wash off till Monday afternoon. You can build color intensity by using several sheer coatings and can even use it to even out your tan.

Cinandre Powdergloss. $6.00. A do-everything product you could become very attached to. A highly versatile, semiprecious gleamer made out of finely milled powder. You can use it anywhere on your face or body to produce an instant gold, silver or copper shine. You can use it over or under your eye color or your cheek color, and you can even add it to your nail enamel for a high-class, understated, blatantly beautiful gloss.

Cinandre Brushes. 7 different styles, $1.00–$3.00. Wood-handled, sable-tipped brushes line your eyes or outline your lips or put on your shadow or fluff on your powder ... AND speaking of powder, Cinandre has a marvelous talcumlike shaker of loose translucent powder to add the finishing touch to the rest of the stuff you've done to your face—$5.00. Cinandre will not only send you a price list but will deliver your products COD. You only have to write:

Linda Christiano
CINANDRE
11 East 57th Street
New York, New York 10022
(Please send a self-addressed stamped envelope.)

What To Do If Your Favorite Product is Discontinued

1. Try other stores and buy as many as you can—and keep them locked in the wall safe so the dog won't eat them.
2. Consider that it might be time for a change and that there might be something better out there. Then ...
3. Get in touch with The Face Factory.

Imagine walking into a giant sample box full of cosmetics. Pots and bottles and jars full of every color imaginable—108 eye shadows, 229 lipsticks, 23 foundations (8 of them for blacks), 60 nail polishes in color gradations from pale to pow.

Imagine being able to have a lipstick custom-made to match a swatch of fabric from your living-room drapes or the color of your favorite pants suit. Imagine 74 offbeat shades with names like Last Mango In Paris ... Traffic Jam ... Nutcracker Sweet ... Track Brown ... Raisin Kane. Imagine all this for less than $2 (per product) and a money-back guarantee—and the ease of shopping by mail—and you've got THE FACE FACTORY.

If there's no Face Factory in your town (check the White Pages) get yourself a price list by sending a self-addressed, stamped envelope to:

Suzanne Grayson
FACE FACTORY
269 Fountain Road
Englewood, New Jersey 07631

Profit is the residual that the consumer allows you to make if you satisfy her. And if you have NOT satisfied her, you do not get the residual. It costs a lot to get her in the first place ... and your profit only comes when you satisfy her. That's when she lets you make a profit ... if you've done a good job. If you HAVEN'T done a good job, she DOESN'T let you make a profit. She goes and buys somebody else's.
—Suzanne Grayson, President,
The Face Factory

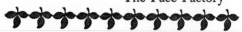

HOORAY FOR HOLLYWOOD!
—IN NEW YORK

Everything from skinheads to assorted handmade noses (which your kids will LOVE come Halloween) to grease paint and professional tele-vision and movie makeup by Lichner of London, Kryolan (from Germany), Mehron, Max Factor—plus—tools, instruction booklets and a beautifully illustrated shop-at-home catalog listing their own On-Stage Makeup Collection. These are the things that have endeared the MAKE UP CENTER to extrabeautiful women like Diana Ross, Catherine Deneuve, Cher Bono, Bette Midler and Mia Farrow. (OK, some of them aren't EXTRAbeautiful, but they're all pretty striking, aren't they?) Anyway, the MAKE UP CENTER has for years made it their business to supply every model and actress around with at least part of her collection of best-kept secrets. You can get in on the action by trying the MAKE UP CENTER's house brand (ON STAGE), which is unscented to minimize your chances of breaking out in bumps ... or, for $5 (products included) you can take a makeup lesson and even get your hair washed and set (for an additional $5). The CENTER also offers brow shaping, eye makeup, facials, and a Build-A-Nail service. It's all by appointment only, so while you're in New York be sure to call ... or write the MAKEUP CENTER and ask for their catalog.

THE MAKE UP CENTER LTD.
150 West 55th Street
New York, New York
(212) 977-9449

GLORIA NATALE (THE MAKEUP LADY) TELLS ALL

Professional makeup people have to deal with things you and I *never* have to deal with. For example, when were you last called on to sit under a very, very hot light for eight or ten hours, or stand under a waterfall or in a shower from breakfast until lunch break, or indulge in the same passionate kiss thirty-eight times until the cameraman and the director and the assistant producer were all happy with the way your makeup looked?

Through grueling tests like the three I've just mentioned, professional makeup people are called upon time and time again to see that the cosmetic part of the picture is picture perfect ... no matter what the conditions are or how adverse the circumstances.

Makeup artist Gloria Natale, who *looks* like Suzy Blakely and who's put a powder puff to almost any famous model you can name from Christina Ford to Liza Minnelli, let me in on several of her trade secrets, and it is with great relish that I will now share them with you.

Oh, yes—the one thing Gloria asked me to mention was that her makeup kit changes about as often as hotels change towels. This means that the products we talked about in 1978 may not be the products she's using or endorsing by the time you read this interview. But the information, and the inside view of what a makeup person has to deal with, is still invaluable.

KTM: Gloria, what sorts of things do professional makeup artists know about cosmetics that civilians don't?

GN: Well, a makeup artist will try something out till he or she finds what works best. If you looked at my makeup kit, you'd find certain brands of foundations, certain brands of lipsticks, certain brands of cheek colors—because I've found that they work the best and that they stay on under extreme circumstances.

KTM: Can you tell us some of the brand names you've found work well in professional situations?

GN: Clinique base (foundations) and Estée Lauder Cream Cheek Colors stay on very well. As a matter of fact, I've found them to stay on all day without disappearing or running or getting clogged up in the pores. Ultima II Powder Eyeshadows seem to stay on everyone and work very easily, and don't irritate models' eyes. They're great for girls who wear contact lenses and have problems with shadows.

Lipsticks and lip glosses—I always use Dior because of the color and the quality. They're always terrifically rich-looking and they seem to stay on exactly the way you put them on. If you look at a Dior color in the tube, that's exactly the way it'll look on the lips ... which is not the case with most products.

Then there's something called Estée Lauder Eye Glaze, which you can put on the lid area before you put the shadow on. The glaze makes the shadow work easier. Oh, yes—I always use a gold dot on the lid, right over the iris of the eye; it's kind of my signature. I put it right next to the lashes, and it makes a really beautiful highlight. In fact, I wear it all the time now, myself. I use a cream that somebody found for me in an old Hollywood drugstore, but you can use Revlon's Pure Gold Powder Shadow, and it'll work just as well.

KTM: As a professional makeup artist, you've got to carry around a lot of supplies. How do you do it?

GN: For years I've been using this black box, which a lot of makeup artists use. It was originally designed as a candy salesman's sample case, and the reason it's good is that you can open it up and lift out four trays of very neatly displayed products. Some people use fishing-tackle boxes. I never did, because after all, I AM a lady, and I didn't think it was quite my image. I preferred the black box—a little ominous, I grant you, but really quite terrific. Besides, I think the black box is pretty marvelous for collecting all your makeup in, anyway, it's so organized ... and you can keep the whole thing neatly in a closet rather than having it nested messily in a drawer someplace.

KTM: How can I get a black box?

GN: They're made by a company called

Ikelheimer-Ernst, Inc. Wait a minute, I have the information here somewhere ... Here it is ... Write to

Ikelheimer-Ernst, Inc.
Fibre Products Division
601 West 26th Street
New York, New York 10001
(212) 675-5820

The case I use is model #763-10. It sells for $20.65. They mail it to you at manufacturer's price plus U.P.S. But you should probably write or call them just to make sure.

KTM: What about applicators ... implements ... special makeup artists' tools?

GN: Brushes are my favorite tools. They're furry and friendly, and I can really relate to them. I use brushes to put loose powder on with, because I think I get a finer coverage than I do with a puff. I get many of my brushes from a Chinese art-supply store. They have fabulous sumi brushes in all sorts of shapes and sizes. Most of them have bamboo handles. They're fat coming out of the handle and come to an incredibly fine point ... and you can get really tiny ones that make superb lip brushes. Sumi is a Japanese art form, you know ... black ink on white rice paper.

KTM: Is there anyplace I can get sumi brushes through the mail?

GN: Sure. Sam Flax has a neat selection of everything from a 3½-inch-wide Hacke brush with flat handle and bristles for about $8.50 to a puffy watercolor mop made of camel hair for $4.50. Flax will send you the brush page from their catalog if you write them at:

SAM FLAX
Customer Service
25 East 28th Street
New York, New York 10016

Just ask for their price and ordering information on artists' and sumi brushes.

Marvin (who handles these things) promises that you'll get fast—almost immediate—attention.

KTM: I've heard a rumor that you'll give private makeup lessons to a privileged few. Is there any truth to that rumor?

GN: Yes, it is true. I will be giving makeup lessons as my schedule permits. They'll be an hour and a half long and cover everything you'll ever have to know about makeup.

KTM: How much will they cost?

GN: $500.

KTM: Thank you, Gloria; will you tell me where to write to set up an appointment?

GN: Gladly. You write:

GLORIA NATALE ENTERPRISES
c/o TWM Management Service
641 Lexington Avenue
New York, New York 10022
(No Phone Calls Please)

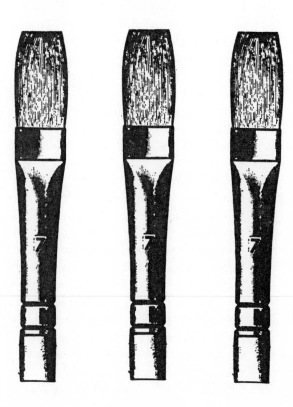

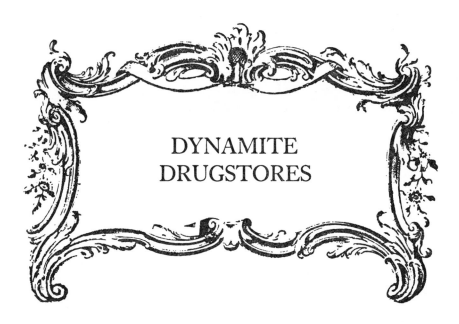

DYNAMITE
DRUGSTORES

Did you know that there was a drugstore smack in the center of the Pentagon? Or that there's another one somewhere in the Dakotas that advertises its famous free glass of iced water on huge billboards that line the highways for hundreds of miles? Have you ever thought of having your latent talent discovered in Schwab's, the famous drugstore in Hollywood? Or would you just like to get your hands on the cosmetic catalogs of two dynamite drugstores—easily—without ever leaving home? If so, here are two addresses to clip out and stick in your wallet:

Boyd's on Madison Avenue specializes in European makeups. They're famous for Evermond from Italy, Garraud from France, Fenjal from Switzerland, Day Dew from Denmark and Renoir (their own brand name, made by chemists especially for Boyd's).

Models and actresses I know swear by Boyd's eye pencils, which (they tell me) stay on for hours and can be used in hundreds of different ways. To get the Boyd's Catalog, Write:

BOYD CHEMISTS
655 Madison Avenue
New York, New York 10021

CASWELL-MASSEY is the oldest pharmacy in the United States. To step through the door at Caswell-Massey is to step out of the twentieth century and into another time. This ancient, venerated apothecary is also famous for it's profusely illustrated catalog. I am NOT overstating the case: If you send for only one thing in this book, it should definitely be the Caswell-Massey catalog. I can't praise it highly enough, nor tell you what a good investment it is, save for telling you that for a *single dollar* you get a two-year subscription, which means TWO catalogs and TWO spring supplements which make marvelous collector's items and terrific reading. To get yours, write:

CASWELL-MASSEY
320 West 13th Street
New York, New York 10014

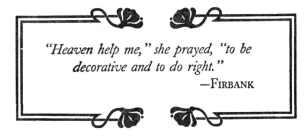

"Heaven help me," she prayed, "to be decorative and to do right."
—FIRBANK

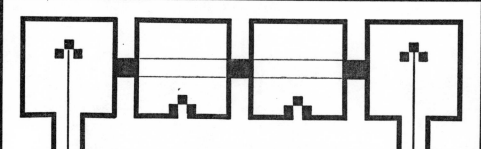

COMPLAINING

WHERE TO TURN
WHEN SOMETHING GOES WRONG

Let's say that it's your birthday and your husband has given you a big, beautiful bottle of your favorite perfume. You're delighted. You quickly rush to the bedroom and spray yourself from head to toe. Then you and your husband dash out to have dinner at the best restaurant in town. So it isn't until sometime the next afternoon that you notice (resting in the bottom of your brand-new birthday perfume) a fly . . . quite dead . . . and obviously sealed in there before they put the aerosol gizmo on the bottle.

After your first moment of shock and nausea, you will (if you are anything at all like I am) go quivering to your typewriter and tap out a long, explicit letter to the XYZ Company, who sealed the fly into your birthday gift.

You will (if you are anything at all like I am) be outraged, unhappy, infuriated and mad as a hornet. You will feel awful. And you will (if we are at all alike) pack every erg of emotional energy you can into your letter. You will clearly explain all your childhood fears of flying insects. You will further detail your shock and surprise at finding one of them in your birthday present.

And you will demand some sort of satisfaction from the XYZ Company.

In short, you will (if you are anything like I am) dump a lot of frustration onto a page of 8½″ × 11″ paper and quickly mail it off to the unsuspecting manufacturer.

Some days later, your letter (and sacks full of other letters like yours) will be delivered to the consumer relations department of the XYZ Company, to a woman named Bea Marker, who will probably be unable to do anything at all about it because (if you are anything at all like I am) you just didn't give her the proper information to work with. For example, you didn't send her your sales slip. Or the bottle with the fly in it. Or your return address. And without these vital components, Bea Marker and her consumer relations department can't do anything except absorb some of your frustration.

Now, if you're anything like I am, you don't *want* to carry on a lengthy correspondence with Bea Marker or the XYZ Company. You want one of two things: your money back, or a new bottle of perfume. Besides, if you are anything like I am, by the time the XYZ Company informs you that you'll have to send them the sales slip or the perfume, or both, you've probably thrown all these items into the trash. So you are now faced with the further frustration of writing another nasty letter or throwing your hands up and calling it quits.

There is no need for this pointless frustration. You never again have to write an ineffective letter of complaint. All you have to do is stop for a minute, consider the problem from the other side, learn a couple of trade secrets and a bit of consumer-relations vocabulary—and you're home free.

Let's stop for a minute and consider Bea Marker's position (Bea, by the way, is not ONE woman, but a composite picture of eighteen different consumer-relations specialists).

Bea Marker and hundreds of other women like her devote eight hours a day five days a week to handling your problems. She is not an impersonal multiphase computer; she's a flesh-and-blood human being. And she really DOES want to help you and all the others of us who occasionally find flies in our perfume or specks in our night cream, or have the hinges of our cream-blusher compact dissolve, or the aerosol sprays on our deodorant go funny. She understands your problem, and if you think *you're* frustrated, you should only know how Bea feels.

On an average day, Bea Marker, consumer relations specialist, will open her mail and find any one of five major types of complaints. These break down into roughly two major categories: those she can do something about and those she can't really help with.

Let's look at the problems Bea can do something about, because these are the letters that get answered and processed most quickly. Just what is it Bea Marker can do for you? For one thing, she can listen intelligently to your problem. You're talking to a professional, after all, who is thoroughly trained to answer any question you might have about her company's products. Chances are your husband will have no idea how that fly got into your perfume ... but Bea will. What's more, Bea will be able to replace the perfume or give you your money back. Or she can tell you how to get the fly out of the bottle and send it to the local museum (if that's what you want to do with it). On the other hand, she can give you technical information on her company's quality-control procedures, so if you were considering doing a term paper on quality control, she can be an invaluable (and inexpensive) research assistant. Bea sees lots of quality-control letters; they're one of the five major complaints she deals with day in and day out. Here, the problem is the product itself or something unexpected within the product. Like perfume that doesn't smell at all, for example. This sort of thing happens when somebody mistakenly packs up a bottle of colored water which was meant to be used for display purposes, but ends up on the regular product line. Unexpected or unwelcome additions to the product itself also qualify as quality-control problems. Wildlife, dirt, cuff links, bridgework or anything else that shouldn't be there—all these things can be the basis of a legitimate complaint. And Bea wants to know about them, not only because they've caused you trouble, but so that she can turn the information over to the quality-control people at XYZ. Enough quality-control letters, and the XYZ people will seriously reexamine their operations for both minor and major flaws. Remember, unless you send the product back to her, Bea can do nothing except write you again.

One of the other prevalent problems Bea has to deal with is packaging. A packaging-problem letter usually starts out like this: "For the fifth time this month, the hinges on my pressed powder compact have fallen apart, scattering powder all over my (handbag) (linen suit) (dog) (Aubusson carpet)." Now, not only can Bea Marker help you here, you can help *her*, because the packaging department at XYZ is just as interested in packages that fall apart or don't work correctly as the quality-control people are at errors in their operation. If the oils in XYZ Creme Blusher, for example, are eating through the polyvinyl chloride of the XYZ compact, something is going to have to be done about that—and quickly. Bea wants to see the problem product (complete with package), so that she can pass it along to her packaging department, tell you what went wrong, replace the product or refund your money and relax in the knowledge that the packaging people are on their phones with suppliers, trying to work things out so that other consumers won't have their compacts dissolve on them (or their suits, or their dogs, or their Aubusson carpets).

In the course of her day, Bea usually gets a number of allergic-reaction letters. They usually start out something like this: "Gentlemen: I've been using Zit-Away for three years now and never had any trouble with it until last week when I broke out in lumps the size of ping-pong balls..." These letters are tricky for Bea and sometimes make her reach for her bottle of Maalox, because while she knows her company's products have been tested and retested to screen out any possible irritants, she also knows that she's not a doctor and will have to do some fancy footwork to find out what actually went wrong.

The first thing she'll do is get an allergic-reaction letter (and product) directly to the XYZ dermatologist or medical expert for review. The medical expert will then ask some searching questions. He'll want to know exactly how the writer used the product, for example. Did she follow the instructions on the label? What other products was she using at the time? Was she taking medication or doing anything else that might have caused her to break out in lumps? You may actually get a personal letter from XYZ's medical person if you have an allergic reaction, or you may simply get an expression of sympathy from Bea, along with some sort of adjustment. Very seldom will Bea or her company be able to pay for your medical bills or for your discomfort, but she may be able to give you some idea of what really *did* cause the lumps (if the product didn't), so that you can continue to use Zit-Away without unhappy aftereffects.

The other area where Bea can really help is in response to the where-can-I-get-it letter. Say, for instance, that you were in New York for the holidays and discovered XYZ's eye shadow at Saks Fifth Avenue. And you loved it. But, when you got back home to Butte, you couldn't find XYZ eye shadow anywhere. Bea can be terrific with this sort of request. After only a few minutes with her computer printout and her world atlas, she'll be able to tell you exactly where to go to find the nearest XYZ dealer.

These are not the problems that bug Bea Marker. No. The problems that distress her, that distress all consumer-relations people, are the problems they can do nothing about. Like the discontinued-product letters Bea gets by the balefull. These start: "Dear Sirs: How *dare* you discontinue my favorite shade of..." Now, Bea knows you're angry. And she knows that you're frustrated. But there's very little she can do for you except (in rare cases) tell you how to blend two other colors to get the same effect or suggest some alternate product for you to try. There's no sense in reviling her or heaping imprecations on XYZ or on fate. The shade or product you liked so well was probably dropped from the line because not enough people felt the way you did about it, and it just didn't sell. Bea can't bring your shade back. She can only feel her stomach knot up as she reads your letter over her morning toast and coffee. She also doesn't keep your favorite shade stocked in her desk drawer, so asking for the remaining stock won't produce anything more than a letter from Bea saying: "Sorry."

The enclosed-is-a-check letter is another major headache for Bea. She usually saves them for after lunch, when she's calmer and she can face them with a fresh flush of benevolent energy. Never—never—ever—send a check (or worse even, cash or coin) to a consumer-relations department. Consumer-relations departments don't deal in mail orders. They have no stock on hand. They can, in fact, do nothing with your money except send it back to you. If you really want to get your hands on a product, send Bea a where-can-I-get-it letter, then send your money to your nearest source of supply.

While checks and discontinued-shade problems bother Bea, the letters that drive her straight up the wallpaper are not so easily categorized. Most often they don't have to do with product at all, but come from people who want to buy large-size dummy bottles or promotional props or the scarves worn by the saleswomen. You'd be surprised at how many requests come in for tester units. Or how many women who attended an XYZ makeup clinic in Florida that was followed by a luncheon are seriously interested in where they can get the seashells the lobster salad was served in. There is no way Bea Marker can deal with this sort of request. Nor should we expect her to.

The thing to remember is that we (as consumers), though we're very often RIGHT, are also (at times) unreasonable and can solve whatever problems we've got very simply and easily on our own. So, in order to cut right through the confusion, here is

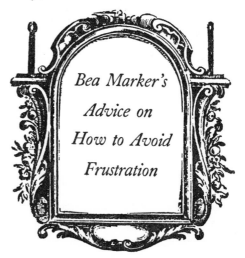

Bea Marker's Advice on How to Avoid Frustration

1. Save your sales slips until you've opened and used the product. Even if you've used the same product before, hang onto the sales slip for at least two weeks. Then, if there's any problem, take the sales slip and go back to the store with it (and the product). Most reputable stores will instantly make an on-the-spot adjustment for you, and you'll never have to write Bea in the first place.

2. If you've got a packaging problem on your hands, a defective atomizer, or a cap that breaks off or a compact that's falling to pieces—and you've already destroyed the sales slip—don't throw the product away and then write an angry protest letter. Simply wrap your product and your letter and send them by registered or insured mail to Bea (or her counterpart). Companies are not being difficult when they ask you to do it this way. They know it's more expensive to send a registered package. But they also know that there's many a slip between the mail room and the right person, and that a registered-mail receipt is the one assurance you have of being able to verify your claim.

Large companies won't accept COD packages, but they will very often reimburse you for the postage if you ask them to.

3. Keep your letter brief and to the point and stick to the facts. Tell the company where you bought its product, when you bought it and exactly what went wrong. Don't just say, "It looks funny"; tell them why. If you've never used the stuff before, say so (you may have been using it incorrectly rather than having problems with the product itself). Also tell the company exactly what you want from them. Do you want a replacement (because you really love the one you bought and just want it exchanged)? Do you want your money back? The clearer you are about what you want, the more easily the company can help you.

4. There are some things a company really can't do for you that you should be aware of before expending a lot of energy writing in about them. The first is personal preference. If you've always used a liquid makeup and for some reason were pressured to try a translucent cream version, and you get home and find out that you hate the cream, don't write in demanding your money back. The trick is not to be pressured into buying the cream in the first place, or if you have been pressured, consider the switch a gamble and be ready to throw the cream away and chalk the whole thing up to experience.

The second area in which the company can do nothing at all to help you is when you ask for a substitution on a prepackaged promotional item. Let's say you were intrigued with an ad that said you could get a three-piece XYZ makeup organizer *and* four XYZ products (a $4,000-value) for only $6.50. Sounds like a good deal. And it IS a good deal, an excellent way to sample a range of XYZ products without spending the money you were planning to use to send the kids to college.

You're getting a three-piece makeup or-

ganizer, a lipstick, a mascara, a blusher and maybe some perfume for $6.50—when without the promotion you'd be investing $5.00 in the mascara alone. The only problem is, if you only use green mascara, black lipstick and mauve rouge, you are never going to find them in a promotional package. If large companies had to pack specific products individually into their promotional packages, they couldn't afford to do them in the first place. So there's no way they can begin to make substitutions for you after the fact. The best thing to do, if you're interested in buying a purchase-with-purchase, is go to the store and look at it first. Then make a decision you can be happy with.

5. Make sure you have an accurate address for the company; then please, please be patient. I know this seems unreasonable, but it sometimes takes two weeks for your package to reach Bea Marker's desk. Once it gets there, she'll do everything in her power to help you as quickly as possible. Give her at least three weeks and, if you haven't heard something in a month . . . write again.

And now, because you've already been so patient, here in three ingeniously planned and executed appendices are the current addresses of America's leading cosmetic companies, fragrance manufacturers and publishers.

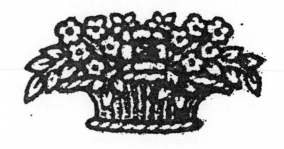

APPENDIX A
—List of Major Cosmetics Manufacturers

ALMAY, INC.
562 Fifth Avenue
New York, New York 10036
(212)869-0500

ELIZABETH ARDEN, INC.
1345 Avenue of the Americas
New York, New York 10019
(212)399-2000

ARMOUR-DIAL, INC.
Greyhound Tower
Phoenix, Arizona 85077
(602)248-2800

AVON PRODUCTS, INC.
9 West 57th Street
New York, New York 10019
(212)593-4017

AZIZA EYE COSMETICS
33 Benedict Place
Greenwich, Connecticut 06830
(203)661-2000

AZUREE, INC.
767 Fifth Avenue
New York, New York 10022
(212)826-3600

BONNE BELL, INC.
18519 Detroit Avenue
Lakewood, Ohio 44107
(216)221-0800

JOHN H. BRECK, INC.
Berdan Avenue
Wayne, New Jersey 07470
(201)831-1234

BRISTOL-MYERS COMPANY
345 Park Avenue
New York, New York 10028
(212)644-2100

CHANEL, INC.
9 West 57th Street
New York, New York 10019
(212)688-5055

CHAP STICK COMPANY
1000 Robins Road
Lynchburg, Virginia 24505
(703)845-7073

CHESEBROUGH-POND'S INC.
33 Benedict Place
Greenwich, Connecticut 06830
(203)661-2000

CLAIROL, INC.
345 Park Avenue
New York, New York 10022
(212)644-3100

CLINIQUE LABORATORIES, INC.
767 Fifth Avenue
New York, New York 10022
(212)826-3600

COLGATE-PALMOLIVE COMPANY
300 Park Avenue
New York, New York 10022
(212)PL1-1200

COSMAIR, INC.-L'OREAL-LANCOME-GUY
LAROCHE-COURREGES
530 Fifth Avenue
New York, New York 10036
(212)697-5115

COTY, Div. of Pfizer, Inc.
235 East 42nd Street
New York, New York 10017
(212)573-3500

HELENE CURTIS INDUSTRIES, INC.
4401 West North Avenue
Chicago, Illinois 60639
(312)292-2121

DANA PERFUMES CORP.
625 Madison Avenue
New York, New York 10022
(212)751-3700

ALEXANDRA DE MARKOFF
Div. of Lanvin-Charles of the Ritz

40 West 57th Street
New York, New York 10019
(212)489-4500

FRANCES DENNEY
5935 Woodland Avenue
Philadelphia, Pennsylvania 19101
(215)729-8200

CHRISTIAN DIOR
9 West 57th Street
New York, New York 10019
(212)759-1840

FABERGÉ, INC.
1345 Avenue of the Americas
New York, New York 10019
(212)581-3500

FACE FACTORY
269 Fountain Road
Englewood, New Jersey 07631
(201)568-5023

MAX FACTOR & CO.
1655 N. McCadden Place
Hollywood, California 90028
(213)462-6131

FASHION FAIR
820 South Michigan Avenue
Chicago, Illinois 60605
(312)786-7607

FULLER BRUSH COMPANY
7400 North Caldwell
Niles, Illinois 60648
(312)775-9300

THE GILLETTE COMPANY
Prudential Tower Building
Boston, Massachusetts 02199
(617)421-7000

DOROTHY GRAY, LTD.
Lehn & Fink Products Co.
225 Summit Avenue
Montvale, New Jersey 07645
(201)391-8500

HOUSE OF WESTMORE, INC.
175 Great Neck Road

Great Neck, Long Island, New York 11021
(516)466-6310

JOHNSON & JOHNSON BABY PRODUCTS
COMPANY
501 George Street
New Brunswick, New Jersey 08903
(201)524-0400

JOVAN, INC.
875 North Michigan Avenue
Chicago, Illinois 60611
(312)787-2929

BOB KELLY COSMETICS, INC.
151 West 46th Street
New York, New York 10036
(212)245-2238

KEY WEST FRAGRANCE & COSMETIC
FACTORY
528 Front Street, P.O. Box 1643
Key West, Florida 33040
(305)294-6661

LANCOME, Div. of Cosmair, Inc.
530 Fifth Avenue
New York, New York 10036
(212)697-5115

LANVIN-CHARLES OF THE RITZ
40 West 57th Street
New York, New York 10019
(212)489-4500

ESTEE LAUDER, INC.
767 Fifth Avenue
New York, New York 10022
(212)826-3600

L'OREAL OF PARIS, Div. of Cosmair, Inc.
530 Fifth Avenue
New York, New York 10036
(212)697-5115

LOVE COSMETICS BY MENLEY & JAMES
1500 Spring Garden Street
Philadelphia, Pennsylvania 19101
(215)854-5000

PRINCE MATCHABELLI
33 Benedict Place
Greenwich, Connecticut 06830
(203)661-2000

GERMAINE MONTEIL COSMETIQUES
40 West 57th Street
New York, New York 10019
(212)582-3010

THE NESTLE-LeMUR COMPANY
902 Broadway
New York, New York 10010
(212)867-8900

MERLE NORMAN COSMETICS, INC.
9130 Bellanca Avenue
Los Angeles, California 90045
(213)641-3000

NOXELL CORPORATION
11050 York Road
Baltimore, Maryland 21203
(301)666-2662

ORLANE
Jean D'Albret-Orlane Cosmetics
680 Fifth Avenue
New York, New York 10019
(212)757-4200

PHYSICIANS' FORMULA COSMETICS, INC.
230 S. Ninth Avenue
City of Industry, California 91746
(213)968-3855

PLOUGH, INC.
3030 Jackson Avenue
Memphis, Tennessee 38151
(901)320-2011

THE PROCTER & GAMBLE COMPANY
P.O. Box 599
Cincinnati, Ohio 45201
(513)562-1100

MARY QUANT COSMETICS, INC.
Div. of Gala Cosmetics
450 Park Avenue
New York, New York 10022
(212)644-1234

REVLON, INC.
767 Fifth Avenue
New York, New York 10022
(212)758-5000

FLORI ROBERTS

907 Embury Avenue
Neptune, New Jersey 07753
(201)774-8844

ROUX LABORATORIES, INC.
Prudential Building
Jacksonville, Florida 32207
(904)396-6161

HELENA RUBINSTEIN, INC.
767 Fifth Avenue
New York, New York 10022
(212)355-2100

SCHOLL, INC.
213 W. Schiller Street
Chicago, Illinois 60610
(312)642-7200

SHISEIDO COSMETICS, INC.
540 Madison Avenue
New York, New York 10022
(212)752-2644

SHULTON, INC.
697 Route 46
Clifton, New Jersey 07015
(201)546-7000

TRUE EARTH COSMETICS
P.O. Box 1328
1275 Bloomfield Avenue
Fairfield, New Jersey 07006
(201)575-7050

TUSSY COSMETICS, INC.
Lehn & Fink Products Co.
225 Summit Avenue
Montvale, New Jersey 07645
(201)391-8500

DIANE VON FURSTENBERG, INC.
530 Seventh Avenue
New York, New York 10018
(212)369-3770

WELEDA, INC.
30 South Main Street
Spring Valley, New York 10977
(914)356-4134

THE WELLA CORPORATION
524 Grand Avenue

Englewood, New Jersey 07631
(201)569-1020

YARDLEY OF LONDON, INC.
40 West 57th Street
New York, New York 10019
(212)582-3010

 APPENDIX B—
List of
Fragrance Manufacturers

ELIZABETH ARDEN
1345 Avenue of the Americas
New York, New York 10019
(212)399-2000

STEPHEN BURROWS FRAGRANCES
40 West 57th Street
New York, New York 10019
(212)489-9521

CHANEL, INC.
9 West 57th Street
New York, New York 10019
(212)688-5055

COTY, Div. of Pfizer, Inc.
235 East 42nd Street
New York, New York 10017
(212)573-3500

DANA PERFUMES CORP.
625 Madison Avenue
New York, New York 10022
(212)PL1-3700

FRANCES DENNEY
630 Fifth Avenue
New York, New York 10022
(212)977-8400

PARFUMS JEAN DESPREZ S.A.
13 rue Ernest Deloison
Neuilly 92, France

FABERGE
1345 Avenue of the Americas
New York, New York 10019
(212)581-3500

GRES
c/o Milton Stern Co.
40 West 57th Street
New York, New York 10019
(212)765-2060

GUERLAIN
444 Madison Avenue
New York, New York 10022
(212)PL1-1870

HALSTON FRAGRANCES, INC.
40 West 57th Street
New York, New York 10019
(212)489-9624

HERMES
745 Fifth Avenue
New York, New York 10022
(212)759-7585

HOUBIGANT
1135 Pleasant View Terrace, West
Ridgefield, New Jersey 07657
(201)941-3400

JOVAN, INC.
875 North Michigan Avenue
Chicago, Illinois 60611
(312)787-2929

PARFUMS LAGERFELD
1345 Avenue of the Americas
New York, New York 10019
(212)399-2000

LANVIN-CHARLES OF THE RITZ
40 West 57th Street
New York, New York 10019
(212)489-4500

LOVE COSMETICS
540 Madison Avenue
New York, New York 10022
(212)751-3822

PRINCE MATCHABELLI
33 Benedict Place
Greenwich, Connecticut 06830
(203)661-2032

MYRURGIA PERFUMES, INC.
1370 Avenue of the Americas

New York, New York 10019
(212)541-5410

NORELL PERFUMES, INC.
767 Fifth Avenue
New York, New York 10022
(212)758-5000

PACO RABANNE
9 West 57th Street
New York, New York 10019
(212)759-5930

RAPHAEL, INC.
767 Fifth Avenue
New York, New York 10022
(212)758-5000

REVLON, INC.
767 Fifth Avenue
New York, New York 10022
(212)758-5000

R.H. COSMETICS
641 Lexington Avenue
New York, New York 10022
(212)758-9440

SHISEIDO COSMETICS, INC.
540 Madison Avenue
New York, New York 10022
(212)752-2644

TUVACHE
40 West 57th Street
New York, New York 10019
(212)582-3010

DIANE VON FURSTENBERG
530 Seventh Avenue
New York, New York 10018
(212)354-8336

WELEDA, INC.
30 South Main Street
Spring Valley, New York 10977
(914)356-4134

YARDLEY OF LONDON, INC.
700 Union Blvd.
Totowa, New Jersey 07511
(201)256-3100

YVES SAINT LAURENT
40 West 57th Street
New York, New York 10019
(212)489-4500

APPENDIX C—
Publishers Whose Books
Appear in These Pages

ATHENEUM PUBLISHERS
122 East 42nd Street
New York, New York 10017
(212)661-4500

BALLANTINE BOOKS
Westminster, Maryland
(301)848-1900

BANTAM BOOKS, INC.
666 Fifth Avenue
New York, New York 10022
(212)765-6500

BERKLEY PUBLISHING CORP.
200 Madison Avenue
New York, New York 10016
(212)883-5500

COWARD, McCANN & GEOGHEGAN, INC.
200 Madison Avenue
New York, New York 10016
(212)883-5500

THOMAS Y. CROWELL CO.
666 Fifth Avenue
New York, New York 10022
(212)489-2200

DELACORTE PRESS
885 Second Avenue
New York, New York 10017
(212)832-7300

DELL PUBLISHING CO., INC.
885 Second Avenue
New York, New York 10017
(212)832-7300

DOUBLEDAY & CO., INC.
245 Park Avenue
New York, New York 10017
(212)953-4561

FARRAR, STRAUS & GIROUX, INC.
19 Union Square
New York, New York 10003
(212)741-6900

FAWCETT PUBLICATIONS, INC.
Fawcett Place
Greenwich, Connecticut 06830
(203)NO1-6700

HARPER & ROW PUBLISHERS, INC.
103 East 53rd Street
New York, New York 10022
(212)593-7000

HOLT RINEHART & WINSTON, INC.
383 Madison Avenue
New York, New York 10017
(212)MU8-9100

ALFRED A. KNOPF, INC.
201 East 50th Street
New York, New York 10022
(212)PL1-2600

J. B. LIPPINCOTT CO.
227 South Six Street
Philadelphia, Pennsylvania 19106
(215)574-4200

DAVID McKAY COMPANY
750 Third Avenue
New York, New York 10017
(212)MO1-1700

NELSON-HALL PUBLISHERS
325 Jackson
Chicago, Illinois 60606
(312)922-0856

PINNACLE BOOKS, INC.
275 Madison Avenue
New York, New York 10016
(212)532-4286

POCKET BOOKS
630 Fifth Avenue
New York, New York 10022
(212)CI5-6400

PRENTICE-HALL, INC.
Englewood Cliffs, New Jersey 17632
(201)592-2000

PYRAMID BOOKS
919 Third Avenue
New York, New York 10022
(212)688-9215

QUADRANGLE/New York Times Book Co.
10 East 53rd Street
New York, New York 10022
(212)593-7800

RANDOM HOUSE, INC.
201 East 50th Street
New York, New York 10022
(212)PL1-2600

ST. MARTIN'S PRESS
175 Fifth Avenue
New York, New York 10010
(212)674-5151

SHERBOURNE PRESS
8063 Beverly Boulevard
Los Angeles, California
(213)658-5444

SIMON & SCHUSTER, INC.
630 Fifth Avenue
New York, New York 10022
(212)CI5-6400

STRAIGHT ARROW BOOKS
78 East 56th Street
New York, New York 10022

W. B. SAUNDERS CO.
West Washington Square
Philadelphia, Pennsylvania 19105
(215)574-4700

WORKMAN PUBLISHING CO., INC.
231 East 51st Street
New York, New York 10022
(212)421-8050